Dr. SEBI BIBLE

21 Books in 1: The Definitive Compendium to Dr. Sebi's Alkaline Mastery. Unlock a Life Free from Disease with Herb Insights, and Time-Tested Cures.

© Copyright 2023 by **Natalia Westbrook** All rights reserved.

The following Book is reproduced below with the goal of providing information that is as accurate and reliable as possible. Regardless, purchasing this Book can be seen as consent to the fact that both the publisher and the author of this book are in no way experts on the topics discussed within and that any recommendations or suggestions that are made herein are for entertainment purposes only. Professionals should be consulted as needed prior to undertaking any of the action endorsed herein.

This declaration is deemed fair and valid by both the American Bar Association and the Committee of Publishers Association and is legally binding throughout the United States.

Furthermore, the transmission, duplication, or reproduction of any of the following work including specific information will be considered an illegal act irrespective of if it is done electronically or in print. This extends to creating a secondary or tertiary copy of the work or a recorded copy and is only allowed with the express written consent from the Publisher. All additional right reserved.

The information in the following pages is broadly considered a truthful and accurate account of facts and as such, any inattention, use, or misuse of the information in question by the reader will render any resulting actions solely under their purview. There are no scenarios in which the publisher or the original author of this work can be in any fashion deemed liable for any hardship or damages that may befall them after undertaking information described herein.

Additionally, the information in the following pages is intended only for informational purposes and should thus be thought of as universal. As befitting its nature, it is presented without assurance regarding its prolonged validity or interim quality. Trademarks that are mentioned are done without written consent and can in no way be considered an endorsement from the trademark holder.

Table of Contents

Foreword 9

The Revolutionary Impact of Dr. Sebi's Teachings 9

Introduction 13

Why Alkalinity Matters in Today's World 13

Book 1: Dr. Sebi – The Man, The Myth, the Legend 19

Childhood and Formative Years 19

The Awakening: Discovering Natural Healing 24

Trials, Tribulations, and Triumphs 29

The Legacy Left Behind: The Inception of a Legacy 33

Book 2: The Alkaline Diet – Beyond Basics 41

The Science of Body pH: A Deep Dive: 41

Alkaline vs. Acidic: What Does It Truly Mean? 48

The Detrimental Effects of an Acidic Diet 55

Transitioning: Steps to Adopt an Alkaline Lifestyle 60

Book 3: Dr. Sebi's Herbal Encyclopedia 71

The power and potency of herbs 71

Detailed Profiles of Dr. Sebi's Top 50 Herbs 78

Crafting Herbal Solutions: From Teas to Tinctures 84

Potential Side Effects and Interactions: 92

Book 4: Disease Eradication and Natural Healing 99

Understanding the Root Causes of Modern Ailments: 99

Dr. Sebi's Approach: A Case-by-Case Analysis –..105

Success Stories: Testimonials of Recovery..112

Book 5: Comprehensive Nutrition Guide... 123

Breaking Down Nutritional Needs by Age and Gender..123

Superfoods: Benefits and Incorporation into Daily Life...129

Supplements: Navigating the Good and the Bad..137

Book 6: Mind, Body, and Spiritual Alignment... 145

The Psychological Benefits of an Alkaline Lifestyle...145

Meditation, Mindfulness, and Alkalinity:..151

Yoga, Physical Activity, and Their Role in Alkaline Living... 158

Book 7: Alkaline Gourmet – A Recipe Book..167

Breakfast: Energizing Alkaline Starters..167

Lunch: Nutrient-Packed Midday Meals... 173

Dinner: Hearty Alkaline Delights... 180

Desserts: Guilt-Free Alkaline Treats.. 184

Book 8: Liquid Nutrition – Beyond Water.. 193

The Science Behind Alkaline Water...193

Crafting Nutrient-Packed Smoothies..199

Herbal Teas: Benefits, Brewing, and Best Practices... 206

Book 9: Women's Health – An Alkaline Approach..215

Nutrition Across Different Life Stages.. 215

Addressing Women's Health Concerns Naturally.. 221

Beauty, skin care and alkaline practices...230

Book 10: Men's Health – Strength and Vitality...239

Unique Nutritional Needs for Men.. 239

Fitness and Muscle Building in Alkalinity.. 245

Addressing Common Male Health Concerns.. 252

BOOK 11: ALKALINE FAMILY – RAISING THE NEXT GENERATION... 261

Introducing Children to Alkaline Foods... 261

Crafting Family-Friendly Alkaline Meals.. 267

Natural Remedies for Common Childhood Ailments... 274

BOOK 12: SOCIAL CHALLENGES IN ALKALINE LIVING..283

Navigating Dining Out and Social Events.. 283

Handling Criticism and Skepticism.. 289

Building a Supportive Alkaline Community.. 296

BOOK 13: MODERN MEDICINE VS. ALKALINE PRACTICES...305

A Comparative Analysis of Treatment Modalities.. 305

How to Integrate Alkaline Practices with Modern Medicine..309

Real-Life Case Studies and Outcomes... 312

BOOK 14: DEBUNKING MYTHS AND MISCONCEPTIONS... 319

Common Criticisms of the Alkaline Diet..319

Scientific Evidence Supporting Alkaline Living..322

Addressing Doubts and Concerns.. 327

BOOK 15: GROW YOUR OWN – THE ALKALINE GARDEN... 331

Basics of Alkaline Farming and Gardening.. 331

Sourcing Seeds and Plants: Organic and Non-GMO... 335

The Joy of Foraging and Wildcrafting.. 339

BOOK 16: DR. SEBI'S GLOBAL FOOTPRINT... 345

How Different Cultures Embraced Dr. Sebi's Teachings..................345

The Spread and Influence of Alkaline Practices Worldwide..................349

Continuing the Legacy: Alkaline Advocates Around the Globe..................353

Book 17: Tools, Resources, and Continued Learning..................359

Dr. Sebi's Product Recommendations and Reviews..................359

Further Reading: Books, Journals, and Research Papers..................363

Online Platforms, Forums, and Communities for Support..................366

Book 18: Personal Transformation Chronicles..................371

Real-Life Journeys of Health and Healing..................371

ChalleOvercoming nges: Personal Stories of Resilience..................374

The Growing Community of Alkaline Advocates..................379

Book 19: The Intersection of Technology and Alkalinity..................385

Digital Tools for Tracking and Promoting Alkaline Living..................385

Online Courses, Webinars, and Workshops..................389

The Future of Alkaline Advocacy in the Digital Age..................392

Book 20: Advocacy, Legacy, and Making a Difference..................399

How to Become an Advocate for Alkaline Living..................399

Organizing Community Events, Workshops, and Seminars..................403

The Path Forward: Spreading Awareness and Education..................407

Book 21: The Future Landscape of Alkaline Living..................413

Predicting Trends in Alkaline Health and Wellness..................413

The Role of Research and Science in Shaping the Future..................417

Your Personal Role in the Global Alkaline Movement..................421

Conclusion..................425

The Lifelong Journey of Alkaline Mastery 425

ACKNOWLEDGMENTS 429

Foreword

The Revolutionary Impact of Dr. Sebi's Teachings

A Paradigm Shift in Health and Wellness: In a world teeming with health fads and quick fixes, Dr. Sebi's teachings stand as a beacon of enduring wisdom. His approach to health isn't just another diet plan or a list of forbidden foods; it's a lifestyle, a philosophy, and for many, a path to redemption. Dr. Sebi's alkaline diet isn't just about what you eat; it's about understanding the fundamental laws of life and how our choices can either align us with nature or lead us down a path of decay.

The Man Who Dared to Challenge the Status Quo: Dr. Sebi, born Alfredo Darrington Bowman, was not just a self-taught herbalist but a visionary. He dared to challenge the medical orthodoxy of his time, questioning the efficacy of conventional treatments for chronic illnesses. His courage to stand against established norms was not without its share of controversies and legal battles, but it was this very audacity that made him a revolutionary figure in the realm of natural healing.

The Essence of Alkalinity: At the core of Dr. Sebi's teachings is the concept of alkalinity. In simple terms, an alkaline body is a healthy body. But Dr. Sebi took this idea further, delving into the intricacies of cellular biology, the role of minerals, and the impact of food choices on our overall well-being. His research led him to develop a list of approved alkaline foods, designed to detoxify the body and restore it to its natural alkaline state.

The Healing Power of Herbs: One of the most groundbreaking aspects of Dr. Sebi's work was his deep understanding of herbs and their medicinal properties. He wasn't just recommending herbs as supplements; he was prescribing them as medicine.

From the deserts of Africa to the rainforests of South America, Dr. Sebi traveled the world to study indigenous plants and their healing properties. His herbal formulas have been credited with curing everything from diabetes to cancer, often in cases where conventional medicine had failed.

Dr. Sebi's teachings go beyond diet and herbs; they encompass a holistic view of health that includes mental, emotional, and spiritual well-being. He understood that the mind and body are interconnected, and one cannot be healed without the other. This is why his approach has been so effective for people from all walks of life, suffering from a myriad of conditions. It's not just about treating symptoms; it's about addressing the root cause of illness and fostering a state of health that is sustainable in the long term.

The Ripple Effect: The impact of Dr. Sebi's teachings has been nothing short of revolutionary. It has empowered individuals to take control of their health, breaking free from the shackles of a medical system that often prioritizes treatment over prevention. His influence has also permeated the cultural fabric, inspiring a new generation of holistic health practitioners, nutritionists, and herbalists who are carrying forward his legacy.

A Legacy of Empowerment: Perhaps the most enduring aspect of Dr. Sebi's impact is the sense of empowerment he has instilled in people. Health is no longer something that happens to you; it's something you actively participate in. This shift in perspective has been life-changing for many, turning them from passive recipients of healthcare into active participants in their own well-being.

As we move forward into an era where health and wellness are at the forefront of global conversations, the teachings of Dr. Sebi serve as a timeless guide. His revolutionary approach has already changed countless lives, and as more people awaken to the power of natural healing, his impact will only continue to grow.

Introduction

Why Alkalinity Matters in Today's World

In today's fast-paced world, we're constantly bombarded with choices that can either enhance our well-being or diminish it. From processed foods to stressful work environments, the modern lifestyle is a breeding ground for acidity. This acidity, both metaphorical and literal, seeps into our bodies and minds, creating an imbalance that can lead to a host of health issues. It's no wonder that chronic diseases like diabetes, heart disease, and cancer are on the rise; our bodies are in a state of constant turmoil, struggling to maintain equilibrium.

Contrary to what the modern lifestyle imposes on us, our bodies thrive in an alkaline state. Alkalinity is not a new-age fad or a dietary trend; it's the natural state of our bodies. When we're born, our bodies are alkaline, and as we grow, various factors like diet, stress, and environmental toxins contribute to increasing acidity. The importance of alkalinity is not just a matter of preventing disease; it's about returning to our natural state of health and well-being.

The Science Behind Alkalinity: While the concept of alkalinity may seem abstract, it's deeply rooted in science. Our body's pH level, a measure of acidity or alkalinity, plays a crucial role in cellular function. Enzymes, the catalysts for every biochemical reaction in our bodies, are highly sensitive to pH levels. A slight deviation from the optimal pH can disrupt these reactions, leading to inefficient metabolism, reduced energy levels, and impaired immune function.

The Domino Effect: How Acidity Affects Your Health: When your body is acidic, it's like a domino effect; one system's inefficiency leads to another's malfunction. For instance, an acidic environment can compromise your digestive system, leading to poor nutrient absorption.

This, in turn, affects your immune system, making you more susceptible to infections and diseases. The impact of acidity is not limited to physical health; it also takes a toll on your mental well-being. An acidic body is a stressed body, and this stress manifests as anxiety, depression, and a general sense of malaise.

The Alkaline Advantage: More Than Just Disease Prevention

While it's essential to understand the detrimental effects of acidity, it's equally important to recognize the benefits of an alkaline state. Alkalinity is not just about disease prevention; it's about enhancing your quality of life. An alkaline body is an energized body, one that is better equipped to handle the stresses of modern life. From improved mental clarity to enhanced physical stamina, the advantages of maintaining an alkaline state are manifold.

The Environmental Connection: Alkalinity and Sustainability

In a world grappling with environmental issues like climate change and pollution, the concept of alkalinity extends beyond individual well-being. An alkaline lifestyle is often synonymous with a sustainable lifestyle. From choosing organic produce to reducing waste, the principles that govern alkalinity are intrinsically linked to environmental stewardship. By adopting an alkaline lifestyle, you're not just improving your health; you're contributing to the well-being of the planet.

The importance of alkalinity is not just a personal matter; it has social implications as well. When you prioritize your health, you set an example for others to follow. Whether it's your family, friends, or co-workers, your commitment to an alkaline lifestyle can inspire change on a larger scale. In a society plagued by health issues, this ripple effect can be revolutionary.

The Path Forward: Alkalinity as a Way of Life: As we navigate the complexities of modern life, the importance of alkalinity becomes increasingly evident. It's not just a dietary choice; it's a way of life, a holistic approach to well-being that encompasses every aspect of human existence.

From the foods we eat to the thoughts we think, every choice we make can either contribute to acidity or promote alkalinity. The path forward is clear: to live a life of optimal health and well-being, alkalinity matters, now more than ever.

The Silent Epidemic: Chronic Inflammation and Acidity

One of the most overlooked aspects of an acidic lifestyle is its role in chronic inflammation. Inflammation is the body's natural response to injury or infection, but when it becomes chronic, it serves as the underlying cause of numerous diseases. An acidic environment in the body exacerbates this inflammation, creating a vicious cycle that is hard to break. The foods we eat, the air we breathe, and even the thoughts we entertain can contribute to this silent epidemic. Alkalinity serves as a natural antidote, helping to quell the inflammatory response and restore balance.

The Mental Toll: Acidity and Cognitive Function

We often underestimate the impact of acidity on our mental faculties. Studies have shown that an acidic environment can impair cognitive function, leading to issues like memory loss, decreased attention span, and even mood disorders. Alkalinity, on the other hand, promotes mental clarity and focus. It's not just about feeling good; it's about optimizing your mental capabilities to navigate the complexities of modern life effectively.

Our emotional well-being is intricately linked to our physical state. An acidic body is a stressed body, and this stress manifests not just as anxiety or depression but also as emotional volatility. Mood swings, irritability, and a general sense of dissatisfaction are common symptoms of an acidic lifestyle. Alkalinity offers emotional stability, providing a sense of calm and peace that is often elusive in today's fast-paced world.

The Physical Rejuvenation: Alkalinity and Cellular Regeneration

Our bodies are in a constant state of renewal and repair. Cellular regeneration is an ongoing process, but it's severely hampered in an acidic environment.

Alkalinity promotes cellular health, enhancing the body's natural repair mechanisms. This has far-reaching implications, from slowing down the aging process to speeding up recovery from physical exertion or even surgery.

The Hidden Costs: Healthcare and Alkalinity

The financial burden of an acidic lifestyle is another aspect that we often overlook. From frequent doctor visits to long-term medication, the costs can add up quickly. Alkalinity offers a preventive approach, reducing the need for medical intervention and thereby lowering healthcare costs. It's an investment in your health that pays dividends in the long run.

In a corporate environment where productivity is prized, the role of alkalinity becomes even more critical. An alkaline body is an energized body, capable of sustained focus and increased output. Employers are beginning to recognize this, and some are even incorporating alkaline diet plans into their employee wellness programs. The benefits are mutual; a healthier employee is a more productive employee.

When a community embraces alkalinity, the effects are transformative. From community gardens that focus on alkaline foods to educational programs that teach the benefits of an alkaline lifestyle, the collective impact is significant. It fosters social cohesion, reduces healthcare costs, and even lowers crime rates, as a healthier community is generally a happier community.

The Global Perspective: Alkalinity as a Universal Need

In a world where healthcare systems are often stretched to their limits, the universal adoption of an alkaline lifestyle could be revolutionary. It transcends cultural, social, and economic barriers, offering a simple yet effective solution to a global problem. As we face the challenges of a rapidly changing world, the need for alkalinity becomes not just a personal priority but a global imperative.

An alkaline diet is often plant-based, which has significant implications for animal welfare. The mass production of meat is not just an environmental concern; it's an ethical issue. By adopting an alkaline lifestyle, you're also making an ethical choice, contributing to a more humane and compassionate world.

Finally, let's not forget the spiritual dimension. Alkalinity is not just about physical or even mental well-being; it's about achieving a state of inner peace and spiritual harmony. In various spiritual traditions, the concept of bodily purity is emphasized, and alkalinity aligns perfectly with this ancient wisdom.

By now, it should be abundantly clear why alkalinity matters so much in today's world. It's a multifaceted issue with far-reaching implications, affecting every aspect of our lives from our physical health to our emotional well-being, from our social interactions to our global responsibilities. The choice is ours to make, and the path forward is clear: to live a life of optimal health and well-being, alkalinity matters, now more than ever.

Book 1: Dr. Sebi – The Man, The Myth, the Legend

Childhood and Formative Years

In the small village of Ilanga, Honduras, a young boy named Alfredo Darrington Bowman—later known to the world as Dr. Sebi—was born into a world of limited means but unlimited potential. His family, like many in the region, relied on the land for sustenance, cultivating crops and raising livestock. The simplicity of this lifestyle, far removed from the complexities of modern medicine, would later serve as the cornerstone of Dr. Sebi's revolutionary approach to health and well-being.

Dr. Sebi's early years were deeply influenced by his grandmother, "Mama Hay." A herbalist and traditional healer, Mama Hay instilled in young Alfredo a profound respect for the natural world. She taught him the names of plants, their uses, and the delicate balance of nature that sustains life. These early lessons were not formal education but a form of ancestral wisdom passed down through generations.

The Curiosity of a Young Mind: Early Signs of a Healer:

As a child, Alfredo was not just content with learning; he was driven by an insatiable curiosity to understand the 'why' behind things. Why did certain herbs have healing properties? Why did some foods make you feel energized while others made you sluggish? These questions were not mere child's play; they were the early stirrings of a mind that would one day challenge the very foundations of modern medicine.

Dr. Sebi never received formal education in the way we understand it today. His school was the vast expanse of nature, his teachers the elders of his community, and his textbooks the plants and herbs that grew abundantly around him. This lack of formal education was never a hindrance; if anything, it freed him from the dogmas that often restrict scientific inquiry.

As he grew into adolescence, the confines of his small village could no longer contain his burgeoning curiosity. With nothing but a few belongings and a heart full of dreams, Alfredo set out to explore the world. His travels took him across Central America, through the Caribbean, and eventually to the United States. Each new place brought new learnings, new perspectives, and new pieces to the puzzle he was subconsciously assembling.

The Struggles of a Young Immigrant: The American Dream or Nightmare?

Arriving in New Orleans and later moving to Los Angeles, Alfredo—now adopting the name Dr. Sebi—faced the harsh realities of life as an immigrant. Jobs were hard to come by, and the ones available were often backbreaking with little pay. But it was during these trying times that Dr. Sebi had an epiphany. He realized that despite the advancements in medicine and technology, people were not healthier. In fact, chronic diseases were on the rise, and the so-called modern lifestyle was anything but conducive to health.

The Catalyst: Personal Health Crisis as a Wake-Up Call

In his early 30s, Dr. Sebi found himself plagued with obesity, asthma, diabetes, and even impotence. The man who had spent his childhood exploring the secrets of nature was now a victim of his neglect of those very principles. This personal health crisis served as a wake-up call. Dr. Sebi knew he had to return to the roots, to the wisdom that had been his foundation. Determined to heal himself, Dr. Sebi began a period of self-experimentation. Drawing upon the knowledge he had gained over the years, both from his grandmother and his travels, he began to make changes in his diet and lifestyle. Slowly but surely, he started to see improvements. His weight stabilized, his asthma symptoms reduced, and his energy levels soared. It was a transformation that

The Awakening: Realizing the Mission

As he stood at the precipice of this newfound health, Dr. Sebi had an awakening. He realized that his journey, with all its trials and tribulations, had prepared him for a larger mission. He was not just meant to heal himself; he was meant to heal the world. And so, armed with the wisdom of his ancestors and the courage of his convictions, Dr. Sebi embarked on a mission to bring the gift of natural healing to the world. Looking back, it's clear that Dr. Sebi's formative years were not just a period of personal growth but a preparation for the path that lay ahead. Every experience, every challenge, and every lesson served to shape the man he would become—a man who would challenge the status quo, inspire a generation, and leave a legacy that continues to transform lives to this day.

In understanding Dr. Sebi's childhood and formative years, we don't just see the making of a legend; we witness the universal human potential for transformation and growth. It serves as a poignant reminder that sometimes the most extraordinary heroes arise from the most ordinary beginnings.

Thus, Dr. Sebi's early years were not just a chapter in his life but the very foundation upon which his revolutionary approach to holistic health was built. It's a testament to the enduring power of curiosity, the resilience of the human spirit, and the transformative potential of returning to one's roots.

Childhood and Formative Years:

In the small village of Ilanga, Honduras, a young boy named Alfredo Darrington Bowman—later known to the world as Dr. Sebi—was born into a world of limited means but unlimited potential. His family, like many in the region, relied on the land for sustenance, cultivating crops and raising livestock. The simplicity of this lifestyle, far removed from the complexities of modern medicine, would later serve as the cornerstone of Dr. Sebi's revolutionary approach to health and well-being.

Dr. Sebi's early years were deeply influenced by his grandmother, "Mama Hay." A herbalist and traditional healer, Mama Hay instilled in young Alfredo a profound respect for the natural world. She taught him the names of plants, their uses, and the delicate balance of nature that sustains life. These early lessons were not formal education but a form of ancestral wisdom passed down through generations.

The Curiosity of a Young Mind: Early Signs of a Healer: As a child, Alfredo was not just content with learning; he was driven by an insatiable curiosity to understand the 'why' behind things. Why did certain herbs have healing properties? Why did some foods make you feel energized while others made you sluggish? These questions were not mere child's play; they were the early stirrings of a mind that would one day challenge the very foundations of modern medicine.

Dr. Sebi never received formal education in the way we understand it today. His school was the vast expanse of nature, his teachers the elders of his community, and his textbooks the plants and herbs that grew abundantly around him. This lack of formal education was never a hindrance; if anything, it freed him from the dogmas that often restrict scientific inquiry.

As he grew into adolescence, the confines of his small village could no longer contain his burgeoning curiosity. With nothing but a few belongings and a heart full of dreams, Alfredo set out to explore the world. His travels took him across Central America, through the Caribbean, and eventually to the United States. Each new place brought new learnings, new perspectives, and new pieces to the puzzle he was subconsciously assembling.

The Struggles of a Young Immigrant: The American Dream or Nightmare?

Arriving in New Orleans and later moving to Los Angeles, Alfredo—now adopting the name Dr. Sebi—faced the harsh realities of life as an immigrant. Jobs were hard to come by, and the ones available were often backbreaking with little pay. But it was during these trying times that Dr. Sebi had an epiphany. He realized that despite the advancements in medicine and technology, people were not healthier. In fact, chronic diseases were on the rise, and the so-called modern lifestyle was anything but conducive to health.

The Catalyst: Personal Health Crisis as a Wake-Up Call

In his early 30s, Dr. Sebi found himself plagued with obesity, asthma, diabetes, and even impotence. The man who had spent his childhood exploring the secrets of nature was now a victim of his neglect of those very principles. This personal health crisis served as a wake-up call. Dr. Sebi knew he had to return to the roots, to the wisdom that had been his foundation.

Determined to heal himself, Dr. Sebi began a period of self-experimentation. Drawing upon the knowledge he had gained over the years, both from his grandmother and his travels, he began to make changes in his diet and lifestyle. Slowly but surely, he started to see improvements. His weight stabilized, his asthma symptoms reduced, and his energy levels soared. It was a transformation that

The Awakening: Realizing the Mission

As he stood at the precipice of this newfound health, Dr. Sebi had an awakening. He realized that his journey, with all its trials and tribulations, had prepared him for a larger mission. He was not just meant to heal himself; he was meant to heal the world. And so, armed with the wisdom of his ancestors and the courage of his convictions, Dr. Sebi embarked on a mission to bring the gift of natural healing to the world.

Looking back, it's clear that Dr. Sebi's formative years were not just a period of personal growth but a preparation for the path that lay ahead. Every experience, every challenge, and every lesson served to shape the man he would become—a man who would challenge the status quo, inspire a generation, and leave a legacy that continues to transform lives to this day.

In understanding Dr. Sebi's childhood and formative years, we don't just see the making of a legend; we witness the universal human potential for transformation and growth. It serves as a poignant reminder that sometimes the most extraordinary heroes arise from the most ordinary beginnings.

Thus, Dr. Sebi's early years were not just a chapter in his life but the very foundation upon which his revolutionary approach to holistic health was built. It's a testament to the enduring power of curiosity, the resilience of the human spirit, and the transformative potential of returning to one's roots.

The Awakening: Discovering Natural Healing

Dr. Sebi's life was a tapestry of experiences, each thread woven meticulously to form the intricate design of his legacy. But even the most beautiful tapestries have their knots and tangles. For Dr. Sebi, this came in the form of a personal health crisis. It was a reckoning, a moment that forced him to confront the dissonance between his ancestral wisdom and the life he was leading.

The crisis was a wake-up call that reverberated through the very core of his being. It was as if the universe itself was urging him to pause, to reflect, and most importantly, to return. Return to what, you ask? To the roots. To the wisdom of the soil, the whispers of the wind, and the songs of the river. To the natural world that had been his first teacher, his first love, and his first sanctuary.

The Rediscovery: Nature as Medicine

Dr. Sebi began to revisit the teachings of his grandmother, "Mama Hay," and the wisdom of his community elders. He delved into the ancient texts and oral traditions that spoke of herbs as medicine, food as nourishment, and nature as the ultimate healer. This was not a mere academic exercise; it was a rediscovery of his own self, a reconnection with his own nature.

Armed with this renewed understanding, Dr. Sebi embarked on a series of experiments that were as audacious as they were revolutionary. He began to test the healing properties of various herbs, not in a sterile lab but in the laboratory of life. He used himself as the subject, meticulously documenting the effects of each herb, each food, and each lifestyle change.

The results were nothing short of miraculous. His asthma symptoms began to subside, his energy levels soared, and his chronic ailments started to wane. But this was not just a physical transformation; it was a spiritual awakening. Dr. Sebi began to realize that healing was not just about curing diseases; it was about restoring balance, about realigning oneself with the natural world.

As he delved deeper into this newfound realm of natural healing, Dr. Sebi began to formulate a philosophy, a healing paradigm that was as ancient as the hills yet as revolutionary as the future. He understood that the body was not a machine to be fixed but a garden to be tended. He realized that diseases were not just random occurrences but symptoms of a deeper imbalance.

The Alkaline Revelation: Balance as the Key

One of the cornerstones of Dr. Sebi's healing philosophy was the concept of alkalinity. He discovered that an alkaline body was a healthy body, a body in balance. But this was not just about the pH level of the blood; it was about the pH level of the soul. It was about creating an environment where diseases could not thrive, where the natural state was not just survival but flourishing.

Dr. Sebi's ideas were radical, and like all radical ideas, they were met with skepticism and criticism. The medical establishment was quick to dismiss his claims, labeling them as pseudoscience. But Dr. Sebi was not deterred. He knew that the proof of the pudding was in the eating, and so he continued to heal, to transform, and to awaken.

The Validation: Healing as Proof

As word spread about Dr. Sebi's miraculous healings, people began to seek him out. They came with their ailments, their skepticism, and their desperation. And they left with their health, their belief, and their liberation. Each healing was a validation, a testament to the power of natural remedies, and a rebuke to the limitations of conventional medicine.

As Dr. Sebi stood on this precipice of transformation, he made a vow. A vow to dedicate his life to healing, to sharing the wisdom that had saved him, and to awakening the world to the power of natural remedies. It was a mission that would take him across continents, into the hearts of millions, and onto the pages of history.

Dr. Sebi may have left this earthly realm, but his awakening continues to ripple through time and space, touching lives and transforming realities. His philosophy of natural healing serves as a beacon, guiding us through the labyrinth of modern ailments toward a sanctuary of holistic well-being.

In understanding Dr. Sebi's awakening to natural healing, we are not just chronicling the life of a man; we are mapping the evolution of a philosophy, the birth of a movement, and the awakening of a collective consciousness. It's a narrative that resonates deeply with anyone navigating the complexities of modern life, offering not just remedies but revelations. It serves as a mirror reflecting our own potential for transformation, inviting us to embark on our own journey of discovery, balance, and awakening.

The Symbiosis: Nature and Human Connection

Dr. Sebi's journey into the realm of natural healing wasn't just a solitary endeavor; it was a symbiotic relationship with the natural world. He understood that the human body is not an isolated entity but a part of the larger ecosystem. This realization was transformative. He began to see the interconnectedness of all life forms, recognizing that the health of the individual is intrinsically tied to the health of the planet.

As Dr. Sebi delved deeper into the world of herbs and natural remedies, he also confronted the ethical dimensions of healing. He was acutely aware of the exploitation that often accompanies the commercialization of natural resources. Dr. Sebi made it a point to source his herbs and ingredients ethically, ensuring that he was not only healing individuals but also contributing to the well-being of the communities that nurtured these natural treasures.

The Emotional Quotient: Mind-Body Synergy

While the physical benefits of Dr. Sebi's natural healing methods were evident, what often goes unnoticed is the emotional and psychological transformation that accompanied it. People who came to him were not just physically sick; they were emotionally drained and mentally fatigued. Dr. Sebi's holistic approach aimed to heal not just the body but also the mind and spirit. He often said that a calm mind leads to a healthy body, and he was living proof of that philosophy.

Dr. Sebi was a cultural bridge, connecting the ancient wisdom of natural healing with the modern quest for well-being. He was as comfortable quoting scientific studies as he was recounting folk tales and ancestral wisdom. This made him incredibly relatable to a diverse audience, ranging from academics to everyday people seeking relief from their ailments. His ability to speak multiple 'languages'—be it scientific jargon or cultural idioms—made his message universally appealing.

One of the most striking aspects of Dr. Sebi's approach was its simplicity. He often said, "Simplicity is the key to brilliance," and his methods were a testament to this belief. He didn't advocate for complicated regimens or expensive treatments. His solutions were straightforward, accessible, and effective. This simplicity was not a sign of naivety but a mark of profound understanding. He knew that the most effective solutions are often the simplest ones.

The Community: A Collective Awakening

Dr. Sebi was not just a healer; he was a catalyst for a collective awakening. He empowered people to take control of their health, to question conventional wisdom, and to seek alternatives. This created a ripple effect, inspiring a community of natural healing practitioners and advocates. His teachings became the foundation for a larger movement, one that transcended geographical boundaries and cultural barriers.

Dr. Sebi's journey was not without challenges. From legal battles to personal attacks, he faced numerous obstacles that would have deterred a lesser person. But Dr. Sebi was resilient. He drew strength from his convictions and the tangible results of his work. Each challenge was an opportunity for growth, a lesson in resilience, and a stepping stone to greater heights.

The Mentorship: Passing the Torch

As Dr. Sebi's work gained recognition, he took on the role of a mentor, guiding the next generation of natural healing practitioners. He understood that his mission was larger than himself, and for it to continue, he needed to pass on his wisdom. Through workshops, seminars, and one-on-one mentorship, Dr. Sebi ensured that his legacy would live on in the hearts and minds of those he inspired.

Dr. Sebi's physical presence may no longer be with us, but his teachings are timeless. They continue to inspire, heal, and awaken people to the possibilities of natural healing. His legacy is not confined to the pages of books or the walls of a clinic; it lives in the lives he touched, the minds he opened, and the world he helped to heal.

The Invitation: Your Personal Awakening

As we delve into the life and philosophy of Dr. Sebi, we are also invited to examine our own beliefs, our own practices, and our own potential for transformation. Dr. Sebi's awakening is not just a historical event but an ongoing invitation. An invitation to each one of us to embark on our own journey of natural healing, to awaken to our own innate power, and to become active participants in a collective movement towards holistic well-being.

In sum, Dr. Sebi's awakening to natural healing was not just a personal transformation but a societal shift. It was a paradigm change that challenged conventional medical practices, offering a more holistic, ethical, and sustainable approach to health and well-being. His life serves as a testament to the transformative power of natural healing, and his legacy offers a roadmap for anyone seeking to embark on their own journey of self-discovery and holistic health.

Trials, Tribulations, and Triumphs

The beginning of trials

Every legend, no matter how great, faces trials that test its mettle. For Dr. Sebi, these trials were not just personal obstacles, but social challenges that challenged the very foundations of his beliefs. When he began advocating the alkaline lifestyle, he encountered skepticism not only from strangers, but often from close acquaintances and even family members. The world he was trying to change was deeply rooted in conventional medical practices, and any deviation was seen as heresy.

Dr. Sebi's first encounters with the medical community were far from welcoming. He often encountered a wall of skepticism so thick that it stifled any lower spirit. The medical world, with its labyrinthine regulations and allegiance to pharmaceutical giants, was not ready for a disruptor. Dr. Sebi was seen as a maverick, something that could destabilize the very foundations of a system built for centuries.

Dr. Sebi's first forays into the world of natural cures were met with a shrug. The medical community, bound by years of traditional practices and pharmaceutical influences, found it difficult to accept a man who claimed that nature, in its purest form, possessed the answers to humanity's most pressing health problems. They questioned his credentials, his methods and his results. But most of all they questioned his audacity to challenge the status quo.

Personal tribulations

But it was not only the outside world that posed challenges. Dr. Sebi's journey was fraught with personal tribulations. There were moments of self-doubt, moments when he questioned the path he had chosen. Was he right to challenge the established norms? Were his methods really superior or was he leading people astray? These internal battles were as intense as the external ones and shaped the man Dr. Sebi would become.

As Dr. Sebi's work began to take hold, the media took notice. While this brought much-needed attention to his revolutionary ideas, it also exposed him to a level of scrutiny that few could have withstood. His every word, his every statement was dissected and analyzed, often with a cynical eye. The media circus became a double-edged sword, amplifying his message but also his challenges.

The emotional toll of these trials was immense. Dr. Sebi found himself walking a tightrope between his beliefs and the skepticism of the world. He was a man torn between the wisdom of ancient traditions and the skepticism of modern science. The nights were long, full of introspection and doubt. Could he really achieve the change he believed in so deeply? Was he a visionary or just a dreamer lost in his idealism?

Despite growing challenges, Dr. Sebi's faith in the power of nature remained unshakable. He delved into ancient texts, seeking confirmation and further knowledge. He traveled to remote parts of the world, learning from indigenous tribes and understanding their relationship with nature. These travels, both literal and metaphorical, strengthened his beliefs and equipped him with a broader perspective on natural healing.

Dr. Sebi faced not only emotional and social trials, but also financial difficulties. Funding research, procuring rare herbs and even maintaining a basic lifestyle became increasingly difficult. Each financial setback tested his commitment, forcing him to question whether his mission was worth the personal sacrifices he was making.

Triumphs begin

As time passed, the results of Dr. Sebi's methods began to speak for themselves. People who had been discarded by conventional medicine found relief and healing through his practices. Chronic ailments were healed and terminal diagnoses were disproved. Testimonies began to pour in, and the world had to stand up and take notice.

At a time when information was not as easily accessible as it is today, word of mouth was the most powerful tool. Stories of Dr. Sebi's miraculous healings spread like wildfire. People from all walks of life, from different parts of the world, began to seek him out. They came with hope in their eyes and faith in their hearts and, more often than not, left with their faith confirmed. But with recognition also came challenges of a different kind.

Just when it seemed that the weight of the world's skepticism would crush him, the first triumphs began to emerge. One patient, long afflicted with a chronic ailment, found relief through Dr. Sebi's methods. Then another. And yet another. The dominoes began to fall and the wall of skepticism began to crack. Each success story was a ray of light that ripped through the darkness of doubt that had clouded his path.

Dr. Sebi's growing popularity threatened the established medical order. Legal battles ensued, with attempts to discredit his work and tarnish his reputation. But each lawsuit, each legal challenge, only strengthened Dr. Sebi's resolve. He faced these battles head-on, armed with evidence, testimony and an unwavering faith in his mission.

Perhaps one of the most significant triumphs occurred not in a clinic, but in a courtroom. Dr. Sebi was dragged into a legal battle, accused of making false statements. Armed only with his unwavering conviction and a mountain of evidence, he stood his ground. When the dust settled, Dr. Sebi emerged victorious, with his methods validated by the most rigorous scrutiny. This victory in court was not only a personal triumph: it was a triumph for alternative medicine and for the countless lives that would be touched by his work.

As the legal battles raged, a global movement was taking shape. Dr. Sebi's teachings were no longer confined to a small community or a single country. They were resonating with people all over the world. From the Americas to Africa, from Europe to Asia, the alkaline lifestyle was gaining followers. It was becoming clear that this was not a passing trend, but a paradigm shift in the way people viewed health and wellness.

The global movement: The tipping point

While legal and social battles raged, something extraordinary was happening. Dr. Sebi's teachings were crossing borders, breaking cultural barriers, and sparking a global movement. From the crowded streets of New York to the remote villages of Africa, his message was resonating. The alkaline lifestyle was no longer a fringe concept, but was becoming a global phenomenon.

Dr. Sebi's life was a testimony to the resilience of the human spirit. He showed the power of conviction and the impact a person can have when he truly believes in his mission. His trials and tribulations were numerous, but so were his triumphs. And these triumphs were not just personal victories: they were victories for humanity, for holistic health and for the timeless wisdom of nature.

The legacy of triumph: an indelible impact

Dr. Sebi's life was a symphony of trials, tribulations and triumphs. Each challenge faced added a new note to this complex composition, and each triumph transformed that note into a melody. His legacy is not only in the lives he has touched, but also in the global shift toward holistic health that he has helped ignite.

Dr. Sebi's journey is a testimony to the resilience of the human spirit. It is a story that shows that when you stand firm on your convictions, even the most insurmountable challenges can be overcome. Her life serves as an inspiration to each of us, reminding us that the path to true change is often fraught with trials, but it is a path worth walking. It is a tale that speaks directly to the heart of anyone seeking to maintain optimal health while navigating the complexities of modern life, offering not just a method but a way of life, not just advice but a philosophy. It is a story that transcends Dr. Sebi, becoming a story about each of us and our potential for triumph in the face of trials and tribulations.

In conclusion, Dr. Sebi It is an inspiration to all, reminding us that true change often comes from challenging established norms and daring to chart one's own path.

The Legacy Left Behind: The Inception of a Legacy

In the vast tapestry of history, few individuals leave an indelible mark that transcends their lifetime. Dr. Sebi was one such individual whose legacy began not with grandeur but with a simple, profound belief: nature holds the key to our well-being.

This belief, rooted in ancient wisdom yet revolutionary in its approach, would set the stage for a journey that would impact millions worldwide.

The Humble Beginnings

Every great legacy has humble beginnings. For Dr. Sebi, it was a personal quest for health and wellness. Born Alfredo Darrington Bowman in the village of Ilanga, Honduras, he was not always the iconic figure the world came to know. As a young man, he grappled with ailments that modern medicine failed to address. It was this personal struggle that led him to the ancient practices of herbal healing, practices that had been passed down through generations but were slowly being overshadowed by modern medicine.

His initial experiments with herbs were for personal healing. But as he delved deeper into the world of natural remedies, he discovered a profound truth: the body, when given the right tools, can heal itself. This revelation was not just a personal epiphany; it was the birth of a philosophy that would challenge the very foundations of modern healthcare.

Challenging the Status Quo

In an era dominated by pharmaceutical solutions, Dr. Sebi's approach was radical. He believed that diseases were primarily caused by mucus buildup in the body, and by eliminating mucus-forming foods and consuming a diet rich in natural, alkaline foods, one could achieve optimal health. This was not just a dietary recommendation; it was a call to return to nature, to embrace the wisdom of our ancestors, and to challenge the commercial interests that had come to dictate healthcare norms.

As Dr. Sebi began to share his discoveries, he faced resistance. The medical community, driven by a combination of skepticism and commercial interests, was quick to dismiss his claims. But Dr. Sebi was undeterred. He had witnessed the transformative power of his methods firsthand, and he knew that this was a truth that needed to be shared.

The Birth of the Dr. Sebi Cell Food Company

Recognizing the need to make his remedies accessible to a larger audience, Dr. Sebi established the Dr. Sebi Cell Food Company. Based in Los Angeles, the company offered a range of herbal products designed to cleanse the body and promote holistic health. But this was not just a commercial venture; it was a mission. Every product, every remedy was a testament to Dr. Sebi's belief in nature's healing power.

The company's success was a testament to the efficacy of Dr. Sebi's methods. As more and more individuals experienced the benefits of his remedies, the word began to spread. From celebrities to everyday individuals, people from all walks of life began to seek out Dr. Sebi's guidance.

The initial phase of Dr. Sebi's legacy was marked by challenges and triumphs. From personal struggles to challenges from the established medical community, he faced numerous hurdles. But with unwavering conviction and a deep belief in nature's wisdom, he laid the foundation for a legacy that would continue to inspire and heal for generations to come. The story of Dr. Sebi is not just a tale of herbal remedies; it is a testament to the power of conviction, the importance of challenging established norms, and the transformative power of nature. As we delve deeper into his legacy, we will discover the profound impact of his teachings and the global movement he inspired.

The Expansion of a Healing Philosophy

The Power of Testimonials. As Dr. Sebi's teachings began to gain traction, something extraordinary happened: people started sharing their stories. These were not just casual endorsements; they were heartfelt testimonials from individuals who had experienced life-altering transformations. The power of these testimonials lay not just in their numbers but in their authenticity. From reversing chronic conditions to achieving a newfound sense of well-being, the stories were as varied as they were compelling.

While Dr. Sebi never sought fame, fame found him, thanks to the high-profile celebrities who became his advocates. Figures like Lisa 'Left Eye' Lopes and Michael Jackson not only sought his advice for their own health but also became vocal supporters of his philosophy. Their endorsements provided a level of visibility that catapulted Dr. Sebi into the mainstream consciousness. However, it's crucial to note that Dr. Sebi never let this newfound fame dilute his message. He remained steadfast in his commitment to natural healing, irrespective of who was listening.

With greater visibility came greater scrutiny. Dr. Sebi found himself embroiled in legal battles, most notably a 1988 case where he was charged with practicing medicine without a license. Armed with testimonials from patients who had been cured of ailments ranging from diabetes to cancer, Dr. Sebi fought the case and won. This legal victory was more than just personal vindication; it was a validation of his life's work and a signal to the world that natural healing was not just folklore but a viable, proven alternative.

As the years passed, Dr. Sebi's influence extended beyond the borders of the United States. His philosophy resonated with people across continents, transcending cultural and linguistic barriers. Workshops, seminars, and healing retreats organized in various parts of the world became platforms for spreading his teachings. The Dr. Sebi Cell Food Company expanded its reach, shipping products globally and making his herbal remedies accessible to people worldwide.

The Digital Age and Its Impact

The advent of the internet and social media platforms gave Dr. Sebi's teachings a new avenue for dissemination. YouTube videos, podcasts, and online courses made it easier for people to access his wisdom. More importantly, these digital platforms allowed for a community to form, a virtual gathering of like-minded individuals who could share experiences, advice, and support.

What started as a personal quest for health had now evolved into a cultural movement. The term 'alkaline diet' became part of the wellness lexicon. Restaurants and cafes started offering 'Dr. Sebi-approved' dishes. Books and documentaries exploring his philosophy and methods began to appear. The legacy of Dr. Sebi was no longer confined to the realm of alternative medicine; it had permeated mainstream culture.

The middle chapter of Dr. Sebi's legacy is characterized by expansion and validation. From legal victories to global outreach, this period marked the transformation of a healing philosophy into a worldwide movement. But beyond the milestones and the accolades, the essence of Dr. Sebi's legacy lies in the lives he touched and transformed. As we delve into the concluding part of his legacy, we will explore how his teachings continue to impact the world today, shaping not just individual health journeys but also influencing the broader discourse on wellness and natural healing.

Lasting impact and the path forward

As Dr. Sebi's teachings reached a crescendo of influence, he remained unyielding in his commitment to authenticity. Unlike many wellness gurus who succumb to the allure of commercialization, Dr. Sebi never compromised the integrity of his message for financial gain. This unwavering commitment is a cornerstone of his enduring legacy. It is a lesson in itself for men and women in their 30s and 50s who find themselves navigating the labyrinth of health advice often clouded by commercial interests. Dr. Sebi's legacy serves as a beacon, illuminating the path to true holistic health.

The Dr. Sebi Foundation: A pillar of continuity

Realizing that his physical presence would not last forever, Dr. Sebi took steps to ensure the continuity of his work. The Dr. Sebi Foundation serves as a repository of his wisdom, a platform for research, and a vehicle for spreading the alkaline lifestyle. For those seeking personal growth and continued learning in the field of holistic health, the Foundation offers a wide range of resources and educational programs.

The ripple effect: inspiring a new generation of healers

Dr. Sebi's influence did not stop with his immediate followers, but spread to inspire a new generation of holistic health professionals. These are people who have picked up the baton from Dr. Sebi, adapting and expanding on his teachings. They are the naturopaths, nutritionists, and wellness coaches who provide better holistic health counseling to their clients, thus extending the reach of Dr. Sebi's philosophy into the future.

For men and women juggling busy lives, stress management and mental well-being are as critical as physical health. Dr. Sebi's teachings offer holistic solutions that are especially relevant in today's fast-paced world. His emphasis on natural foods, herbal remedies, and mental clarity provides a comprehensive toolkit for those seeking to manage stress and maintain optimal health in a fast-paced lifestyle.

Perhaps the most tangible aspect of Dr. Sebi's legacy is the way it manifests itself in people's daily choices. From preferring herbal teas to caffeinated beverages to incorporating more green leafy vegetables into meals, the legacy is alive in the micro-decisions that collectively contribute to improved health and well-being.

Community: A living testament

The community that has formed around Dr. Sebi's teachings is a living testament to his impact. Online forums, social media groups, and real-world communities offer support and guidance, serving as platforms where people share their success stories, challenges, and tips for maintaining an alkaline lifestyle. This community is not just a fan base, but a dynamic ecosystem that continues to evolve, learn, and support its members.

The future: A legacy not bound by time

Looking to the future, it is clear that Dr. Sebi's legacy is not bound by the constraints of time. His teachings have been validated by emerging research in the field of holistic health, and his philosophy continues to gain traction. The future landscape of the alkaline lifestyle is poised to grow, driven by a collective desire for natural and sustainable wellness solutions.

Dr. Sebi's legacy is not just the story of a man who revolutionized holistic health; it is a story of resilience, authenticity, and transformative impact. It is a legacy that serves as a roadmap for anyone committed to personal growth, continuous learning, and optimal wellness. It is a legacy that does not merely remain in the annals of history, but thrives in the choices we make every day, the communities we build, and the lives we touch.

As we close this first part, let us not see it as the end of a story, but as an invitation to become part of an ongoing journey: a journey toward better health, deeper understanding, and a life lived in harmony with the laws of nature. Dr. Sebi's legacy is not only his but also ours to live, nurture and pass on to future generations.

Book 2: The Alkaline Diet – Beyond Basics

The Science of Body pH: A Deep Dive:

Imagine for a moment that your body is like an intricate symphony. Each organ, each cell, plays its part in a grand orchestral performance that happens every second of every day. Now, what if I told you that the conductor of this symphony is something as simple yet complex as pH levels? Yes, the scale that measures the acidity or alkalinity of a substance is the maestro of your bodily functions. It's a concept that often goes unnoticed, yet its implications for our health are monumental.

The pH Scale: More Than Just Numbers

The pH scale ranges from 0 to 14. A pH of 7 is considered neutral, below 7 is acidic, and above 7 is alkaline. But these aren't just numbers; they're indicators of a state of balance or imbalance in the body. When we talk about body pH, we're delving into the core of cellular function, metabolic processes, and overall well-being. It's not just a topic for science geeks; it's a subject that holds the key to understanding how to achieve optimal health in a world that constantly throws us off balance.

Why Body pH Matters

You might wonder why something as seemingly trivial as body pH could have such a significant impact on your health. The answer lies in the delicate balance that our bodies strive to maintain. Every biochemical reaction, from digesting food to thinking, is pH-sensitive. Even a slight deviation from the ideal pH range can disrupt these processes, leading to health issues that range from minor annoyances to severe conditions.

The Cellular Perspective

At the cellular level, pH plays a crucial role in energy production. The mitochondria, often referred to as the "powerhouses" of the cell, function optimally at a specific pH level. When this balance is disrupted, it can lead to decreased energy, fatigue, and eventually, the deterioration of cell health. For those of us navigating the demands of a hectic lifestyle, understanding the role of pH in cellular energy production is not just academic; it's a practical approach to maintaining vitality.

The Metabolic Angle

Metabolism is another area profoundly affected by pH levels. Enzymes, the catalysts for metabolic reactions, are sensitive to pH changes. An imbalance can slow down metabolic rates, affecting everything from weight management to mental clarity. For men and women in their 30s to 50s who are juggling careers, families, and personal growth, a sluggish metabolism due to pH imbalance can be a significant setback.

The Immune System: A pH-Sensitive Fortress

Our immune system is remarkably pH-sensitive. A body that's too acidic becomes a breeding ground for bacteria and viruses, while an overly alkaline body can inhibit the immune system's ability to fight off infections. The key is balance. Achieving the right pH levels enhances the body's natural defense mechanisms, making it easier to fend off illnesses.

The Mind-Body Connection

The influence of pH doesn't stop at the physical body; it extends to mental well-being. Neurotransmitters, the chemicals responsible for our mood and mental state, are affected by pH levels. An imbalance can lead to mood swings, anxiety, and depression. For those seeking holistic ways to manage stress and improve mental health, understanding the role of pH is invaluable.

The Environmental Factor

Our environment plays a significant role in affecting our body's pH. From the food we eat to the air we breathe; external factors can easily throw our internal balance off-kilter. This is especially true in today's world, where processed foods and pollution are the norms rather than the exceptions. Being aware of how these factors affect our body's pH is the first step in reclaiming control over our health.

The Journey Ahead

As we delve deeper into the science of body pH, we'll explore how to maintain this delicate balance through diet, lifestyle, and mindfulness. We'll examine the myths and realities surrounding alkalinity and acidity, providing you with the knowledge you need to make informed decisions about your health.

Understanding the science of body pH is not just an intellectual exercise; it's a journey into the heart of what makes us tick. It's about empowering ourselves to take control of our health in a way that's grounded in scientific understanding and holistic wisdom. So, let's take this journey together, diving deep into the science of body pH, and unlocking the secrets to a balanced, healthy life.

The Mechanisms and Milestones of pH Balance

As we continue our journey through the labyrinth of body pH, let's delve into the mechanisms that govern this delicate balance. It's not just about avoiding certain foods or following a particular diet; it's about understanding the intricate systems that keep us in equilibrium. This knowledge is not just for the health-conscious; it's for anyone who wants to live a fuller, more vibrant life.

Our bodies are incredibly resilient, equipped with buffer systems that act as safety nets, neutralizing excess acidity or alkalinity. These systems—comprising bicarbonate, phosphate, and proteins—work tirelessly to maintain the pH within a narrow range. When you're running a marathon or pulling an all-nighter, these buffers are the unsung heroes that keep you going. Understanding how they work can give you a new appreciation for your body's innate wisdom.

The Role of Organs in pH Management

The kidneys and lungs play pivotal roles in managing body pH. The kidneys excrete or retain hydrogen ions and bicarbonate to balance acidity, while the lungs regulate the amount of carbon dioxide—a key component of the body's acid-base balance—by adjusting the rate and depth of breathing. It's a harmonious dance, finely tuned to respond to the body's ever-changing needs. For those of us who are always on the go, recognizing the importance of these organs can be a wake-up call to prioritize their health.

Nutrition: The Building Blocks of Balance

The foods we consume have a direct impact on our body's pH. Alkaline-forming foods like fruits and vegetables contribute to a more balanced pH, while acidic foods like processed meats can tip the scale in the other direction. But it's not just about what you eat; it's about the quality of the food. Organic, non-GMO produce not only supports a balanced pH but also provides essential nutrients that boost overall health. For those seeking to maintain optimal health amid a busy lifestyle, making informed food choices is crucial.

The Stress Connection

Stress is an often-overlooked factor that can affect body pH. The stress hormone cortisol can lead to a cascade of physiological responses that make the body more acidic. This is why holistic stress management techniques, such as mindfulness and meditation, are not just good for the mind but also beneficial for the body. For those grappling with the pressures of modern life, incorporating stress-reducing practices can be a game-changer in achieving pH balance.

Hydration: More Than Just Quenching Thirst

Water is the medium in which all biochemical reactions occur, and its quality can significantly impact body pH. Alkaline water, rich in minerals like magnesium and calcium, can help neutralize acidity. But beware of the marketing hype; not all alkaline waters are created equal. It's essential to choose a reputable source to ensure you're getting the benefits without the drawbacks.

The Exercise Equation

Physical activity is another key factor in maintaining a balanced body pH. Exercise helps to improve respiratory function, which in turn aids in regulating pH. However, it's essential to strike a balance. Over-exercising can lead to lactic acid build-up, making the body more acidic. For those juggling work, family, and personal growth, finding the right exercise regimen can be a balancing act in itself.

The Environmental X-Factor

We can't ignore the impact of our environment on body pH. Pollutants in the air and chemicals in our food and water supply can contribute to acidity. While we may not have control over all environmental factors, being aware of their potential impact can empower us to take proactive steps, such as using air purifiers or choosing organic products.

As we've seen, achieving a balanced body pH is not a one-size-fits-all endeavor. It requires a personalized approach, taking into account individual lifestyle factors, health conditions, and even emotional well-being. For those committed to personal growth and holistic health, understanding the science of body pH can be a transformative experience.

The Road Ahead

As we move forward, we'll explore practical ways to apply this knowledge in our daily lives. We'll look at how to make sustainable changes that not only balance our body's pH but also enhance our overall quality of life. It's a journey worth taking, filled with insights, challenges, and ultimately, the promise of a healthier, more harmonious existence.

By understanding the mechanisms that govern body pH, we're not just gaining scientific knowledge; we're acquiring tools for a lifetime of well-being. It's an investment in ourselves, one that pays dividends in the form of better health, greater vitality, and a deeper connection with our bodies.

The culmination of balance and well-being

Having reached the culmination of our exploration of the science of body pH, it is essential to reflect on the profound implications of this knowledge. We have delved into the mechanisms, organs involved, and lifestyle factors that contribute to our body's pH balance. Now, let's try to put it all together, synthesizing what we have learned into actionable insights that can transform our lives.

Understanding the science of body pH is not just an intellectual exercise, but a call to action. It invites us to take a more holistic approach to health, one that goes beyond diet and exercise to include stress management, emotional well-being, and environmental awareness. This is not a fad or a quick fix. It is a lifelong commitment to understanding one's body and taking proactive measures to maintain its delicate balance.

The power of knowledge

Knowledge gives power. When you understand the science behind body pH, you are better equipped to make informed decisions. You can choose foods that contribute to a balanced pH, practice physical activities that improve your well-being, and adopt stress management techniques that not only calm your mind but also balance your body. It's not just about avoiding disease; it's about improving your quality of life.

The benefits of maintaining a balanced body pH go far beyond the individual. Optimal health has a positive impact on relationships, work and emotional well-being. You become a better partner, a more effective worker, and a more empathetic friend. You not only improve your life, but contribute to a healthier and more harmonious world.

The pH balance of our bodies is a microcosm of the interconnectedness of all things. It reminds us that we are not isolated entities, but part of a larger ecosystem. The air we breathe, the water we drink and the food we eat all have a ripple effect on our health and well-being. This interconnectedness requires a more conscious approach to life that respects not only our bodies but also the world we inhabit.

One of the keys to understanding body pH is the wisdom of moderation. Extreme diets, excessive exercise, and chronic stress can alter the body's natural balance. The path to optimal health is not about extremes, but balance. It is about listening to one's body, understanding its signals, and making choices that bring us closer to balance

The future of pH science

Looking to the future, ongoing research promises to shed even more light on the complexities of body pH. From the possibility of personalized pH management plans to the development of new diagnostic tools, the future is bright for those committed to understanding and achieving pH balance. It is an exciting time to be at the forefront of this scientific frontier.

As we conclude this in-depth look at the science of body pH, the call to action is clear: take charge of your health. Don't wait for disease to strike or for stress to overwhelm you. Be proactive. Use the knowledge you gain to make informed choices that contribute to a healthy, balanced life.

Understanding the science of body pH is not a destination, but the beginning of a journey. It is the first step in a lifelong commitment to health, wellness and personal growth. It is about embracing the complexities of the human body and marveling at its innate ability to heal, adapt and thrive.

In concluding this point, let us not forget that the science of body pH is not just a topic of academic interest, but is a vital component of our daily lives. It is the undercurrent that influences our health, our emotions and our interactions with the world. Understanding it means not only acquiring scientific knowledge, but also a set of tools for a life of well-being. It is an investment in ourselves that pays off in the form of better health, increased vitality and a deeper connection with our bodies and the world around us.

So, as you move into the rest of your life, take this knowledge with you. Let it guide, empower and inspire you to live a life of balance, health and holistic well-being. This is not the end; it is only the beginning. Welcome to the lifelong journey toward alkalinity mastery.

Alkaline vs. Acidic: What Does It Truly Mean?

As we embark on this enlightening journey through the labyrinth of alkalinity and acidity, let's start with a fundamental question: What does it truly mean to be alkaline or acidic? It's a question that has intrigued scientists, nutritionists, and health enthusiasts alike. But more importantly, it's a question that holds the key to unlocking a higher state of well-being, a state where the body, mind, and soul are in harmonious balance.

At its core, the concept of alkalinity and acidity is about balance. It's about the equilibrium of ions and molecules in our bodily fluids, tissues, and organs. But it's not just a biochemical phenomenon; it's a holistic experience that permeates every aspect of our lives. From the food we eat to the thoughts we think, everything contributes to our internal pH environment.

The Language of pH

The term "pH" stands for "potential of hydrogen," a measure of the hydrogen ion concentration in a solution. In layman's terms, it's a scale that tells us how acidic or alkaline a substance is. The pH scale ranges from 0 to 14, with 7 being neutral. Anything below 7 is acidic, and anything above 7 is alkaline. But here's the kicker: the human body operates in a very narrow pH range, usually between 7.35 and 7.45. Even a slight deviation from this range can have profound implications for our health.

Think of your body as a finely tuned orchestra. Each organ, each cell, each molecule is like a musical instrument, playing its unique role in creating a harmonious symphony. The conductor of this orchestra is the pH level. When the pH is balanced, the music is sweet, and the body functions optimally. But when the pH is off, the music turns discordant, and the body begins to suffer.

The Culinary Connection

Let's talk about food, the fuel that powers this incredible machine we call the human body. The food we consume has a direct impact on our internal pH levels. Foods like fruits, vegetables, and certain grains are alkaline-forming, meaning they help to maintain a balanced pH. On the other hand, foods like meat, dairy, and processed sugars are acid-forming, contributing to an acidic internal environment.

But it's not just about what's on your plate; it's also about what's in your heart and mind. Emotions like stress, anger, and fear can trigger a cascade of biochemical reactions that lead to increased acidity. On the flip side, emotions like joy, love, and gratitude promote alkalinity. It's a fascinating interplay between the emotional and the biochemical, a dance that shapes our internal pH landscape.

We can't discuss alkalinity and acidity without acknowledging the role of our environment. The air we breathe, the water we drink, even the thoughts we entertain are influenced by the environment we inhabit. Pollution, toxins, and negative energy can all contribute to an acidic state, both physically and emotionally.

The Wisdom of Ancestral Practices

Long before the advent of modern science, ancient civilizations understood the importance of balance. Practices like Ayurveda and Traditional Chinese Medicine have emphasized the concept of balance for thousands of years. They may not have used the term "pH," but they understood the essence of what it means to be alkaline or acidic.

As we delve deeper into this topic, consider this chapter an invitation to explore the fascinating world of alkalinity and acidity. It's an invitation to question, to learn, and to grow. It's an invitation to take charge of your health and well-being, to become the master of your internal universe.

So, let's take this journey together, a journey that promises to be as enlightening as it is empowering. Let's unravel the mysteries of alkalinity and acidity, and in doing so, let's unlock the doors to a higher state of well-being, a state where the body, mind, and soul are in perfect harmony. Welcome to the genesis of understanding what it truly means to be alkaline or acidic.

ALKALINE/ACID PH CHART

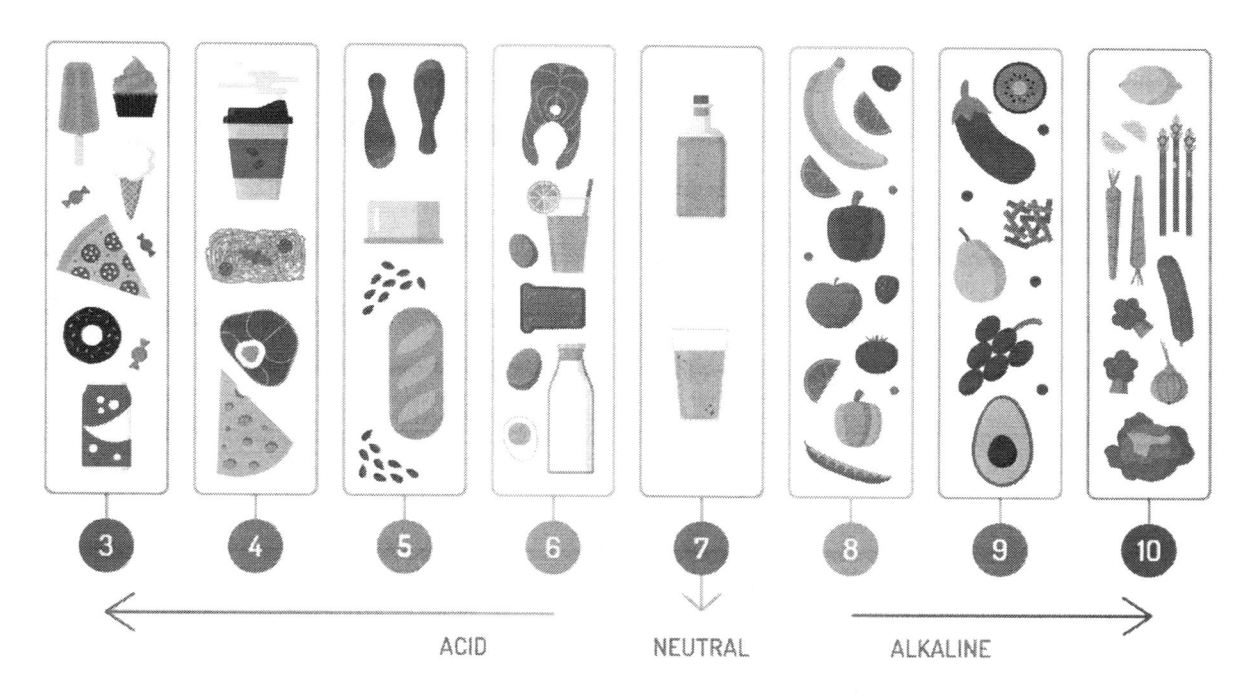

3 — 4 — 5 — 6 — 7 — 8 — 9 — 10

← ACID — NEUTRAL — ALKALINE →

The Heart of the Matter

As we delve deeper into the heart of this topic, let's consider the alchemy of transformation. The shift from an acidic to an alkaline state isn't just a change; it's a metamorphosis. It's akin to the caterpillar becoming a butterfly. The caterpillar doesn't merely grow wings; it undergoes a profound transformation that affects its very essence. Similarly, when we transition from an acidic to an alkaline state, we're not just altering our diet or lifestyle; we're transforming our entire being.

To truly understand alkalinity, we must first understand its opposite: acidity. Imagine your body as a garden. In an acidic state, this garden is overrun with weeds, pests, and disease. The soil is depleted, and the plants are struggling to survive. This is the state many find themselves in—bogged down by fatigue, stress, and chronic ailments. Acidity is the soil in which disease thrives.

Now, envision transforming that garden into an oasis of vitality. The soil is rich and fertile, the plants are robust, and there's a natural balance between all living things. This is what an alkaline state looks like at the cellular level. It's a state of optimal health, where the body's systems function in harmony, and the mind is clear and focused.

At the cellular level, alkalinity and acidity play a symphonic role. Each cell in our body is like a tiny orchestra, with ions and molecules playing the instruments. In an alkaline state, these cellular orchestras are in harmony. The cells can efficiently produce energy, repair themselves, and communicate with each other. In an acidic state, however, this cellular symphony turns into a cacophony, leading to dysfunction and disease.

Beyond the cellular level, there's a biochemical ballet taking place. Enzymes, hormones, and neurotransmitters—all are influenced by the body's pH level. For instance, digestive enzymes function best in a specific pH range. When we're too acidic, digestion suffers, leading to a cascade of health issues like bloating, gas, and nutrient deficiencies.

The Mind-Body Connection: A Two-Way Street

We've talked about how emotions like stress and anger can contribute to acidity, but it's a two-way street. An acidic body can also affect our emotional state, leading to mood swings, anxiety, and depression. It's a vicious cycle that can only be broken by restoring alkaline balance.

The benefits of an alkaline state extend beyond physical health. It's about mental clarity, emotional resilience, and spiritual alignment. When you're alkaline, you're not just surviving; you're thriving. You're better equipped to handle life's challenges, and you're more in tune with your inner self.

The most empowering aspect of understanding alkalinity and acidity is realizing that you have a choice. Every meal, every thought, every action is an opportunity to either contribute to acidity or promote alkalinity. It's a series of choices that shape your internal landscape and, by extension, your external reality.

As we each make these choices, we contribute to a collective shift. Imagine a world where the majority are operating from an alkaline state. It's a world of enhanced creativity, compassion, and conscious living. It's not just a personal transformation; it's a societal evolution.

So here we are, at the heart of the matter. Understanding the true meaning of alkaline versus acidic is not just an intellectual exercise; it's a call to action. It's an invitation to take responsibility for your own health and well-being, to be an active participant in your own healing journey. As we transition to the final phase of this exploration, let's carry with us the wisdom and insights we've gained. Let's move forward with a sense of purpose, armed with the knowledge that we have the power to transform not just our bodies, but our lives and, ultimately, our world.

The alkaline epiphany: A moment of clarity

Now consider the moment when the fog clears: the alkaline epiphany. It is that moment when you realize that the power to transform your health and well-being is within you. It's not just about changing your diet; it's about changing your life. It is about realizing that every choice you make, from the foods you eat to the thoughts you have, has a profound impact on your inner and outer world.

In a society obsessed with quick fixes and instant gratification, the sour lifestyle often seems easier. Fast food, stress-driven decisions and lack of mindfulness can create an illusion of comfort. But it is only an illusion. The long-term consequences of these choices can be dire and lead to a life of hardship, disease and dissatisfaction.

The alkaline commitment: A lifelong journey

Embracing an alkaline lifestyle is not a one-time event, but a lifelong commitment. It is about making conscious choices every day, even when it is difficult. It is about valuing one's health and well-being enough to make sacrifices and take the road less traveled. This commitment is not only to oneself, but also to one's loved ones, the community and the planet. It is a commitment to a higher quality of life.

Never underestimate the power of one person to make a difference. When you commit to an alkaline lifestyle, you become a beacon of health and well-being. Your energy changes and people notice. You inspire others to make healthier choices, creating a ripple effect that can transform communities and ultimately the world.

What will your alkaline legacy be? Will you be remembered as someone who took control of their health and lived life to the fullest? Or will you be another statistic, a cautionary tale of what happens when we neglect our well-being? The choice is yours and it starts with understanding the true meaning of alkaline and acid.

Imagine your life as a tapestry, where each thread represents a choice, you have made. An alkaline lifestyle is about weaving a tapestry of well-being, where each thread is a conscious decision that contributes to a beautiful and vibrant life. It is about creating a masterpiece to look back on with pride and satisfaction.

To conclude this exploration, let us return to the metaphor of the cellular symphony. The final movement is a crescendo, a culmination of all the choices made. It is a harmonious blend of physical, emotional and spiritual well-being. It is the magnum opus of your life, a testimony to the power of alkalinity.

The Alkaline Manifesto: A Declaration of Independence

Let this be your alkaline manifesto, a declaration of independence from the acidic lifestyle that has held you captive. Free yourself from the chains of poor health, chronic stress and emotional turmoil. Declare your sovereignty and take control of your destiny.

When the curtain falls on this chapter, give yourself a standing ovation. You have taken the first step on a transformational journey, a journey that will lead you to unparalleled health, happiness and harmony. You have armed yourself with knowledge and insight to make conscious choices, to be masters of your destiny and captains of your soul.

But remember that this is not the end; it is only the beginning. The journey to alkalinity is continuous, full of challenges and triumphs, setbacks and victories. It is a journey that requires courage, commitment and, above all, awareness.

When you step off the stage and into the world, take the wisdom you have gained with you. Let it guide you in moments of doubt and give you strength in moments of challenge. Let it be the compass that guides you through the labyrinth of life, leading you to a state of optimal health and holistic well-being.

And so, as we close this chapter, we open a new one, full of endless possibilities and infinite potential. We enter a future where alkalinity is not just a concept but a way of life, a future where the true meaning of alkaline and acid is not just understood but experienced.

Here is your alkaline journey, may it be as transformative as it is enlightening. Cheers to a life well lived, a life in balance, a life in harmony. Cheers to you.

The Detrimental Effects of an Acidic Diet

Imagine you are walking through a dense forest. The air is thick, the path is unclear, and you are not sure where you are going. This forest represents the maze of food choices that we walk through on a daily basis. In this maze, there is a silent culprit lurking in the shadows, often unnoticed but with a profound impact: the acid diet.

At first glance, an acid diet may seem harmless. After all, it often includes foods that are widely considered delicious and satisfying. But don't be fooled. This diet is a wolf in sheep's clothing, offering short-term pleasure at the expense of long-term health. It is like a siren's song, luring you in with the promise of instant gratification, only to leave you stranded on the rocks of poor health.

The acid diet has found a comfortable home in our modern, fast-paced, high-stress lifestyle. We are always on the move and juggling work, family and social commitments. In this maelstrom, convenience often trumps health. Fast food, processed snacks and sugary drinks become the preferred options. These choices, though seemingly harmless, are the building blocks of an acid diet.

When we consume acidic foods, we are essentially creating a breeding ground for disease within our bodies. The acidic environment weakens our immune system, making us more susceptible to disease. It is like planting the seeds of disease and watering them daily with poor food choices. Over time, these seeds germinate into various health problems, ranging from minor ailments to chronic conditions.

Acidic diet and emotional health: A vicious cycle

The impact of an acidic diet is not limited to physical health, but also extends to emotional well-being. Consuming acidic foods can lead to mood swings, irritability, and increased stress levels. This creates a vicious cycle: we eat badly because we are stressed, and we are stressed because we eat badly. It is a self-perpetuating vicious cycle that can be difficult to break.

One of the most insidious effects of an acidic diet is the acceleration of aging. The acidic environment in our bodies accelerates cell wear and tear, leading to premature aging. It is like adding miles to the biological clock at an alarming rate. The result? Wrinkles, decreased energy levels, and a host of age-related health problems show up earlier than they should.

The acid diet affects not only you, but also those around you. When you are not feeling your best, interactions with family, friends, and colleagues are affected. Decreased energy levels and mood swings can put a strain on relationships, creating a domino effect that extends far beyond the circle of your loved ones.

The acid diet: A cultural phenomenon

The acid diet has become a cultural phenomenon, deeply embedded in our social norms. It is celebrated in advertisements, social gatherings, and even family traditions. This makes it even more difficult to break free from its grip. It is not just a food choice, but a cultural mindset that needs to be challenged and changed.

As we delve deeper into this chapter, we will explore the various ways in which the acid diet acts like an invisible hand, subtly shaping our lives. It affects our health, our emotional well-being, our relationships and even our social structures. It is a pervasive force operating under the radar, and it is time to bring it to light.

We have just scratched the surface of the harmful effects of an acid diet. But awareness is the first step toward change. Moving forward, we will delve into the science, the symptoms and the solutions. It is a journey that promises to open eyes, enlighten and ultimately empower.

The Hidden Culprits: Everyday Foods and Habits

As we delve deeper into the topic of acidic diets, it's crucial to understand that the foods we consume daily are often the hidden culprits behind our body's acidic state. It's not just the obvious offenders like soda or processed snacks; even foods that are generally considered healthy can contribute to an acidic environment within the body. For instance, lean meats, whole grains, and dairy products can all tip the scale toward acidity when consumed in excess.

An acidic diet doesn't just affect your digestive system; it has a domino effect on your entire body. Your kidneys, for example, work overtime to filter out excess acids, which can lead to kidney stones or even chronic kidney disease over time. The liver, another vital organ, can also suffer from the strain of metabolizing acidic foods, potentially leading to liver disorders.

The Mental Toll: Stress and Acidity

It's not just what you eat; it's also how you feel. Stress is a significant contributor to acidity. Cortisol, the "stress hormone," can cause a cascade of physiological responses that make your body more acidic. This is a two-way street: an acidic body can also contribute to stress and anxiety, creating a vicious cycle that's hard to break.

The Silent Scourge: Inflammation

One of the most insidious effects of an acidic diet is inflammation. Chronic inflammation is linked to a host of diseases, from arthritis to cancer. When your body is acidic, it creates an environment where inflammation can thrive. This is not just a theory; numerous studies have shown a direct link between acidic diets and inflammatory markers in the blood.

Let's talk about weight. Obesity is a growing concern worldwide, and while many factors contribute to weight gain, an acidic diet is a significant player. Acidic foods can disrupt the body's ability to regulate insulin, leading to weight gain and even diabetes. Moreover, an acidic environment can slow down metabolism, making it harder to shed those extra pounds.

The Skin as a Mirror

Your skin often reflects what's happening inside your body. Conditions like acne, eczema, and premature aging can all be exacerbated by an acidic diet. The skin is one of the body's primary detoxification pathways, and when you're consuming too many acidic foods, it has to work harder to expel toxins, often leading to breakouts and other skin issues.

The Energy Drain

Feeling tired all the time? Your diet might be to blame. Acidic foods can sap your energy by disrupting your body's natural pH balance. This imbalance can affect your cells' ability to produce energy, leaving you feeling perpetually drained.

The Risk of Osteoporosis

There's a common misconception that osteoporosis is solely a result of calcium deficiency. However, an acidic diet can leach calcium from your bones to neutralize the acid, weakening them over time. This is particularly concerning for women, who are already at higher risk for osteoporosis.

The Heart of the Matter

Last but not least, let's talk about heart health. An acidic diet has been linked to increased cholesterol levels, high blood pressure, and a higher risk of developing heart disease. The inflammation caused by acidic foods can also damage blood vessels, leading to plaque buildup and, eventually, heart issues.

In summary, the detrimental effects of an acidic diet are far-reaching, affecting both physical and mental health. It's not just a matter of avoiding certain foods; it's about creating a balanced, holistic approach to health that considers the body's natural pH level as a cornerstone of well-being. The good news is that these effects are reversible. By making conscious choices and adopting an alkaline diet, you can restore your body's natural balance and pave the way for optimal health.

The Unseen Consequences: The Long-Term Impact of Acidic Diets

As we reach the final stretch of our exploration into the detrimental effects of an acidic diet, it's essential to focus on the long-term consequences that often go unnoticed until it's too late. These aren't just temporary setbacks; they are life-altering conditions that can significantly reduce the quality of your life.

One of the most overlooked aspects of an acidic diet is its impact on longevity. While it's easy to dismiss the immediate discomforts like bloating or fatigue, the long-term effects can be far more severe. Studies have shown that chronic acidity can lead to a shorter lifespan, primarily due to the increased risk of chronic diseases like cancer, heart disease, and diabetes.

The Emotional Quagmire: Mental Health and Acidic Diets

We've touched upon how stress can contribute to an acidic body environment, but let's delve deeper into the emotional and psychological toll. Chronic acidity can lead to mood swings, depression, and even cognitive decline. The brain, like any other organ, functions optimally in a balanced pH environment. An acidic diet can disrupt neurotransmitter functions, leading to emotional instability and reduced mental acuity.

The Social Costs: Relationships and Acidic Lifestyles

Your diet doesn't just affect you; it affects everyone around you. Chronic health issues can strain relationships, leading to emotional distance and, in extreme cases, isolation. The constant fatigue and irritability can make social interactions challenging, affecting your personal and professional life.

The Economic Burden: Healthcare Costs and Lost Opportunities

Let's talk numbers for a moment. The healthcare costs associated with managing chronic diseases stemming from an acidic diet can be astronomical. From frequent doctor visits to long-term medications and potential surgeries, the financial burden can be overwhelming for many families. Moreover, the lost opportunities in terms of career growth and personal development can't be quantified but are equally significant.

While it may seem unrelated, the environmental impact of an acidic diet is worth mentioning. Foods that contribute to acidity are often produced in unsustainable ways, contributing to environmental degradation. By choosing an alkaline diet, you're not just improving your health; you're also making an eco-friendly choice.

The Wake-Up Call: Recognizing the Signs

The body has a remarkable way of signaling when something is amiss. Frequent illnesses, unexplained fatigue, skin issues, and digestive problems are often the body's way of sounding an alarm. Ignoring these signs can lead to irreversible damage. It's crucial to listen to your body and take corrective action before it's too late.

The silver lining in all of this is that the body is incredibly resilient. The detrimental effects of an acidic diet are reversible to a large extent. By making conscious choices, you can restore your body's natural pH balance and significantly improve your quality of life. The first step is awareness, followed by action.

The Final Word: Your Health is Your Wealth

In conclusion, the detrimental effects of an acidic diet are far-reaching, affecting every facet of your life, from your physical and mental health to your relationships and even your financial stability. However, the power to change lies within you. By understanding the risks and taking proactive steps, you can break free from the shackles of an acidic lifestyle and embark on a journey towards holistic well-being.

The choices you make today will shape your tomorrow. Don't let an acidic diet dictate the course of your life. Take control, make informed decisions, and pave the way for a healthier, happier future. After all, your health is your greatest wealth, and it's time to invest in it wisely.

Transitioning: Steps to Adopt an Alkaline Lifestyle

So, you've come to the realization that your current dietary habits are not serving you well. You've read about the science of body pH, understood the difference between alkaline and acidic foods, and you're now fully aware of the detrimental effects of an acidic diet. The question that looms large is, "What's next?" The answer is transition—a thoughtful, deliberate shift towards adopting an alkaline lifestyle. This chapter is your roadmap, your guide to making that transition as smooth as possible.

Before we delve into the nitty-gritty of dietary changes, it's crucial to prepare your mind. Transitioning to an alkaline lifestyle is not just a physical endeavor; it's an emotional journey as well. You'll be bidding farewell to some of your favorite comfort foods, and that's not easy. It's essential to approach this transition with a sense of purpose and commitment. Understand that you're not depriving yourself; you're empowering yourself. You're making choices today that your future self will thank you for.

The Importance of Timing: When to Start?

One of the most common pitfalls in transitioning to a new lifestyle is the "I'll start tomorrow" syndrome. Tomorrow turns into next week, next week turns into next month, and before you know it, you're back to square one. The best time to start is now. Not after the holidays, not after your birthday, but now. There's a certain magic in the immediacy, a momentum that can carry you through the initial challenges.

While it's tempting to go all-in and make drastic changes overnight, experience tells us that a gradual approach is more sustainable in the long run. Start by incorporating one or two alkaline foods into your meals. Pay attention to how your body responds. You'll likely notice an increase in energy and a sense of well-being. These positive reinforcements will motivate you to continue on this path.

The Role of Education: Know What You're Eating

Ignorance is not bliss when it comes to your health. Take the time to educate yourself about the foods you're consuming. Learn to read labels, understand nutritional information, and be aware of misleading marketing terms like "all-natural" or "low-fat." The more you know, the better choices you'll make.

The Support System: You Don't Have to Do It Alone

Transitioning to an alkaline lifestyle can be challenging, but you don't have to do it alone. Seek out a community of like-minded individuals, whether it's online forums, social media groups, or local meetups. Share your challenges and triumphs, ask for advice, and offer support to others. The journey is more enjoyable—and sustainable—when you have company.

Let's address the elephant in the room—cost. Many people are deterred from adopting an alkaline lifestyle due to perceived financial constraints. While it's true that organic, fresh produce can be more expensive than processed foods, think of it as an investment in your health. Moreover, as you become more adept at sourcing and preparing alkaline foods, you'll find ways to make it more budget-friendly.

For many, food is closely tied to cultural identity, and the idea of giving up traditional dishes can be emotionally challenging. The key is to find a balance. You don't have to forsake your cultural heritage to adopt an alkaline lifestyle. Many traditional dishes can be modified to fit into an alkaline diet, allowing you to honor your roots while prioritizing your health.

The Trial and Error: Finding What Works for You

Finally, understand that transitioning to an alkaline lifestyle is a process of trial and error. What works for one person may not work for you, and that's okay. The goal is to find a sustainable, enjoyable way of living that also happens to be alkaline. It's a journey of self-discovery, of learning to listen to your body and respond to its needs.

Transitioning to an alkaline lifestyle is not a one-size-fits-all endeavor. It's a deeply personal journey that requires emotional readiness, timely action, gradual changes, continuous education, a strong support system, financial planning, cultural sensitivity, and a willingness to experiment. As you embark on this transformative journey, remember that the road may be long and fraught with challenges, but the destination—a healthier, happier you—is well worth the effort.

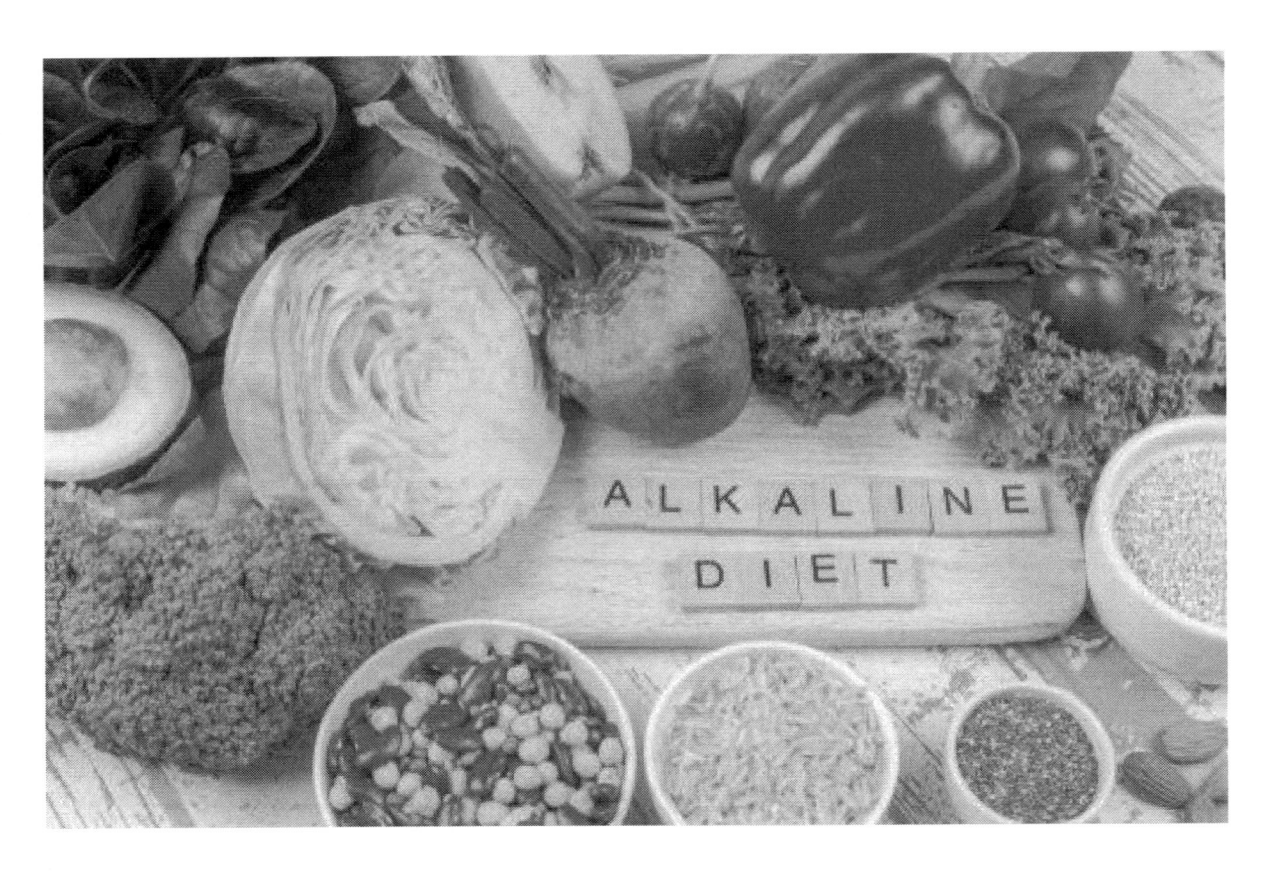

The Alkaline Kitchen: Your Culinary Sanctuary

As you embark on this journey toward alkalinity, your kitchen will become your sanctuary. It's where you'll prepare the foods that nourish not just your body, but also your soul. The first step in making your kitchen alkaline-friendly is a pantry overhaul. Out with the processed snacks, sugary cereals, and canned goods high in sodium. In their place, stock up on fresh fruits, vegetables, and whole grains that are the cornerstone of an alkaline diet. But remember, it's not just about what you bring into your kitchen; it's also about what you do with it. Cooking methods matter. Opt for steaming, grilling, or raw preparations to maintain the integrity of your alkaline foods. In our fast-paced world, meals are often rushed affairs, consumed in front of screens or on the go. Transitioning to an alkaline lifestyle invites you to slow down and savor your food.

Make mealtime a ritual. Set the table, even if it's just for you. Chew your food thoroughly, appreciating the flavors and textures. This practice of mindful eating not only enhances your dining experience but also aids in digestion and nutrient absorption.

Let's walk through what an average day might look like as you transition into an alkaline lifestyle. Start your morning with a glass of warm lemon water to kickstart your metabolism and balance your pH levels. For breakfast, opt for a smoothie packed with alkaline fruits like berries and kiwi, along with a handful of leafy greens. Lunch could be a hearty salad with a variety of colorful vegetables, topped with a homemade alkaline dressing made from olive oil, lemon juice, and herbs. Dinner might feature grilled tempeh or tofu, steamed vegetables, and a side of quinoa. Notice the absence of processed foods, dairy, and meat. It's a day rich in nutrients, flavors, and colors, leaving you satiated and energized.

It's not all smooth sailing. As you transition, you may experience cravings for the acidic foods you've left behind. You might even encounter detox symptoms like headaches or fatigue as your body adjusts. It's essential to listen to your body during this time but also to differentiate between a genuine need and a fleeting craving. When the urge for a sugary snack hit, reach for a piece of alkaline fruit instead. If you're feeling lethargic, try a brisk walk or a few minutes of deep breathing. These are your body's ways of communicating with you; it's up to you to respond in a manner that aligns with your new lifestyle.

Your dietary choices don't exist in a vacuum; they're part of a broader social context. Friends and family may question your new lifestyle, especially if it disrupts shared meals or traditions. Be prepared to explain your choices without being defensive or judgmental. Offer to bring an alkaline dish to gatherings, or suggest restaurants that cater to various dietary needs. It's an opportunity for dialogue and perhaps even inspiring others to consider their own dietary choices.

The Accountability Factor: Tracking Your Progress

One of the most effective ways to stay on course is to track your progress. Keep a food diary, noting what you eat and how you feel afterward. Take regular pH tests to monitor your body's acidity levels. Celebrate the small victories—a day without cravings, a noticeable increase in energy, or a positive comment from a loved one. These milestones, no matter how minor, serve as affirmations that you're on the right path.

The Resilience: Overcoming Setbacks

Setbacks are inevitable. You might slip up and indulge in a non-alkaline treat, or find yourself feeling discouraged by the pace of change. It's crucial to approach these setbacks with resilience rather than self-criticism. Understand that transitioning to an alkaline lifestyle is a marathon, not a sprint. Each day offers a new opportunity to make choices that bring you closer to your goal.

While this chapter focuses on transitioning to an alkaline diet, it's worth noting that an alkaline lifestyle extends beyond what you eat. It encompasses your physical activity, your mental well-being, and your emotional health. As you become more attuned to your body's needs, you'll find that this holistic approach becomes second nature. You'll not only eat better but live better.

In sum, transitioning to an alkaline lifestyle is a multifaceted endeavor that requires a commitment to change, a willingness to adapt, and the resilience to overcome challenges. It's a journey that promises not just better health, but a better quality of life. And that, dear reader, is a promise worth striving for.

The Alkaline Lifestyle: A Commitment to Wholeness

As you stand on the threshold of embracing an alkaline lifestyle, it's essential to recognize that this isn't a mere diet; it's a holistic approach to living. It's about making choices that align with your body's natural state, choices that not only nourish you but also enrich your life in countless ways.

One of the most significant challenges people face when transitioning to a new lifestyle is maintaining consistency. It's easy to be enthusiastic in the beginning, fueled by the excitement of new discoveries and initial improvements in well-being. However, the real test lies in sustaining this momentum. Consistency is the cornerstone of any successful transition, and it's particularly crucial when adopting an alkaline lifestyle.

The beauty of consistency is that it creates a self-reinforcing cycle. The more consistently you make alkaline choices, the better you'll feel, and the better you feel, the more motivated you'll be to continue making those choices. It's a virtuous circle that propels you toward ever-greater levels of health and happiness.

The Role of Mindfulness: Being Present in Your Choices

Mindfulness is often associated with meditation or yoga, but its application is far more extensive. It's about being fully present in the moment, aware of your actions and their consequences. When it comes to transitioning to an alkaline lifestyle, mindfulness plays a pivotal role.

Being mindful means paying attention to what you eat, how you prepare it, and even how you consume it. It means being aware of how different foods make you feel and adjusting your choices accordingly. It's about listening to your body and honoring its needs, rather than following the whims of your taste buds or the dictates of convenience.

The Emotional Connection: Food as a Source of Joy, Not Guilt

In many cultures, food is deeply intertwined with emotion. We eat to celebrate, to commiserate, and sometimes, to alleviate stress or boredom. This emotional connection to food can be both a blessing and a curse when transitioning to an alkaline lifestyle.

The key is to shift the emotional narrative around food. Instead of viewing alkaline foods as a form of deprivation, see them as a source of nourishment and joy. Relish the vibrant colors, the rich flavors, and the complex textures. Take pleasure in the act of preparing a meal, savoring the aromas and anticipating the feast to come. Make eating an act of self-love, not a source of guilt or stress.

The Community Aspect: Finding Your Tribe

No man is an island, as the saying goes, and this is particularly true when making significant lifestyle changes. The support of like-minded individuals can be invaluable in helping you stay on track. Whether it's a friend who shares your passion for alkaline foods, a family member who joins you in your journey, or an online community where you can exchange tips and recipes, finding your tribe can make all the difference.

The Lifelong Journey: Beyond the Transition

Transitioning to an alkaline lifestyle is not a destination but a journey—a lifelong journey. It's about continually evolving, learning, and growing. It's about listening to your body and making adjustments as needed. It's about extending the principles of alkalinity beyond your plate to encompass every aspect of your life; from the products you use to the thoughts you think.

As you fully embrace this alkaline journey, you're not just improving your life; you're also impacting those around you. Your choices serve as a silent testimony to the power of living in harmony with your body's natural state. You become a living example of what's possible, inspiring others to embark on their own journeys toward better health and greater well-being.

In conclusion, transitioning to an alkaline lifestyle is a profound commitment to yourself. It's a commitment to honor your body, to nourish your soul, and to enrich your life in ways you've yet to imagine. It's a challenging journey, fraught with obstacles and temptations, but it's also an incredibly rewarding one. And as you navigate this path, remember: you're not alone. Your part of a growing community of individuals who have chosen to live life at a higher octave, to tune into a frequency of wellness that resonates with the very core of who they are. Welcome to the tribe. Welcome to a life well-lived. Welcome to the lifelong journey of alkaline mastery.

Book 3: Dr. Sebi's Herbal Encyclopedia

The power and potency of herbs

Imagine walking through a lush forest, with the air tinged with the earthy aroma of foliage and the subtle sweetness of blooming flowers. Every step you take is a step into a living pharmacy, a treasure trove of potential remedies used for millennia. This is the world of herbs, a world that Dr. Sebi has passionately explored and brought to the forefront. But what makes herbs so powerful? What is it about these simple plants that can bring about profound changes in health and well-being?

Herbs are not simply plants, but concentrated containers of complex biochemical compounds. Alkaloids, flavonoids, and essential oils are just some of the components that give herbs their unique properties. These compounds interact with the human body in intricate ways, often mimicking the effects of synthetic drugs, but without the side effects. The power of herbs lies in their complexity, in the synergistic way their compounds interact to produce effects greater than the sum of their parts.

The wisdom of ancestral practices

Long before the advent of modern medicine, our ancestors relied on herbs to heal themselves. They were the original pharmacists, able to intuitively understand the benefits of different plants and use them in a variety of applications. From poultices to tinctures, teas to medicinal baths, herbs were the cornerstone of traditional medicine. This ancestral wisdom has been passed down for generations and forms the foundation of Dr. Sebi's herbal philosophy.

The alkaline lifestyle is not only about the foods you eat, but also about the herbs you incorporate into your regimen. Many herbs are naturally alkaline, meaning they help balance the body's pH levels, creating an environment in which disease cannot thrive. This is a crucial aspect of herbal medicine that is often overlooked in traditional practices. Focusing on alkaline herbs not only treats symptoms, but creates the foundation for long-term health.

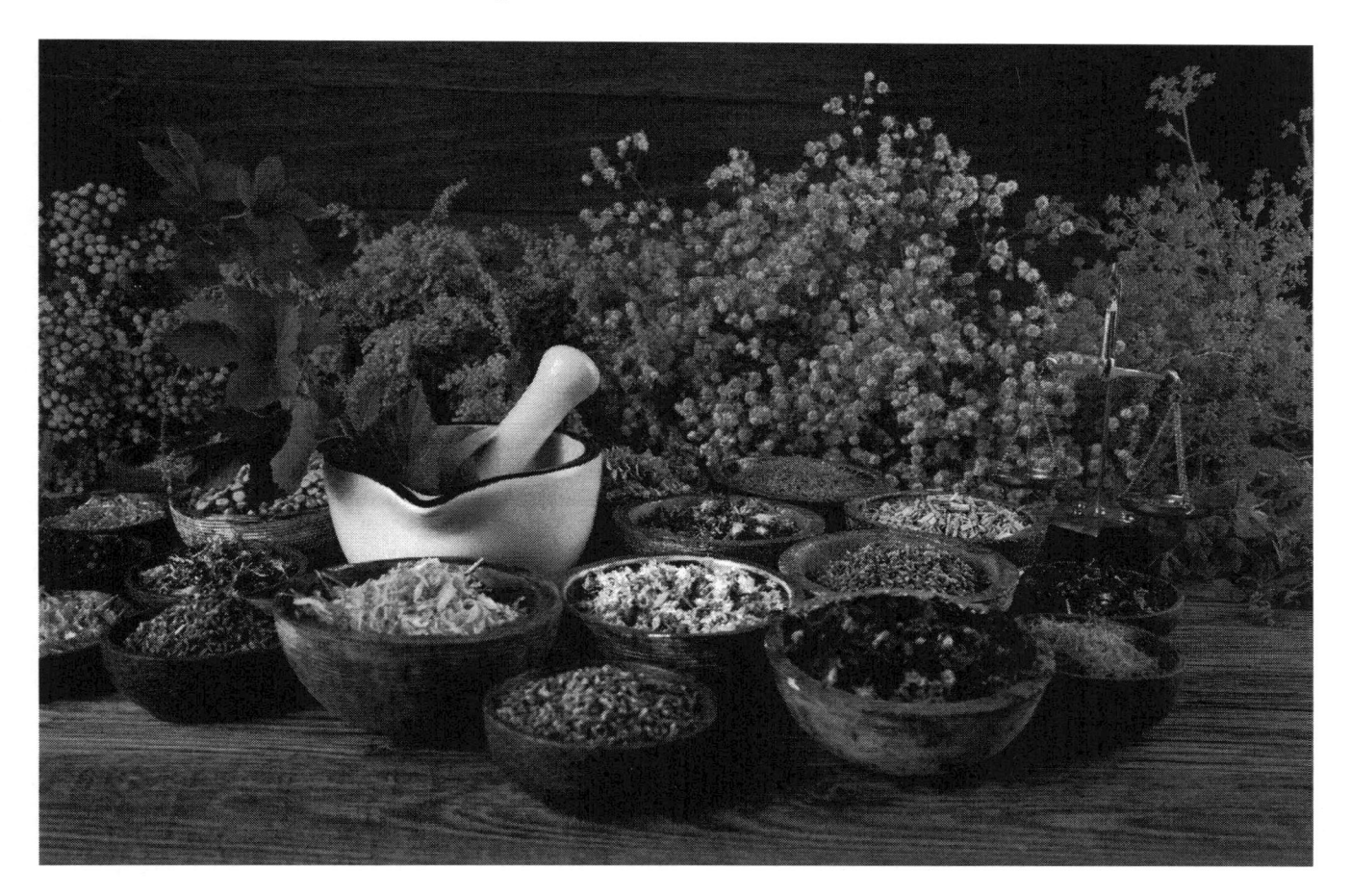

The mind-body-spirit triad

Herbs not only act on the body, but also have a profound impact on the mind and spirit. Take for example the calming effects of chamomile or the mental clarity conferred by ginkgo biloba. These are not mere coincidences, but the result of complex interactions between herbal compounds and human physiology. In this way, herbs offer a holistic approach to health that takes into account the interconnectedness of mind, body and spirit.

As we enter the world of herbal medicine, it is essential to approach it with a sense of responsibility. Increased interest in natural remedies has led to overharvesting of some species, putting them at risk of extinction. Ethical sourcing and sustainable practices are not just buzzwords-they are imperatives for anyone who is serious about herbalism. If we are careful about where our herbs come from, we can ensure that this ancient wisdom is preserved for future generations.

Embarking on a herbal path is a deeply personal journey, requiring intuition, knowledge and a willingness to experiment. No two bodies are the same, and what works for one person may not work for another. It is about listening to one's body, understanding its signals and responding with the appropriate herbal remedies. It is a journey of trial and error, successes and setbacks, but in the end it is a journey to a more authentic and holistic way of living.

The road ahead

As we delve deeper into this chapter, we will explore the specific herbs recommended by Dr. Sebi, their uses and how to incorporate them into daily life. We will also delve into the science behind herbal medicine, demystifying the complex interactions that give these simple plants their extraordinary power.

In essence, herbs are not just an adjunct to the alkaline lifestyle; they are an integral part of it. They offer a way to deepen the connection with the body, to sharpen intuition and to tap into a reservoir of ancestral wisdom. So when you turn the page, do so with an open mind and heart, for you are about to embark on one of the most rewarding journeys of your life. Welcome to the world of the power and potency of herbs. Welcome to the pharmacy of nature. Welcome to Dr. Sebi's herbal encyclopedia.

The Heart of Herbal Wisdom

As we delve deeper into the heart of herbal wisdom, it's crucial to understand the concept of synergy. In the realm of herbs, synergy is the magical process where the sum of the parts becomes greater than the individual components. It's not just about one active ingredient doing all the work; it's about a multitude of compounds working in harmony to produce a more potent effect. This is the alchemy that turns simple plants into powerful medicines.

One of the most fascinating aspects of herbal medicine is the practice of combining different herbs to enhance their effectiveness. This is not a haphazard process but a fine art backed by centuries of empirical knowledge and increasingly, by modern science. For example, turmeric and black pepper are often combined because the piperine in black pepper enhances the absorption of curcumin in turmeric. This is a perfect illustration of how understanding the nuances of herbal interactions can significantly amplify their healing power.

In our fast-paced world, stress is an unavoidable reality. Adaptogens, a unique class of herbs, have gained prominence for their ability to help the body adapt to stress. Herbs like ashwagandha, holy basil, and ginseng don't just tackle one issue; they bring a sense of balance and resilience to the entire system. For the modern individual juggling work, family, and personal commitments, adaptogens offer a holistic approach to managing stress and enhancing overall well-being.

The Herbal Impact on Emotional Health

While much focus is given to the physical benefits of herbs, their impact on emotional health is equally compelling. Plants like lavender and chamomile have been revered for their calming effects, often used to combat anxiety and insomnia. St. John's Wort is another example, frequently utilized as a natural alternative to antidepressants. The emotional tranquility that these herbs offer is not merely a side effect but a testament to their multifaceted healing capabilities.

Nature operates in cycles, and so does the human body. Traditional herbalism often aligns the use of herbs with the seasons, tapping into the natural rhythms of the earth for optimal health. For instance, immune-boosting herbs like echinacea and elderberry are most effective during the winter months, while detoxifying herbs like dandelion and milk thistle are better suited for spring. This seasonal approach to herbalism is not just poetic; it's a practical way to harness the most potent healing energies at the right time.

In our globalized world, exotic herbs from far-off lands are easily accessible. However, there's a growing movement advocating the use of local herbs. The philosophy behind this is simple yet profound: the plants that grow in your immediate environment are best suited to treat the health conditions prevalent there. While it's tempting to seek out rare, exotic herbs, sometimes the most potent medicine is growing right in your backyard.

As we embrace the power of herbs, it's our responsibility to do so sustainably. Wildcrafting, the practice of harvesting wild herbs, must be done with the utmost care and respect for the ecosystem. Overharvesting not only depletes resources but also disrupts the local flora and fauna. Ethical wildcrafting guidelines, such as taking only what you need and leaving enough for natural regeneration, are not optional; they are a moral imperative for anyone committed to the herbal path.

The Empowerment of Home Herbalism

One of the most empowering aspects of herbal medicine is that it puts the power back into the hands of the individual. You don't need a lab full of chemicals to create effective remedies; often, a simple kitchen will do. The act of preparing your herbal teas, tinctures, and salves is not just a form of self-care; it's a radical act of reclaiming your health autonomy.

As we transition into the final part of this chapter, we'll delve into the practical aspects of using herbs, from preparation methods to potential side effects. But for now, let's pause and appreciate the profound wisdom encapsulated in these humble plants. They are not just adjuncts to our wellness journey; they are active participants, offering their healing gifts freely and abundantly. In embracing the power and potency of herbs, we're not just tapping into ancient wisdom; we're also charting a course for a more sustainable, holistic, and empowered future.

The Power and Potency of Herbs: A Conclusive Exploration

As we reach the culmination of our exploration into the power and potency of herbs, it's essential to recognize that herbalism is not just a science; it's also an art and a spiritual practice. The herbs we use are not merely commodities to be exploited but living beings that share our planet. When we approach them with respect and reverence, we not only honor their intrinsic value but also open ourselves to a deeper level of healing that transcends the physical realm.

One of the most empowering aspects of herbal medicine is its adaptability to individual needs. Unlike the one-size-fits-all approach often seen in conventional medicine, herbalism allows for a highly personalized treatment plan. This is particularly important in our era of personalized medicine, where understanding one's unique genetic makeup and lifestyle factors is becoming increasingly relevant. Herbs offer a plethora of active compounds that can be tailored to address specific health conditions, making them an invaluable tool in personalized healthcare.

The Importance of Quality and Source

The efficacy of herbal medicine is highly dependent on the quality of the herbs used. Factors such as soil quality, growing conditions, and harvesting methods can significantly impact the potency of an herb. As consumers, it's crucial to be discerning about the source of our herbs. Opting for organic, sustainably harvested, and ethically sourced products is not just a matter of personal health but also a statement about the kind of world we want to live in.

Herbal medicine has the potential to democratize healthcare in a profound way. Many potent herbs are easily grown at home or found in the wild, making them accessible to communities that may not have easy access to conventional medical treatments. This is particularly relevant in a world where healthcare costs are soaring, and access to quality medical care is increasingly becoming a privilege rather than a right. Herbalism offers a way to take back control of our health and well-being, leveling the playing field in a healthcare system that often favors the wealthy.

While herbal medicine is often seen as a 'traditional' form of healthcare, it's important to recognize that tradition and modernity are not mutually exclusive. Many of the principles of herbal medicine are now being validated through scientific research, and there's a growing body of evidence supporting the efficacy of various herbs. This integration of ancient wisdom and modern science is one of the most exciting developments in the field of herbal medicine, offering a holistic approach that respects both empirical evidence and experiential knowledge.

The Lifelong Journey of Herbal Mastery

Understanding the power and potency of herbs is not a destination but a lifelong journey. As we deepen our knowledge and experience, we become more attuned to the subtle nuances that make each herb unique. This is a path of continuous learning and growth, where each step brings us closer to a state of holistic well-being. It's a journey that not only enriches our lives but also connects us to the natural world in a meaningful way.

When we embrace the power of herbs, the impact is not limited to our personal health. It creates a ripple effect that can influence our families, communities, and even the world at large. By choosing to support sustainable and ethical practices in herbal medicine, we contribute to a more just and equitable global healthcare system. And by sharing our knowledge and experience, we empower others to take control of their health, creating a community of informed and conscious consumers.

The Legacy of Herbal Wisdom

As we conclude this chapter, let's take a moment to honor the legacy of herbal wisdom that has been passed down through generations. This wisdom is a collective heritage that belongs to all of humanity, and it's our responsibility to preserve and propagate it for future generations. In a world that's increasingly disconnected from nature, the power and potency of herbs serve as a poignant reminder of the intricate web of life that sustains us all.

In embracing the profound wisdom encapsulated in these humble plants, we're not merely consumers or even practitioners; we're stewards of an ancient tradition that has the power to heal not just our bodies, but also our souls and our planet. And so, as we move forward, let us do so with a sense of reverence and responsibility, fully aware of the incredible power and potential that these natural allies offer us. It's not just about adding years to our life, but life to our years, enriching each moment with the vitality and well-being that is our birthright.

Detailed Profiles of Dr. Sebi's Top 50 Herbs

An In-Depth Introduction

Imagine walking into a pharmacy where the shelves are lined not with synthetic drugs, but with nature's own bounty. Each herb, root, and leaf has its own story, its own unique healing properties, and its own role in the grand symphony of holistic health. This is not a dream; it's a reality that Dr. Sebi brought to the forefront of modern consciousness. His work has illuminated the path for those seeking to harmonize not just the body, but also the mind and spirit, through the use of herbs.

Dr. Sebi's approach to herbal medicine is deeply rooted in ancestral knowledge. It's a wisdom that has been passed down through generations but has often been overshadowed by the rise of modern medicine. However, as we face an increasing number of health challenges that conventional medicine struggles to address effectively, the wisdom of our ancestors is making a resounding comeback. Dr.

Sebi's top 50 herbs are not just plants; they are time-tested solutions that have stood the test of centuries.

The Alchemy of Herbal Combinations

One of the most fascinating aspects of Dr. Sebi's herbal encyclopedia is the focus on not just individual herbs but also their synergistic combinations. It's akin to culinary alchemy, where the combination of individual ingredients creates a dish far greater than the sum of its parts. Similarly, when specific herbs are combined in the right proportions, their healing properties can be amplified exponentially. This is a nuanced art, one that Dr. Sebi mastered through years of research and practice.

In a world where stress has become the norm and where the side effects of synthetic drugs often rival the ailments they're supposed to treat, the relevance of herbal medicine has never been more pronounced. The herbs that Dr. Sebi championed are not just relics of a bygone era; they are vital tools for navigating the complexities of modern life. Whether it's the stress-busting properties of Ashwagandha or the immune-boosting power of Elderberry, these herbs offer tangible solutions for real-world problems.

As we delve into the detailed profiles of Dr. Sebi's top 50 herbs, it's crucial to approach this subject with an ethical lens. The herbs we discuss are not just commodities to be bought and sold; they are living entities that deserve our respect. Ethical sourcing and sustainable harvesting are not just buzzwords; they are imperatives for anyone serious about practicing herbal medicine. By choosing to engage with herbs in an ethical manner, we not only preserve these precious resources for future generations but also honor the intricate web of life that sustains us all.

The Personal Journey of Herbal Discovery

Embarking on the journey of herbal medicine is akin to setting sail on a vast ocean of discovery. Each herb you encounter is like an undiscovered island, rich with unique landscapes, hidden treasures, and untapped potential. As we navigate through the profiles of Dr. Sebi's top 50 herbs, consider this your personal voyage of discovery. It's a journey that will not only deepen your understanding of herbal medicine but also enrich your life in ways you can't yet imagine.

The Invitation to Transformative Healing

As we prepare to delve into the heart of this chapter, consider this an invitation. An invitation to transformative healing, to a deeper connection with the natural world, and to a life imbued with balance, harmony, and vitality. Dr. Sebi's top 50 herbs are not just a list; they are a gateway to a more fulfilling, more authentic, and more vibrant life.

So, as we turn the page to explore each herb in its intricate detail, remember that you're not just reading a book; you're stepping into a new paradigm of health and well-being. One that honors the wisdom of the past, addresses the challenges of the present, and offers hope for a healthier, happier future.

The Art of Herbal Storytelling

As we delve deeper into the heart of this chapter, it's essential to understand that each herb in Dr. Sebi's top 50 list is a character in a grand narrative. These herbs are not just biological entities; they are storied elements of a rich tapestry that weaves together culture, history, and medicine. Each herb has its own tale to tell, its own unique healing properties, and its own role in the grander scheme of holistic wellness.

The Healing Spectrum: From Detoxification to Rejuvenation

The range of healing properties among Dr. Sebi's top 50 herbs is nothing short of astounding. Some herbs are detoxifiers, purging the body of toxins and impurities. Others are rejuvenators, breathing life into tired cells and worn-out tissues. Yet others serve as balancers, helping to maintain the delicate equilibrium of bodily systems. This spectrum of healing is a testament to the richness of nature's pharmacy and the depth of Dr. Sebi's understanding of herbal medicine.

The Personalization of Herbal Medicine

One of the most empowering aspects of Dr. Sebi's herbal approach is the emphasis on personalization. While the herbs have general properties that can benefit everyone, their effects can be tailored to meet individual needs. For instance, someone dealing with chronic stress might find solace in the calming effects of Lavender, while another person battling digestive issues might turn to the soothing properties of Peppermint. The key is to listen to your body, to tune into its subtle signals, and to select herbs that resonate with your unique physiological and emotional landscape.

The Seasonality of Herbal Wisdom

In a world driven by instant gratification, it's easy to forget that nature has its own rhythms and cycles. Many of Dr. Sebi's top 50 herbs are seasonal, their potency varying with the cycles of the Earth. This seasonality is not a limitation but a feature, a reminder that we are part of a larger ecological tapestry. By aligning our herbal practices with the natural rhythms of the Earth, we not only optimize the efficacy of the herbs but also deepen our connection with the world around us.

Dr. Sebi's top 50 herbs are not confined to any single geographical or cultural context. They are a global ensemble, representing the collective wisdom of humanity's interaction with the plant kingdom. From the Ayurvedic treasures of India to the Native American herbs of North America, this list is a celebration of cultural diversity and global unity. It's a reminder that, despite our differences, we all share the same fundamental need for healing and well-being.

The Science Behind the Magic

While Dr. Sebi's approach is deeply rooted in ancestral wisdom, it's also supported by modern scientific research. Phytochemical analyses have confirmed the presence of potent compounds in these herbs, providing empirical validation for their traditional uses. This marriage of ancient wisdom and modern science is a powerful testament to the enduring relevance of herbal medicine.

As we explore the detailed profiles of these herbs, it's crucial to remember that their healing properties extend beyond the physical realm. Many of Dr. Sebi's herbs have psycho-spiritual benefits, affecting not just the body but also the mind and spirit. Whether it's the mood-enhancing effects of St. John's Wort or the spiritual clarity offered by Sage, these herbs serve as bridges between the material and ethereal dimensions of our existence.

Last but not least, let's not forget the culinary aspect of these herbs. Many of Dr. Sebi's top 50 herbs are not just medicinal; they are also culinary delights. Incorporating these herbs into your daily meals is not just a health strategy; it's a culinary adventure, a celebration of flavors, aromas, and textures that make the journey towards holistic health a joyous experience.

As we prepare to delve into the profiles of each individual herb, remember that this is not just an academic exercise; it's a transformative experience. Each herb you encounter is an invitation to expand your horizons, to deepen your understanding of yourself and the world, and to embark on a lifelong journey towards holistic well-being. Welcome to the living encyclopedia of Dr. Sebi's herbal wisdom.

The culmination of herbal wisdom: A journey beyond the leaves

As we come to the conclusion of this detailed exploration of Dr. Sebi's top 50 herbs, it is important to recognize that we have participated in a symphony of healing. Each herb, with its unique properties and applications, is like a musical note. Alone it is beautiful and powerful, but when combined with others it creates a harmonious melody that can heal the body, mind and spirit.

Although each herb in Dr. Sebi's list is a power in its own right, the real magic often occurs when they are combined. It is a kind of alchemy, in which the sum becomes greater than the individual parts. For example, combining anti-inflammatory herbs with those rich in antioxidants can create a blend that not only reduces inflammation but also strengthens the immune system. This alchemy is no accident: it is the result of years of research, experimentation, and deep knowledge of herbal synergies.

Ethical considerations: Sustainability and fair trade

In our enthusiasm for herbal remedies, it is crucial to remember the ethical dimensions. Increasing demand for these powerful herbs must not lead to unsustainable harvesting practices that endanger plant species and the ecosystems in which they live. Dr. Sebi has been a strong advocate of ethical sourcing, emphasizing the importance of fair trade and sustainability. As consumers, our choices can contribute to the problem or be part of the solution.

Although herbs offer a plethora of health benefits, they do not replace the advice of a medical professional. Self-education is essential. Know the herbs, understand their effects and be aware of potential interactions with the medications you are taking. The journey into herbalism is an empowering experience, but it also comes with the responsibility to be well-informed and cautious.

In addition to the physical benefits, these herbs often resonate on an emotional and psychological level. They can be catalysts for emotional healing, helping to relieve stress, anxiety, and even mild forms of depression. This emotional resonance is not a "side effect" but a fundamental feature of holistic healing, which views the emotional and physical self as deeply interconnected.

The Spiritual Dimension: Herbs as Teachers

In indigenous cultures around the world, herbs are often regarded not only as medicines but also as teachers. They have spirits, wisdom and lessons to impart. Whether it is the rooting energy of sage or the heart-opening qualities of rosemary, these herbs invite us to deepen our understanding of ourselves and the world around us. They are not just substances to consume, but allies to engage with.

In a culture obsessed with quick fixes and instant gratification, it is easy to view herbs as just another item on the shopping list. But the relationship with these herbs is not transactional, but transformational. It is a lifelong journey that evolves over time as we tune into our bodies, learn from our experiences, and adapt our herbal strategies to meet our changing needs.

Your journey into the world of Dr. Sebi's herbs not only impacts you, but has a ripple effect that can affect the lives of those around you. Whether it's sharing an herbal recipe with a friend, recommending a calming tea to a stressed family member, or simply radiating health and positivity, your choices can inspire others to embark on their own journey to holistic wellness.

The final note: an invitation to a lifelong odyssey

In closing this point, we remind you that this is not the end, but only a pause, an invitation to continue exploring, learning and growing. The world of Dr. Sebi's 50 Most Important Herbs is rich and expansive and offers endless possibilities to those willing to venture into its depths. Let this be your springboard to a lifelong odyssey of health, healing and holistic wellness. The journey is as rewarding as the destination, and the best is yet to come.

In the words of Dr. Sebi himself, "The Earth has everything you need to heal yourself." And so, armed with this new knowledge and perspective, we can take our steps toward a world that promises holistic health and limitless vitality. Welcome to your new beginning.

Crafting Herbal Solutions: From Teas to Tinctures

The Dawn of a New Alchemy

Imagine walking into your kitchen and seeing it not just as a place to prepare meals but as an alchemist's laboratory, a sacred space where you can craft elixirs that nourish the body, mind, and spirit. This is the essence of crafting herbal solutions, a practice that goes beyond mere consumption and enters the realm of transformation.

Crafting herbal solutions is both an art and a science. It's an art because it requires intuition, creativity, and a deep connection with the herbs you're working with. It's a science because it demands precision, understanding of herbal properties, and the ability to create effective formulations. This delicate balance between art and science is what makes herbal crafting a fulfilling and empowering practice.

The journey from plant to potion is a transformative one. It begins with the selection of high-quality herbs, each chosen for its unique properties and potential synergies with other herbs. The next step is the method of extraction, which can range from simple teas to more complex tinctures and salves. Each method has its own set of rules, its own alchemy, that transforms the raw herb into a potent solution.

The Intimacy of Handcrafting

There's an intimacy in handcrafting your own herbal solutions. When you measure each herb, when you stir the pot, when you strain the liquid, you're not just following steps; you're infusing the solution with your energy, your intention. This is what sets handcrafted solutions apart from mass-produced ones. They carry a piece of you, a piece of your healing intention.

The practice of crafting herbal solutions is not new; it's as old as human civilization itself. Our ancestors knew the power of herbs and used them in various forms to heal, nourish, and enhance well-being. They were the original herbal alchemists, and their wisdom has been passed down through generations. When you engage in herbal crafting, you're not just making a product; you're participating in an ancient lineage of healers.

As modern-day alchemists, we have a responsibility to source our herbs ethically. The surge in interest in herbal remedies has led to overharvesting and endangerment of certain plant species. Ethical sourcing is not just about sustainability; it's about respecting the plant, the farmer, and the ecosystem. It's about creating a chain of goodness that starts from the earth and ends in your herbal solution.

The Personal Touch: Crafting for Individual Needs

One of the most empowering aspects of herbal crafting is the ability to tailor solutions to individual needs. Unlike one-size-fits-all commercial products, handcrafted herbal solutions can be customized. If you're dealing with stress, you can create a blend that not only addresses the physical symptoms but also calms the mind. If you're struggling with digestive issues, you can craft a solution that targets the root cause rather than just alleviating symptoms.

The Community Aspect: Sharing is Caring

Herbal crafting is not a solitary endeavor; it's a community activity. Whether you're sharing recipes, exchanging herbs, or gifting your crafted solutions, you're participating in a community of like-minded individuals who value natural, holistic health. This sense of community not only enriches your own experience but also contributes to a collective consciousness that values sustainability, ethical practices, and holistic well-being.

Crafting herbal solutions is not a skill you master overnight. It's a lifelong learning curve that requires continuous education, experimentation, and refinement. Each crafting session is an opportunity to learn, to improve, and to deepen your connection with the herbs and with yourself.

The Invitation to Transformation

As we delve deeper into the nuances of crafting herbal solutions, from teas to tinctures, let this chapter serve as an invitation to transformation. You're not just making a product; you're crafting a better version of yourself. You're not just following recipes; you're participating in an age-old tradition of healing and empowerment. Welcome to the world of herbal alchemy, where each crafting session is a step toward holistic health, self-empowerment, and transformative well-being.

The Alchemy of Transformation

In the heart of herbal crafting lies the concept of synergy. It's not just about the individual herbs but how they interact with each other to create something greater than the sum of their parts. The alchemy of transformation occurs when you understand the synergistic relationships between herbs. For example, combining turmeric with black pepper enhances the bioavailability of curcumin, the active compound in turmeric. This is not mere happenstance; it's the result of understanding the intricate dance of herbal interactions.

While the allure of complex formulations can be tempting, there's an elegance in simplicity. Sometimes, a single herb, prepared with care and intention, can offer profound healing. Take chamomile, for instance. A simple cup of chamomile tea can offer a range of benefits from easing digestive discomfort to promoting relaxation. The key is to honor each herb for its unique gifts and not to overshadow it with unnecessary complexity.

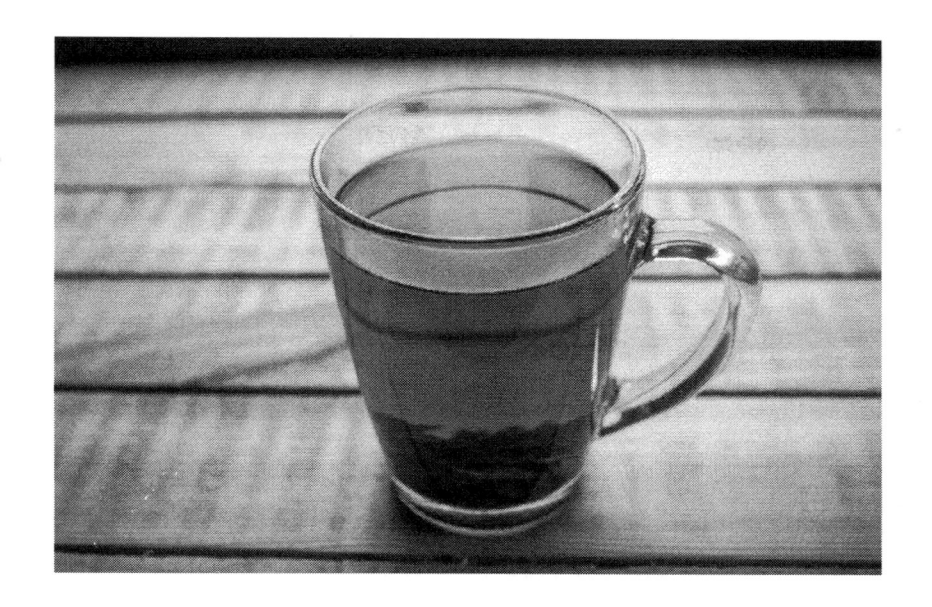

The act of crafting herbal solutions is a ritual in itself. From the initial stages of sourcing herbs to the final steps of bottling a tincture, each phase is imbued with significance. The ritualistic aspect elevates the practice from mere preparation to a form of meditative art. As you pour hot water over a blend of herbs to make tea, visualize the water extracting the essence, the life force, of the plants. As you shake a jar of herbs steeping in alcohol to make a tincture, imagine the liquid becoming more potent with each shake.

Herbal solutions come in various forms, each with its own set of advantages and applications. Teas are gentle, hydrating, and ideal for daily consumption. Tinctures are concentrated, long-lasting, and offer a more potent form of herbal medicine. Salves and balms provide topical relief and are excellent for skin conditions. The form you choose depends on your needs, your lifestyle, and your personal preferences.

One of the most empowering aspects of herbal crafting is the ability to preserve the healing properties of plants for future use. A well-made tincture can last for years, providing a long-term solution for chronic conditions. Herbal oils and salves, when stored correctly, can offer immediate relief for acute issues long after the plant has been harvested. Preservation is not just practical; it's a way to capture the essence of a moment, the peak potency of a plant, for future healing.

The Nuances of Dosage

Determining the right dosage is a crucial part of herbal crafting. Too little, and the solution may not be effective. Too much, and you risk potential side effects. The art of dosing requires a deep understanding of each herb's potency, the individual's constitution, and the specific ailment being addressed. It's a delicate balance that comes with experience and intuition.

Herbal crafting is not a rigid practice; it's fluid and adaptable. As you grow in your understanding of herbs and their properties, you'll find yourself tweaking recipes, experimenting with new combinations, and adapting solutions to meet specific needs. This adaptability is one of the most rewarding aspects of herbal crafting. It allows for personal growth and continuous learning, making each crafting session a new adventure.

Beyond the physical components and the scientific aspects, there's an ethereal element in herbal crafting: the power of intention. When you craft with intention, you're not just mixing herbs; you're infusing them with a specific purpose, whether it's healing, relaxation, or spiritual connection. This intention amplifies the efficacy of the herbal solution, making it more than just a sum of its parts.

Herbal crafting fosters a deep connection with nature. As you work with herbs, you begin to understand the cycles of growth and decay, the rhythms of the earth that govern the potency of each plant. This symbiotic relationship enriches not just your herbal practice but your life as a whole.

The Gift of Empowerment

Ultimately, the practice of crafting herbal solutions is a gift of empowerment. It puts the power of healing back into your hands, allowing you to take charge of your health and well-being. It's a liberating experience that transcends the boundaries of conventional medicine, offering a holistic approach that honors the complexity of human health.

As we continue to explore the world of herbal crafting, let this section serve as your guide to the transformative alchemy that awaits. Each herb, each blend, each crafted solution is a step closer to holistic health and personal empowerment. Welcome to the heart of herbal alchemy, where each crafting session is a journey of discovery, healing, and transformation.

The Culmination of Craftsmanship

The act of crafting isn't just a mechanical process; it's a ritualistic journey that connects us to the essence of life itself. When you steep a cup of herbal tea, you're not just making a beverage; you're participating in a timeless ritual that has been passed down through generations. The resonance of these rituals is what makes herbal crafting a transformative experience, one that transcends the boundaries of time and culture.

Herbal crafting teaches us the wisdom of wholeness. In a world fragmented by the hustle and bustle of modern life, the act of crafting herbal solutions serves as a reminder of the interconnectedness of all things. When you blend herbs to create a tincture, you're not just mixing ingredients; you're harmonizing elements of the earth, water, and air. This wisdom of wholeness is a guiding light, illuminating the path to holistic health and well-being.

Authenticity is the cornerstone of effective herbal crafting. When you craft with authenticity, you're not just following a recipe; you're expressing your unique essence through the medium of herbs. This alchemy of authenticity transforms the act of crafting from a mundane task into a sacred practice. It's this authenticity that makes each herbal solution uniquely potent, imbued with the energy and intention of the crafter.

Herbal crafting is a multisensory experience that engages all our senses. The aroma of lavender calms the mind, the taste of ginger warms the soul, the texture of a salve soothes the skin, and the vibrant colors of herbs delight the eyes. This symphony of the senses is what makes herbal crafting a deeply enriching experience, one that nourishes not just the body but also the soul.

One of the most rewarding aspects of herbal crafting is the legacy of learning it leaves behind. Each crafting session is an opportunity for growth and discovery, a chance to deepen your understanding of the intricate world of herbs. This legacy of learning is a treasure trove of wisdom, one that you can pass down to future generations, enriching their lives just as it has enriched yours.

The Harmony of Healing

At its core, herbal crafting is about healing—physical, emotional, and spiritual. Each crafted solution is a harmonious blend of healing energies, carefully balanced to address the complexities of human health. This harmony of healing is what sets herbal crafting apart from conventional approaches, offering a holistic alternative that honors the dignity and divinity of each individual.

The Tapestry of Tradition and Innovation

Herbal crafting is a tapestry woven from the threads of tradition and innovation. While it's essential to honor the wisdom of ancient practices, it's equally important to embrace the possibilities of modern innovation. This balance between tradition and innovation is what keeps herbal crafting vibrant and relevant, ensuring its continued evolution in the ever-changing landscape of health and wellness.

The Gift of Gratitude

As we conclude this journey through the art and science of herbal crafting, let us pause to express our gratitude. Gratitude for the earth that nourishes the herbs, for the water that brings them to life, for the air that carries their fragrance, and for the fire that transforms them into healing solutions. This gift of gratitude is the final touch, the sealing essence that completes the alchemy of herbal crafting.

Herbal crafting is not a destination; it's a journey—a journey that invites you to explore the infinite possibilities of health and healing. As you continue to craft, experiment, and discover, remember that each step is a part of a larger dance, a cosmic choreography that weaves together the threads of life and death, health and disease, joy and sorrow. It's this invitation to infinity that makes herbal crafting a lifelong adventure, one that promises endless opportunities for growth, healing, and transformation.

In the end, herbal crafting is a symphony of souls—a harmonious blend of human intention and natural wisdom, orchestrated by the unseen hand of the divine. As you sip your herbal tea or apply your herbal salve, know that you're not just consuming a product; you're partaking in a symphony, a celestial celebration of life's beauty, complexity, and mystery.

May each crafted solution be a stepping stone on your path to wellness, and may your life be enriched by the alchemy of herbs, the resonance of rituals, and the harmony of healing. Thank you for joining us on this transformative journey. The path ahead is bright, and the possibilities are endless.

Potential Side Effects and Interactions:

The Unseen Dance of Herbal Dynamics

As we delve into the world of herbal remedies, it's crucial to understand that while nature offers a plethora of healing options, it also presents complexities that deserve our attention. The herbs we celebrate for their curative properties are not isolated entities; they are part of a broader ecosystem of biochemical interactions, both within the plant itself and within our bodies. This chapter aims to shed light on the often-overlooked aspects of herbal medicine: the potential side effects and interactions that can arise when we integrate these natural wonders into our health regimen.

Herbs are potent, and that's precisely why they work. Their potency is a double-edged sword, however. On one side, it offers the promise of relief and healing, but on the other, it carries the risk of adverse reactions and interactions with other substances. The same biochemical compounds that make herbs effective can also make them potentially hazardous if not used wisely. It's akin to a dance, where each step must be carefully choreographed to avoid missteps that could lead to a fall.

When we consume herbs, either as teas, tinctures, or in other forms, they don't act in isolation. They interact with each other and with other substances we may be taking, whether those are pharmaceutical drugs, supplements, or even foods. These interactions can be synergistic, where the effect of the combination is greater than the sum of its parts, or antagonistic, where the substances counteract each other's effects. Understanding this symphony of synergy and antagonism is crucial for anyone looking to make the most out of herbal remedies while minimizing risks.

The Unseen Landscape of Individual Biochemistry

Another layer of complexity arises from our individual biochemistry. Each of us is a unique biochemical entity, and what works wonders for one person might have little effect or even cause harm to another. Factors like genetics, metabolism, and gut microbiota play a significant role in how we respond to herbs. This individual variability makes it all the more essential to approach herbal remedies with a sense of humility and caution.

The Ethical Responsibility of Knowledge

As consumers and practitioners of herbal medicine, we bear an ethical responsibility to be well-informed about both the benefits and the risks. This responsibility is not just to ourselves but also to the broader community. Misinformation can spread like wildfire, especially in the age of social media, and the consequences can be dire. A single adverse reaction can cast a shadow over the entire field of herbal medicine, undermining public trust and potentially leading to restrictive regulations that limit our access to these natural treasures.

Navigating the potential side effects and interactions of herbs requires a dance of discernment. It's about knowing when to step forward and when to hold back, when to embrace the potency of an herb and when to acknowledge its limitations. This discernment comes from a combination of scientific knowledge, personal experience, and intuitive wisdom. It's a dance that we all must learn to perform if we are to integrate herbal medicine into our lives in a way that is both effective and safe.

The Role of Professional Guidance

While self-education is invaluable, there's also a place for professional guidance in the realm of herbal medicine. Herbalists, naturopaths, and even some forward-thinking medical doctors can offer insights that are rooted in both scientific research and clinical experience. Their guidance can help us avoid the pitfalls that come from a lack of understanding of herbal dynamics.

As we move forward in this chapter, we will delve deeper into specific examples of potential side effects and interactions, offering practical advice on how to navigate these complexities. The aim is not to instill fear but to empower you with the knowledge you need to make informed decisions. After all, knowledge is not just power; it's also the foundation of wisdom. And wisdom is what we need to navigate the intricate, beautiful, but sometimes challenging landscape of herbal medicine.

In the end, the goal is not to shy away from the incredible healing potential that herbs offer but to approach them with the respect and understanding they deserve. It's a journey of balance, of weighing the risks against the benefits, and of making choices that align with our unique needs and circumstances. So let's embark on this journey together, with open minds and cautious optimism, as we explore the unseen dance of herbal dynamics.

The Herbal Paradox: Healing and Harm

As we continue our exploration into the potential side effects and interactions of herbal remedies, it's essential to recognize a paradox that exists in the heart of herbal medicine. The same herbs that can heal can also harm. This paradox isn't a flaw in the system but a reflection of the intricate balance that governs all life forms. The key to unlocking the healing potential of herbs lies in understanding this balance and learning how to navigate it skillfully.

Side effects from herbal remedies can range from mild to severe. Mild side effects might include temporary digestive discomfort or a slight rash, while severe side effects could involve liver toxicity or dangerous drops in blood pressure. The severity often depends on various factors, such as dosage, duration of use, and individual sensitivities. It's not just about the herb itself but how it interacts with the unique biochemical landscape of your body.

The Role of Dosage: Less Is More

One of the most common mistakes people make when using herbal remedies is assuming that if a little is good, more must be better. This couldn't be further from the truth. The principle of "less is more" often applies in herbal medicine. A small, carefully measured dose can offer therapeutic benefits, while an excessive dose can lead to toxicity. The wisdom of ancient herbal traditions, which often advocate for minimalism in dosing, holds valuable lessons for us in this regard.

Another area that demands our attention is the use of multiple herbs simultaneously. While some herbs work synergistically to enhance each other's effects, others can interact negatively, neutralizing benefits or exacerbating side effects. The concept of an "herbal cocktail" may sound appealing, but it requires a deep understanding of herbal interactions to avoid unintended consequences.

The timing of herbal consumption can also influence its effects. Some herbs are best taken on an empty stomach, while others require a meal to buffer their impact. Some herbs work better in the morning, aligned with our natural circadian rhythms, while others are more effective in the evening. The field of chronobiology, which studies the timing of biological events, offers intriguing insights into this aspect of herbal medicine.

The Hidden Variables: Lifestyle and Environment

Your lifestyle and environment can also influence how you respond to herbs. Factors like stress levels, sleep quality, and even the air you breathe can modulate the effects of herbal remedies. For instance, if you're living in a polluted environment, certain herbs that detoxify the body might become more crucial but also potentially more taxing on your system.

For those who are already on pharmaceutical medications, the stakes are even higher. Certain herbs can interact with medications in ways that either enhance or diminish their effects. For example, some herbs like St. John's Wort can interfere with the efficacy of birth control pills or anticoagulants. It's crucial to consult healthcare professionals when combining herbs with medications.

Lastly, the source of your herbs matters. The rise in demand for herbal remedies has led to issues of sustainability and quality. Overharvesting threatens not only the plants but also the ecosystems they belong to. Additionally, the market is rife with low-quality, adulterated products. Ethical sourcing and quality assurance are not just buzzwords; they are imperatives for anyone serious about herbal medicine.

The Road to Empowerment: Knowledge as Your Compass

As we navigate the nuanced landscape of potential side effects and interactions, our best ally is knowledge. Not just the knowledge found in books or research papers, but the experiential wisdom gained through mindful observation and listening to our bodies. It's an ongoing journey of discovery, requiring both intellectual rigor and intuitive sensitivity.

In the next section, we will delve into practical strategies for minimizing risks and maximizing benefits, offering you the tools you need to navigate this complex terrain with confidence and wisdom. The aim is to empower you to make informed choices, so you can harness the healing power of herbs while minimizing the risks. After all, the ultimate goal is not just to live longer but to live better, fully aligned with the natural world that sustains us.

Book 4: Disease Eradication and Natural Healing

Understanding the Root Causes of Modern Ailments:

As we embark on this journey to understand the root causes of modern ailments, let's first acknowledge the invisible web that envelops us. This web is woven from the threads of our fast-paced lives, environmental toxins, emotional stressors, and societal pressures. It's a complex tapestry that often obscures the underlying factors contributing to our health issues. But fear not, for the purpose of this chapter is to illuminate these hidden elements, to pull back the veil and offer you a clearer perspective on what's truly affecting your well-being.

Imagine your body as a finely tuned orchestra. Each organ, each cell, plays its part in a grand symphony of life. But what happens when one section of the orchestra is out of tune? The entire performance suffers. Similarly, when one aspect of our health is compromised, it can set off a chain reaction, affecting other systems and ultimately leading to various ailments. The root causes of these ailments are often not isolated incidents but the result of a series of imbalances that have thrown our internal orchestra into disarray.

The Environmental Quagmire

We live in an age of unprecedented technological advancement, but this progress comes at a cost. Our environment is rife with pollutants, from the air we breathe to the water we drink. These environmental toxins can accumulate in our bodies over time, leading to chronic conditions like inflammation, hormonal imbalances, and immune system dysfunction. It's not just the visible pollution; it's also the invisible electromagnetic fields from our gadgets, the synthetic chemicals in our household products, and even the genetically modified organisms in our food.

Our emotional well-being is intrinsically linked to our physical health. Stress, anxiety, and depression can manifest as physical symptoms, from digestive issues to chronic fatigue. The mind-body connection is not some New Age philosophy; it's a scientific fact backed by decades of research. Our emotional landscape serves as fertile ground where the seeds of various ailments can take root. The stress of juggling work, family, and personal life can wear us down, making us susceptible to diseases we might otherwise fend off with ease.

The Nutritional Paradox

In a world of abundance, malnutrition seems like an oxymoron. Yet, here we are, overfed but undernourished. Our diets are laden with processed foods, high in sugar and low in nutrients, setting the stage for a host of health issues, from obesity to diabetes. The irony is that we have more access to food than ever before, but the quality of that food has deteriorated. We've traded convenience for health, and our bodies are paying the price.

Our perception of health is largely shaped by societal norms and cultural biases. We live in a society that glorifies youth, speed, and productivity, often at the expense of health and longevity. The societal pressure to conform to certain body standards or to achieve professional success can lead us down a path of unhealthy choices. We skip meals to meet deadlines, we sacrifice sleep to climb the corporate ladder, and we ignore the warning signs until it's too late.

The Medicalization of Life

Modern medicine has made incredible strides in treating acute conditions and emergencies. However, when it comes to chronic ailments, the conventional approach often falls short. We've become a pill-dependent society, looking for quick fixes to complex problems. This medicalization of life has led us to treat symptoms rather than addressing the root causes. It's like putting a band-aid on a bullet wound; it might stop the bleeding temporarily, but it won't remove the bullet.

As we delve deeper into this chapter, we will explore each of these root causes in detail, offering insights and solutions to help you reclaim your health. This is not just about treating diseases; it's about understanding the intricate web of factors that contribute to them. It's a quest for wholeness, for a life where your body, mind, and spirit are in harmonious alignment.

In the sections that follow, we will equip you with the knowledge and tools to navigate this complex terrain. We will look at case studies, delve into scientific research, and most importantly, listen to the stories of individuals who have successfully overcome their ailments by addressing these root causes. So, buckle up; it's going to be an enlightening ride.

The Dance of Hormones: A Delicate Balance

Let's begin by diving into the world of hormones. These chemical messengers are the unsung heroes of our bodily functions, orchestrating everything from our metabolism to our mood. When this delicate balance is disrupted, it can lead to a cascade of health issues, including thyroid disorders, adrenal fatigue, and even mental health conditions like depression and anxiety. The triggers for these imbalances can range from environmental toxins to chronic stress, and they often operate in the background, unnoticed until symptoms become severe.

The Gut-Brain Connection: A Two-Way Street

The gut is often referred to as the "second brain," and for good reason. The gut and the brain are in constant communication, sending signals back and forth that influence our digestion, mood, and overall well-being. When the gut is compromised—perhaps due to an unhealthy diet, antibiotic use, or chronic stress—it can lead to a host of ailments, including irritable bowel syndrome, autoimmune diseases, and even cognitive issues like brain fog and depression. Understanding this connection is crucial for holistic health, as it underscores the importance of a balanced diet and stress management in maintaining both mental and physical well-being.

The Silent Killer: Chronic Inflammation

Inflammation is the body's natural response to injury or infection, but when it becomes chronic, it turns into a silent killer. Chronic inflammation is a common thread linking various modern ailments, from heart disease to diabetes and cancer. It's often fueled by lifestyle factors such as poor diet, lack of exercise, and stress. The insidious part is that it often goes undetected until it manifests as a full-blown disease. By addressing the root causes of inflammation, we can prevent or mitigate its damaging effects.

We often underestimate the impact of emotional health on our physical well-being. Emotional baggage, unresolved traumas, and chronic stress can manifest as physical ailments over time. The body stores emotional pain in much the same way it stores physical pain, and this can lead to chronic conditions that are difficult to diagnose and treat. Emotional well-being is not a luxury; it's a necessity for holistic health. Therapies like counseling, mindfulness, and even certain physical activities can help release this emotional baggage, leading to improved physical health.

The Vicious Cycle of Lifestyle Diseases

Modern life comes with its conveniences, but it also brings along lifestyle diseases like obesity, diabetes, and cardiovascular issues. These are often the result of a sedentary lifestyle, poor dietary choices, and stress. The vicious cycle starts when one ailment leads to another, creating a complex web of health issues that are difficult to untangle. Breaking this cycle requires a multi-faceted approach that addresses diet, physical activity, and emotional well-being.

While genetics play a role in our susceptibility to certain diseases, they are not the sole determinant. Epigenetics, the study of how environmental factors can change the way our genes are expressed, has shown that lifestyle choices can significantly impact our health outcomes. In essence, genetics may load the gun, but lifestyle pulls the trigger. This empowering perspective gives us the agency to influence our health destiny through conscious choices.

The Overlooked Importance of Sleep

In our hustle culture, sleep is often sacrificed at the altar of productivity. However, lack of sleep is a significant contributor to various health issues, including hormonal imbalances, weakened immune system, and even increased risk of chronic diseases. Quality sleep is not a luxury; it's a non-negotiable aspect of holistic health.

Lastly, let's not forget the environmental factors that often go unnoticed. From the quality of air we breathe to the water we drink, these external factors can have a profound impact on our health. Even the products we use for cleaning or personal care can contain harmful chemicals that contribute to chronic ailments.

Understanding the root causes of modern ailments is not about instilling fear but about empowering you with the knowledge to make informed choices. It's about shifting the focus from symptom management to root cause resolution. As we move forward, we'll delve into actionable strategies to address these root causes, offering a roadmap to reclaim your health and vitality.

The Power of Personal Responsibility

As we reach the conclusion of this exploration into the root causes of modern ailments, it's crucial to emphasize the role of personal responsibility. While external factors like environmental toxins and societal stressors undoubtedly play a role, the choices we make every day significantly impact our health outcomes. The power to change lies within us, and it starts with acknowledging that we are the architects of our own well-being.

Understanding the root causes of your ailments is akin to embarking on a journey of self-discovery. It's about peeling back the layers of your life to uncover the hidden triggers affecting your health. This journey may require you to confront uncomfortable truths, but it's a necessary step in reclaiming your health. It's not just about treating symptoms; it's about understanding why those symptoms exist in the first place. This deeper level of understanding can be transformative, offering you a renewed sense of agency over your health.

The Role of Mindfulness: Tuning into Your Body

One of the most powerful tools you can employ on this journey is mindfulness. By tuning into your body and paying attention to its signals, you can gain invaluable insights into the root causes of your ailments. Whether it's recognizing the early signs of inflammation or identifying the emotional triggers that lead to stress eating, mindfulness allows you to be proactive rather than reactive. It shifts the paradigm from disease management to disease prevention.

No man is an island, and this holds true in the realm of health and wellness. The support of a like-minded community can be invaluable in helping you navigate the complexities of modern ailments. Whether it's sharing resources, discussing strategies, or simply offering emotional support, a strong community can make the journey less daunting. It's about collective wisdom, the kind that comes from shared experiences and mutual support.

The Interconnectedness of All Things

As you delve into the root causes of your ailments, you'll come to appreciate the interconnectedness of all things. Your emotional well-being is intrinsically linked to your physical health, just as your lifestyle choices are connected to your mental state. This interconnectedness is not a curse but a blessing, for it means that positive changes in one area can have a ripple effect, leading to improvements in other areas of your life.

Understanding the root causes of modern ailments is ultimately about empowerment. It's about equipping you with the knowledge and tools you need to take control of your health. It's about moving away from a model of healthcare that treats the body like a machine, fixing isolated parts when they break down. Instead, it's about embracing a holistic model that treats the body, mind, and spirit as an integrated whole.

It's important to recognize that understanding the root causes of your ailments is not a one-time event but a lifelong commitment. It's a continuous process of learning, adapting, and growing. The road ahead may be fraught with challenges, but each challenge presents an opportunity for growth and transformation. And remember, you're not alone on this journey. Whether it's the support of loved ones or the guidance of healthcare professionals, help is always available. All you need to do is take the first step.

The Legacy You Leave

Finally, let's talk about legacy. The choices you make today will not only impact your health but also set an example for future generations. By taking the time to understand the root causes of your ailments, you're not just improving your life; you're contributing to a broader cultural shift towards holistic health and well-being. It's a legacy of empowerment, one that can inspire others to take control of their health and, in doing so, transform their lives.

As we close this chapter, remember that the choice is yours. You can continue down the path of symptom management, or you can choose the path of empowerment by addressing the root causes of your ailments. The journey may be challenging, but the rewards are immeasurable. It's not just about adding years to your life; it's about adding life to your years. Choose wisely, for your health is the most precious asset you have.

Dr. Sebi's Approach: A Case-by-Case Analysis –

As we delve into the heart of Dr. Sebi's approach to disease eradication and natural healing, it's crucial to recognize that each individual is a unique tapestry of experiences, genetics, and environmental exposures. This uniqueness calls for a tailored approach to healing, one that respects the individuality of each person's journey. Dr. Sebi understood this deeply, and it's this understanding that forms the cornerstone of his approach to natural healing.

In a world that often seeks quick fixes and easy answers, the allure of a one-size-fits-all solution is undeniable. However, Dr. Sebi's approach challenges this notion head-on. He believed that each case of ailment or disease is a complex interplay of multiple factors, and treating it as such requires a nuanced, case-by-case analysis. This isn't about slapping on a band-aid; it's about delving deep into the root causes and addressing them at their core.

One of the most striking aspects of Dr. Sebi's approach is the role of empathy. He didn't just treat diseases; he treated people. He listened to their stories, understood their struggles, and took into account the emotional and psychological factors that contribute to physical ailments. This empathetic approach is not just a 'nice-to-have'; it's a critical component of effective healing. It acknowledges that the mind and body are intrinsically linked, and that emotional well-being is a vital part of overall health.

The Power of Observation

Dr. Sebi was a keen observer, not just of scientific studies and medical literature, but of people and their behaviors. He paid close attention to how different foods, environments, and lifestyles affected individuals differently. This power of observation allowed him to make connections that were often overlooked in traditional medical settings. It's this observational acumen that enabled him to tailor his treatments to suit the individual needs of each patient.

The Courage to Challenge Conventional Wisdom

Dr. Sebi was not one to shy away from challenging the status quo. His approach often raised eyebrows in the medical community because it dared to question long-held beliefs and practices. But it's this very courage to challenge conventional wisdom that led to some of his most groundbreaking work. He wasn't constrained by dogma; he was driven by results. And time and again, his case-by-case approach yielded results that were nothing short of remarkable.

While Dr. Sebi was deeply rooted in scientific research, he also understood the value of intuition in the healing process. He recognized that each individual is the best judge of their own body and encouraged people to listen to their inner wisdom. This blend of science and intuition is a defining feature of his approach, allowing for a more holistic understanding of disease and healing.

The Importance of Context

Context is everything when it comes to health and well-being. Factors like cultural background, socioeconomic status, and even geographical location can have a profound impact on how diseases manifest and how individuals respond to treatment. Dr. Sebi took all these factors into account in his case-by-case analysis, ensuring that his treatments were not just effective but also culturally sensitive and socially equitable.

As we proceed to explore the intricacies of Dr. Sebi's case-by-case approach to disease eradication and natural healing, keep in mind that this is a journey of discovery. It's about breaking free from the limitations of a one-size-fits-all mindset and embracing the complexity and beauty of individualized healing. It's a challenging journey, no doubt, but it's also an incredibly rewarding one. For at the end of the day, what could be more empowering than reclaiming your health on your own terms?

As we set the stage for diving deeper into specific case analyses that embody Dr. Sebi's approach, it's essential to carry with us the principles that make this approach so transformative. It's not just about what's happening in the body; it's about the person in whom that body resides. It's about treating people, not just diseases. And most importantly, it's about empowering each individual to become an active participant in their own journey to health and well-being. With this foundation firmly in place, we are now ready to delve into the fascinating world of case-by-case analyses that bring Dr. Sebi's approach to life.

The Core Exploration

When Dr. Sebi embarked on a case-by-case analysis, he wasn't merely looking at symptoms or diagnoses. He was peeling back layers, digging deep into the individual's history, lifestyle, and even their emotional state. This comprehensive analysis allowed him to identify the root causes of ailments, which often eluded conventional medical diagnostics. It's this meticulous attention to detail that sets Dr. Sebi's approach apart from mainstream healthcare.

The Art of Listening

Dr. Sebi was an exceptional listener. He believed that the first step in healing was to listen to the patient's story. This wasn't just about medical history; it was about understanding the person's life journey, their struggles, and their aspirations. This empathetic listening provided invaluable insights into the emotional and psychological factors that often play a significant role in physical health.

Once Dr. Sebi had a comprehensive understanding of the individual case, he would often prescribe customized herbal treatments. These weren't generic herbal supplements; they were carefully selected blends of herbs that targeted the specific imbalances in the individual's body. The herbs were not just symptom relievers; they were catalysts for systemic change, aimed at restoring the body's natural balance.

Diet played a pivotal role in Dr. Sebi's case-by-case approach. He was a firm believer in the adage, "You are what you eat." But he took it a step further by customizing dietary recommendations based on the individual's unique needs. This wasn't about following a trendy diet; it was about understanding how different foods interacted with the individual's body and making informed choices accordingly.

The Emotional and Psychological Component

Dr. Sebi never underestimated the power of the mind in the healing process. He often incorporated emotional and psychological healing techniques, such as mindfulness and stress management, into his treatment plans. He understood that emotional well-being was not a separate entity but an integral part of overall health.

Dr. Sebi's commitment to his patients didn't end with a prescription or a treatment plan. He believed in the importance of follow-up, not just to monitor progress but to make necessary adjustments to the treatment. This iterative approach ensured that the healing process was dynamic and responsive to the individual's evolving needs.

Dr. Sebi was well aware that healing doesn't happen in isolation. He often encouraged his patients to seek support from like-minded communities, be it family, friends, or support groups. This sense of community provided the emotional sustenance that is often crucial for long-term healing.

One of the most commendable aspects of Dr. Sebi's approach was his commitment to making natural healing accessible to all, regardless of their socio-economic status. He often provided free consultations and treatments to those who couldn't afford them, underlining his belief that healthcare is a basic human right, not a privilege.

The Transformative Impact of Individualized Healing

As we delve deeper into the case-by-case analyses that embody Dr. Sebi's approach, it becomes increasingly clear that this is not just a method; it's a movement. It's a call to shift from a mechanistic, one-size-fits-all model of healthcare to a more compassionate, individualized, and holistic approach. It's about recognizing that each person is a unique universe of experiences, needs, and aspirations, and that healing must honor this uniqueness.

As we navigate through the complexities and nuances of Dr. Sebi's case-by-case approach, it's important to remember that this is an ongoing journey. It's a commitment to continuous learning, adaptation, and growth. It's about being open to new insights, willing to make adjustments, and committed to the lifelong journey of health and well-being.

The Lasting Impact of Individualized Care

As we reach the conclusion of our exploration into Dr. Sebi's case-by-case approach, it's crucial to recognize the lasting impact this methodology has had on countless lives. Unlike conventional healthcare systems that often treat patients as mere numbers or diagnoses, Dr. Sebi saw each individual as a unique tapestry of experiences, emotions, and aspirations. This profound respect for human complexity is what made his approach not just effective but transformative.

Dr. Sebi's case-by-case approach didn't just stop at individual healing; it created a ripple effect that extended to families, communities, and even societies. When one person found their path to wellness, it often inspired others to embark on similar journeys. This multiplier effect is one of the most potent aspects of Dr. Sebi's methodology, turning individual success stories into communal revolutions of health and well-being.

The Ethical Imperative: A New Paradigm for Healthcare

Dr. Sebi's approach challenges us to rethink the very foundations of healthcare. It raises ethical questions about the current state of medicine, where profit often trumps patient well-being. Dr. Sebi's case-by-case methodology serves as a clarion call for a more ethical, compassionate, and individualized form of healthcare, one that places the patient's holistic well-being at the center of all decisions.

One of the most enduring legacies of Dr. Sebi's case-by-case approach is the empowerment it offers. Patients are not passive recipients of care but active participants in their healing journey. This empowerment extends beyond the clinic or the herbal shop; it infiltrates every aspect of life, encouraging individuals to take charge of their health, their choices, and ultimately, their destiny.

The Symbiosis of Mind, Body, and Spirit

Dr. Sebi's methodology reminds us that health is not just the absence of disease but a harmonious balance between mind, body, and spirit. This triad is not a theoretical construct but a lived reality, experienced anew by each individual who walks the path of Dr. Sebi's teachings. The case-by-case approach is a testament to the intricate interplay between these three dimensions of human existence, each influencing and being influenced by the other.

As we look to the future, Dr. Sebi's case-by-case approach serves as a beacon of hope and a model for what healthcare can and should be. It's not just about treating symptoms or managing diseases; it's about nurturing the innate healing capacities that reside within each of us. It's about recognizing that each person's journey to health is as unique as their fingerprint and honoring that uniqueness with customized, compassionate care.

As we conclude this chapter, the question that looms large is, "What now?" The answer is both simple and profound: The baton has been passed to you. You have the tools, the knowledge, and the inspiration to be not just a beneficiary of Dr. Sebi's wisdom but also a torchbearer of his healing revolution. Whether you're a healthcare provider, a patient, or someone who simply cares about the well-being of humanity, you have a role to play in this transformative movement.

The Final Word: A Tribute to a Visionary

In closing, it's only fitting to pay tribute to Dr. Sebi, the visionary who dared to challenge the status quo, who had the courage to look beyond the surface, and who had the compassion to treat each patient as a unique individual deserving of holistic care. His case-by-case approach was not just a methodology; it was a philosophy, a way of life, and a beacon of hope for a world in desperate need of healing.

Dr. Sebi's approach to healing, rooted in individualized care, serves as a timeless lesson for all of us. It's a lesson in humility, reminding us that we don't have all the answers but that each individual holds a piece of the puzzle. It's a lesson in compassion, urging us to see the person behind the patient. And most importantly, it's a lesson in hope, assuring us that no matter how dire the diagnosis or how chronic the condition, there is always a path to healing, if only we dare to walk it.

As you turn the page, carry these lessons with you, for they are the essence of Dr. Sebi's case-by-case approach, a gift that keeps on giving, from one individual to another, from one generation to the next, in an unending cycle of healing, empowerment, and transformation.

Success Stories: Testimonials of Recovery

As we delve into the heart of this transformative chapter, "Success Stories: Testimonials of Recovery," it's essential to recognize the profound impact that personal stories can have on our understanding of health and healing. These are not just tales of triumph over adversity; they are living proof of the efficacy of Dr. Sebi's teachings, a testament to the resilience of the human spirit, and a beacon of hope for those still navigating their way through the labyrinth of chronic ailments.

What makes these testimonials so compelling is their emotional resonance. They touch a chord deep within us, reminding us of our shared vulnerability, our collective yearning for wellness, and our innate capacity for renewal. These stories are not just about the eradication of disease; they are about the reclamation of life, the rediscovery of joy, and the rekindling of hope. They are about ordinary people who, through their extraordinary journeys, illuminate the path for others, offering both inspiration and insight.

In a world saturated with quick fixes and miracle cures, the authenticity of these testimonials stands out like a lighthouse in a stormy sea. These are not scripted endorsements or paid promotions; they are heartfelt accounts from real people who have walked the walk, who have experienced firsthand the transformative power of an alkaline lifestyle and Dr. Sebi's herbal remedies. This authenticity lends credibility to their narratives, making them not just relatable but also deeply inspiring.

The Diversity of Experience

One of the most striking aspects of these success stories is their diversity. They come from people of all ages, backgrounds, and walks of life, each with their unique set of challenges and triumphs. This diversity is not just a reflection of the universal applicability of Dr. Sebi's teachings; it's also a powerful reminder that there is no one-size-fits-all approach to health and healing. Each story is a case study in personalized medicine, a vivid illustration of how Dr. Sebi's case-by-case methodology can be adapted to meet the specific needs of each individual.

As we explore these testimonials, you'll notice a recurring theme: the transformative arc. Each story begins with a struggle—be it physical, emotional, or spiritual—but ends with a transformation that goes beyond mere symptom relief. It's about a fundamental shift in perspective, a radical reorientation of priorities, and a newfound sense of purpose and meaning. This transformative arc is what elevates these testimonials from mere anecdotes to profound life lessons, offering valuable insights into the mechanics of change and the dynamics of healing.

The Ripple Effect: Families and Communities

It's important to note that the impact of these success stories extends far beyond the individuals who share them. They have a ripple effect, touching the lives of families, friends, and communities. When one person finds their path to wellness, it often serves as a catalyst for collective change, inspiring others to take charge of their health and well-being. This ripple effect is a testament to the far-reaching impact of Dr. Sebi's teachings, underscoring the interconnectedness of individual and communal health.

As you read these testimonials, I invite you to approach them with an open heart and an empathetic mind. These are not just stories to be read; they are experiences to be felt, lessons to be absorbed, and wisdom to be integrated into your own life journey. Let the courage of these individuals inspire you, let their resilience fortify you, and let their transformations enlighten you.

The Invitation to Your Own Journey

As we embark on this exploration of success stories, consider it an invitation to your own journey of health and healing. These testimonials are not just endpoints; they are starting points, catalysts for your own transformation. They offer both a roadmap and a moral compass, guiding you through the complexities of disease eradication and natural healing, and inspiring you to write your own success story.

In the pages that follow, you will meet remarkable individuals whose lives have been irrevocably changed by their commitment to an alkaline lifestyle and Dr. Sebi's herbal remedies. Their stories are a living testament to the power of holistic health, and they offer a glimpse into what's possible when we take charge of our well-being, one choice, one step, and one day at a time. Welcome to the transformative world of "Success Stories: Testimonials of Recovery."

The Anatomy of a Success Story

As we delve deeper into the core of "Success Stories: Testimonials of Recovery," it's crucial to understand the anatomy of a success story. Each narrative is a tapestry woven from threads of struggle, resilience, and triumph. The individuals in these stories are not superheroes; they are everyday people who faced seemingly insurmountable challenges. Yet, they emerged victorious, not by some stroke of luck, but through a conscious commitment to an alkaline lifestyle and Dr. Sebi's herbal remedies.

The struggle is not merely about overcoming physical ailments; it's a battle for one's soul, a fight for reclaiming one's life. The individuals in these stories often start with debilitating conditions that rob them of their vitality and joy. But the struggle is not just physical; it's emotional and spiritual too. The weight of chronic illness often brings along a heavy emotional toll, affecting relationships, self-esteem, and mental well-being.

In each story, there comes a turning point, a moment of epiphany when the individual realizes that they hold the power to change their destiny. This turning point often comes after years of suffering, failed treatments, and shattered hopes. It's the moment when they encounter Dr. Sebi's teachings and decide to take the plunge into an alkaline lifestyle. This decision is not just a dietary change; it's a life-altering commitment.

The Journey: A Road Less Traveled

The journey towards recovery is a road less traveled, filled with obstacles, setbacks, and moments of despair. Yet, it's also a journey of self-discovery, of learning to listen to one's body, and of finding harmony with nature. It's a path that demands discipline, perseverance, and an unwavering belief in the body's innate ability to heal itself. Along this journey, individuals often discover hidden reservoirs of strength and resilience they never knew they had.

The triumph in these stories is not just about symptom relief or medical reports confirming the absence of disease. It's about a holistic transformation that permeates every aspect of life. It's about rediscovering the joy of living, the pleasure of eating nourishing foods, and the serenity that comes from a balanced mind and body. The triumph is both personal and universal, serving as a beacon of hope for others in similar predicaments.

The wisdom gained from these journeys is not just about the do's and don'ts of an alkaline lifestyle. It's about the profound understanding of the interconnectedness of mind, body, and spirit. It's about the realization that healing is not an isolated event but a continuous process that requires ongoing commitment. This wisdom becomes a guiding light, not just for the individuals but also for their families and communities.

These success stories leave behind a legacy that transcends the individuals themselves. They serve as living proof that it's possible to break free from the shackles of chronic illness and lead a fulfilling life. This legacy is not just an inspiration for those who are suffering but also a call to action for healthcare practitioners, policy-makers, and society at large. It challenges us to rethink our approach to healthcare, to move away from symptom-based treatments and towards holistic well-being.

The most remarkable aspect of these testimonials is their potential to act as a catalyst for collective transformation. When one person heals, it creates a ripple effect, inspiring others to embark on their own journeys of recovery. It challenges societal norms and questions the status quo, pushing us towards a more sustainable and holistic approach to healthcare.

In summary, the central part of "Success Stories: Testimonials of Recovery" serves as the heart and soul of this chapter. It's where the struggle, the journey, and the triumph come alive, offering a panoramic view of what's possible when we take control of our health and well-being. These stories are not just testimonials; they are manifestos for a new way of living, a new way of healing, and a new way of being. They are the living, breathing embodiments of Dr. Sebi's teachings, and they offer each one of us a roadmap for our own journey towards holistic health and wellness.

The Final Word on Success Stories

As we reach the conclusion of "Success Stories: Testimonials of Recovery," it's essential to recognize the profound impact a single story can have. One person's journey can serve as a catalyst for change, not just for themselves but for an entire community. The ripple effect of one individual's success story can be the turning point for someone else who is on the brink of giving up hope. It's a testament to the transformative power of an alkaline lifestyle and Dr. Sebi's herbal remedies.

While scientific studies and clinical trials provide valuable insights into the efficacy of an alkaline lifestyle, they often lack the human element. These success stories fill that gap. They offer a window into the lived experiences of real people who have walked the path of recovery. These narratives are not just data points; they are deeply personal accounts that capture the emotional, psychological, and spiritual dimensions of healing.

The emotional resonance of these stories is what makes them so compelling. They touch the soul, stir the heart, and awaken the spirit. They evoke empathy, compassion, and a sense of shared humanity. This emotional connection is what drives people to take action, to make lifestyle changes, and to embark on their own journeys of recovery. It's the emotional resonance that turns these stories from mere testimonials into powerful agents of change.

The Universality of Experience: A Common Thread

Despite the diversity of conditions, backgrounds, and life circumstances, there's a common thread that runs through all these stories—the universality of human experience. Whether it's a young mother battling postpartum depression or a middle-aged man grappling with diabetes, the core struggles and triumphs are universally relatable. This universality makes these stories accessible, breaking down barriers of age, gender, and socio-economic status.

These success stories are not just inspirational tales; they are an ethical imperative. They challenge us to rethink our approach to healthcare and to question the status quo. They call upon healthcare providers to consider holistic alternatives, policy-makers to enact supportive legislation, and individuals to take responsibility for their own health. This ethical imperative extends beyond the realm of personal well-being to encompass social justice, environmental sustainability, and global health.

The Legacy of Hope: Lighting the Path for Others

Each success story leaves behind a legacy of hope. It lights the path for others, offering a roadmap for navigating the complex terrain of chronic illness. This legacy is not confined to the pages of this book; it lives on in the hearts and minds of those who read these stories, in the communities that are transformed, and in the generations that are yet to come.

The transformative potential of these stories lies in their ability to serve as a blueprint for collective healing. They offer practical strategies, emotional support, and spiritual guidance for those who are ready to take the plunge into an alkaline lifestyle. They demonstrate that recovery is not an isolated event but a communal endeavor that requires collective action, mutual support, and shared wisdom.

The Final Word: An Invitation to Join the Movement

As we close this chapter, let this be an invitation to join the movement—a movement that is redefining the landscape of healthcare, challenging conventional wisdom, and pioneering new pathways to holistic well-being. Let these success stories serve as your inspiration, your guide, and your call to action. Let them remind you that you are not alone, that healing is possible, and that a better future awaits us all.

In the grand tapestry of life, each success story is a vibrant thread, adding color, texture, and richness to the overall design. These stories are not the end; they are just the beginning. They are the opening chapters in an ongoing saga of human resilience, courage, and transformation. So, as you turn the page, know that your story could be the next one, the one that adds another layer of depth, another shade of brilliance, and another dimension of meaning to this ever-evolving tapestry.

And so, we conclude "Success Stories: Testimonials of Recovery," not as an end, but as a new beginning—a beginning that holds the promise of healing, the potential for transformation, and the hope for a brighter, healthier future for us all.

The Intricacies of Individuality: Breaking Down Nutritional Needs by Age and Gender

As we delve into the heart of "Breaking Down Nutritional Needs by Age and Gender," it's crucial to acknowledge that each of us is a unique composition—a symphony of life, if you will. Just as a symphony requires different instruments to create a harmonious melody, our bodies require a tailored blend of nutrients to function optimally. This chapter aims to serve as your personal conductor, guiding you through the complexities of individual nutritional needs.

Biology has a fascinating way of choreographing our lives. From the moment we are born, our bodies undergo a series of transformations, each requiring a specific set of nutrients. As we age, these needs evolve, influenced by factors such as hormonal changes, metabolic rate, and physical activity. Gender adds another layer to this intricate dance, dictating unique requirements that can't be generalized. Understanding these nuances is the first step toward achieving holistic well-being.

Imagine life as a series of seasons, each with its own beauty and challenges. Childhood is the spring of life, a time of rapid growth and development. Adolescence is the summer, marked by the heat of hormonal changes. Adulthood is the autumn, a period of maintenance and potential harvest. Finally, old age is the winter, requiring special care to weather its challenges. Each season demands a different nutritional focus, and failing to adapt can lead to discord in the body's natural rhythm.

The Gender Equation: Beyond Societal Norms

In a world that often reduces gender to societal norms and expectations, it's vital to recognize the biological implications of gender on nutritional needs. Men and women have distinct metabolic rates, muscle mass, and hormonal profiles, all of which influence their nutritional requirements. For instance, women may need more iron during their menstrual cycles, while men might require more protein to maintain muscle mass. These aren't just cultural constructs; they're biological necessities that warrant attention.

The Interplay of Lifestyle: The Modern Dilemma

Our modern lifestyle often throws a wrench into the biological machinery. The frenetic pace of life, coupled with easy access to processed foods, can lead to nutritional imbalances that exacerbate age and gender-specific vulnerabilities. For example, the stress of a high-powered job might deplete essential nutrients more quickly, requiring a more focused nutritional strategy. Or the sedentary nature of modern work could lead to weight gain, necessitating adjustments in caloric intake.

While age and gender dictate specific nutritional needs, the principles of an alkaline lifestyle offer a unifying theme. Alkaline foods are naturally rich in essential nutrients, providing a balanced spectrum that can adapt to individual requirements. Whether you're a young woman needing more calcium for bone health or a middle-aged man focusing on heart health, alkaline foods offer a versatile palette to meet these needs.

The Quest for Balance: A Lifelong Journey

Nutrition is not a one-size-fits-all endeavor; it's a lifelong journey of discovery and balance. It's about listening to your body, understanding its unique language, and responding with love and care. This chapter aims to equip you with the knowledge and tools to embark on this journey, to navigate the ever-changing landscape of your body's needs as you age and as you live.

As we move forward, this chapter will serve as a roadmap, charting the terrain of age and gender-specific nutritional needs. It will provide you with the insights to make informed choices, to adapt and evolve as life unfolds its myriad experiences. But remember, this is just the beginning. Your body is an ever-changing landscape, and your nutritional needs are the compass guiding you through this journey.

So, let's embark on this exploration together, with open minds and willing hearts, as we break down the complexities of nutritional needs by age and gender. Let this chapter be your guide, your mentor, and your companion in this intricate dance of life. Because when it comes to nutrition, one size doesn't fit all; it's a tailored fit, designed by the unique symphony that is you.

Book 5: Comprehensive Nutrition Guide

Breaking Down Nutritional Needs by Age and Gender

The Intricacies of Individuality: Breaking Down Nutritional Needs by Age and Gender

As we delve into the heart of "Breaking Down Nutritional Needs by Age and Gender," it's crucial to acknowledge that each of us is a unique composition—a symphony of life, if you will. Just as a symphony requires different instruments to create a harmonious melody, our bodies require a tailored blend of nutrients to function optimally. This chapter aims to serve as your personal conductor, guiding you through the complexities of individual nutritional needs.

Biology has a fascinating way of choreographing our lives. From the moment we are born, our bodies undergo a series of transformations, each requiring a specific set of nutrients. As we age, these needs evolve, influenced by factors such as hormonal changes, metabolic rate, and physical activity. Gender adds another layer to this intricate dance, dictating unique requirements that can't be generalized. Understanding these nuances is the first step toward achieving holistic well-being.

Imagine life as a series of seasons, each with its own beauty and challenges. Childhood is the spring of life, a time of rapid growth and development. Adolescence is the summer, marked by the heat of hormonal changes. Adulthood is the autumn, a period of maintenance and potential harvest. Finally, old age is the winter, requiring special care to weather its challenges. Each season demands a different nutritional focus, and failing to adapt can lead to discord in the body's natural rhythm.

The Gender Equation: Beyond Societal Norms

In a world that often reduces gender to societal norms and expectations, it's vital to recognize the biological implications of gender on nutritional needs. Men and women have distinct metabolic rates, muscle mass, and hormonal profiles, all of which influence their nutritional requirements. For instance, women may need more iron during their menstrual cycles, while men might require more protein to maintain muscle mass. These aren't just cultural constructs; they're biological necessities that warrant attention.

The Interplay of Lifestyle: The Modern Dilemma

Our modern lifestyle often throws a wrench into the biological machinery. The frenetic pace of life, coupled with easy access to processed foods, can lead to nutritional imbalances that exacerbate age and gender-specific vulnerabilities. For example, the stress of a high-powered job might deplete essential nutrients more quickly, requiring a more focused nutritional strategy. Or the sedentary nature of modern work could lead to weight gain, necessitating adjustments in caloric intake.

While age and gender dictate specific nutritional needs, the principles of an alkaline lifestyle offer a unifying theme. Alkaline foods are naturally rich in essential nutrients, providing a balanced spectrum that can adapt to individual requirements. Whether you're a young woman needing more calcium for bone health or a middle-aged man focusing on heart health, alkaline foods offer a versatile palette to meet these needs.

The Quest for Balance: A Lifelong Journey

Nutrition is not a one-size-fits-all endeavor; it's a lifelong journey of discovery and balance. It's about listening to your body, understanding its unique language, and responding with love and care. This chapter aims to equip you with the knowledge and tools to embark on this journey, to navigate the ever-changing landscape of your body's needs as you age and as you live.

As we move forward, this chapter will serve as a roadmap, charting the terrain of age and gender-specific nutritional needs. It will provide you with the insights to make informed choices, to adapt and evolve as life unfolds its myriad experiences. But remember, this is just the beginning. Your body is an ever-changing landscape, and your nutritional needs are the compass guiding you through this journey.

So, let's embark on this exploration together, with open minds and willing hearts, as we break down the complexities of nutritional needs by age and gender. Let this chapter be your guide, your mentor, and your companion in this intricate dance of life. Because when it comes to nutrition, one size doesn't fit all; it's a tailored fit, designed by the unique symphony that is you.

The Biological Clock: Nutritional Milestones in the Journey of Life

As we traverse the path of life, our biological clock ticks in harmony with our nutritional needs. It's as if each decade unfurls a new chapter in our nutritional storybook. In our 30s, for example, the focus might be on optimizing fertility or building bone density.

Fast forward to the 40s, and the spotlight shifts to maintaining muscle mass and combating the onset of metabolic slowdown. The 50s bring about a focus on heart health and hormonal balance. Each decade is a unique tapestry, woven with threads of age-specific nutritional requirements.

The Feminine Mystique: The Nutritional Ballet of Womanhood

Women are not just men with different reproductive systems; they are biologically distinct beings with unique nutritional needs. From the onset of menstruation to the menopausal transition, a woman's life is a ballet of hormonal fluctuations. These hormonal dances dictate different nutritional needs at various life stages. For instance, the increased iron needs during menstruation, the heightened demand for folic acid in pregnancy, and the shifting requirements for calcium and Vitamin D during menopause are all choreographed by the body's innate wisdom.

The Masculine Equation: Fueling the Engine of Manhood

Men, too, have their own set of nutritional intricacies. While they may not experience the same cyclical hormonal changes as women, they do have specific needs that evolve with age. Testosterone, the hormone often associated with masculinity, plays a significant role in determining a man's nutritional needs. As men age and testosterone levels decline, the need for nutrients that support hormone balance, such as zinc and Omega-3 fatty acids, becomes crucial. Additionally, men are generally more prone to certain conditions like heart disease, making nutrients that support cardiovascular health exceedingly important.

The Middle Ground: Nutritional Synergies and Overlaps

While men and women have their unique nutritional requirements, there's also a middle ground where needs overlap. Both genders benefit from antioxidants to combat aging, fiber for digestive health, and proteins for muscle maintenance. This common ground serves as a reminder that despite our differences, we share the same fundamental need for balanced nutrition to thrive.

In a society that often glorifies busyness, stress has become an unwelcome companion for many. Stress doesn't just take a toll on your mental well-being; it also depletes essential nutrients at an accelerated rate. For example, stress can quickly drain your body's reserves of magnesium, a mineral crucial for relaxation and muscle function. Both men and women, especially those in the 30-50 age bracket, need to be mindful of this and may need to adjust their nutritional intake accordingly.

Nutrition is not just about feeding the body; it's about nourishing the mind and soul as well. Foods rich in Omega-3 fatty acids, for example, are not only good for your heart but also beneficial for your brain and mental health. The holistic approach to nutrition considers the interconnectedness of physical health, emotional well-being, and spiritual balance. It's not just about what's on your plate; it's also about how those choices resonate with your entire being.

The Personalization Paradigm: Your Nutritional Blueprint

As we delve deeper into the age of personalized medicine, the one-size-fits-all approach to nutrition is becoming increasingly obsolete. Advances in science are making it possible to tailor nutritional recommendations based on genetic makeup, lifestyle, and even gut microbiota. This personalization paradigm is particularly relevant when considering the nutritional needs dictated by age and gender.

As we navigate through the complexities of age and gender-specific nutrition, it's essential to remember that balance is the key. It's about orchestrating a symphony where each nutrient plays its part, each life stage has its melody, and each gender brings its unique rhythm. This chapter serves as your conductor's baton, guiding you through the intricate yet beautiful symphony that is your nutritional life.

In this ever-evolving journey, your body is your most loyal companion, whispering its needs through subtle signs and signals. Learning to listen and respond to these cues is the essence of a balanced, holistic approach to nutrition. And as you harmonize these elements, you create a life that is not just longer but richer in quality, resonating with the truest notes of well-being.

The art of listening: Tuning in to your body's nutritional orchestra

To conclude this point, let's review the concept of listening. Your body is an intricate symphony: each cell is a musician, each organ a section of the orchestra, and each nutrient a note. The music they create is the soundtrack of your life and changes with each passing year and each unique stage of your gender journey. The art of listening to this symphony is the key to understanding your nutritional needs. It is about tuning in to the subtle signals, quiet whispers, and loud cries that your body emits to tell you what it needs to thrive.

Life is a sea of constant change, and your nutritional needs are the compass that guides you through these waters. As you age, this compass can point you in new directions. For women, the compass may direct you to nutrients that support hormonal balance during the transition to menopause. For men, it might point you toward nutrients that maintain cardiovascular health and muscle mass. The key is to keep your compass well-tuned, adjusting your course as you go through the different seasons of life.

The nutritional alchemist: Turning knowledge into gold

Knowledge is power, but it is only useful if you apply it. Becoming a nutritional alchemist is about turning acquired knowledge into the gold of optimal health. It involves taking the theoretical concepts of age- and gender-specific nutrition and turning them into practical, everyday choices. Whether it's choosing a nutrient-rich smoothie over sugary milk or preferring a heart-healthy fat over a trans fat, these are the alchemical processes that convey knowledge into wellness.

The nutritional gatekeeper: Protecting one's fortress

In a world filled with stress, pollution, and hectic lifestyles, your body is a fortress to be protected. Nutrition is your armor, your shield and your sword. It is what protects you from the external assaults and internal imbalances that life throws at you. Stress, for example, is an insidious invader that can deplete your nutritional reserves. Being a nutritional guardian means fortifying your fortress with the right nutrients to resist these invasions, especially when dealing with the complexities of age and gender.

The nutritional sage: wisdom in every bite

As we age, every morsel can be a morsel of wisdom. It is an opportunity to nourish not only the body, but also the mind and soul. Antioxidant-rich foods, for example, are like wise old men teaching cells how to age gracefully. Omega-3 fatty acids are the philosophers that brighten the brain and improve mood. The act of eating becomes a ritual of wisdom accumulation, a practice that deepens with each passing year and each unique stage of life.

Your life is a story, and nutrition is the ink with which you write it. Each meal is a sentence, each day a paragraph, and each decade a chapter. As you progress through the ages and stages of sex-specific needs, you build a narrative that is uniquely yours. Whether it is the pregnancy chapter for women or the muscle maintenance chapter for men, these are the pages where your nutritional choices tell your story. And like any good story, it is full of twists and turns, challenges and triumphs, but most of all growth and transformation.

When you master the art of age- and gender-specific nutrition, you are not only improving your life, you are also creating a legacy. You are passing the baton to the next generation, teaching them by example how to listen to their bodies, how to be nutritional alchemists, guardians, sages and storytellers. You are contributing to a collective wisdom that transcends age and gender, a wisdom that enriches not only individual lives but the fabric of society as a whole.

Final note: a lifelong overture

In conclusion, understanding your nutritional needs as they relate to age and gender is not a one-time event, but a lifelong overture. It is a piece of music that you will continue to compose until your final days. And as you do so, you will discover that it is not just about longevity, but about improving the quality of every moment you are given. It is about living a life that is not only longer, but richer, deeper and infinitely more harmonious.

So as you close this point and move on to the next, remember that the best is yet to come. Your nutritional symphony is still unfolding, and the most beautiful notes are the ones you have yet to play.

Superfoods: Benefits and Incorporation into Daily Life

The Dawn of Superfoods: A New Era in Nutritional Enlightenment

Imagine walking into a grand concert hall, the air tinged with anticipation. The musicians are tuning their instruments, each contributing a unique note to a harmonious melody that fills the room.

This is the world of superfoods—a diverse, vibrant, and harmonious assembly of nature's finest nutritional offerings. Each superfood is like a musician in this grand orchestra, playing its unique note in the symphony of your health. As we embark on this exploration of superfoods, consider this your VIP ticket to the most transformative concert of your life—one that promises not just auditory delight but a sensory, intellectual, and spiritual feast.

The term "superfood" has become a buzzword in the health and wellness community, often thrown around with little understanding of its profound implications. At its core, a superfood is a nutrient-dense food that provides a multitude of health benefits. But let's not trivialize it. A superfood is not just a food; it's an alchemical substance, a magical element that has the power to transmute the ordinary into the extraordinary. It can turn a mundane meal into a nutritional elixir, a simple snack into a potent potion for well-being.

Incorporating superfoods into your daily life is like weaving golden threads into a tapestry. Each thread represents a different superfood, and as you weave them together, they form a radiant fabric that not only beautifies your life but also fortifies it. Imagine weaving threads of chia seeds into your morning smoothie, strands of goji berries into your afternoon snack, and fibers of turmeric into your evening tea. Each thread contributes its unique texture, color, and strength to the tapestry, making it more resilient, vibrant, and beautiful.

Superfoods are nature's pharmacy, a veritable Garden of Eden brimming with healing herbs, fruits, vegetables, and grains. Each superfood is a natural remedy, a medicinal plant, a healing herb that has been used for centuries, if not millennia, to treat various ailments. But more than just treating diseases, superfoods are preventive medicine. They are the guardians of your health, the sentinels that stand at the gates of your body, protecting you from the onslaught of environmental toxins, stress, and diseases that are an inevitable part of our modern lifestyle.

The Culinary Artist: Painting Your Plate with Superfoods

Incorporating superfoods into your daily life doesn't have to be a chore or a clinical exercise. It can be an art, a culinary adventure that allows you to paint your plate with vibrant colors, intricate textures, and complex flavors. Imagine your plate as a canvas, and each superfood as a color on your palette. A splash of blueberries here, a stroke of avocado there, a dab of quinoa in the corner. As you mix and match these colors, you're not just creating a visual masterpiece; you're also crafting a nutritional symphony that nourishes your body, mind, and soul.

As we delve deeper into the world of superfoods, it's crucial to approach it with mindfulness and discernment. The market is flooded with products claiming to be "superfoods," but not all are created equal. Being a mindful consumer means doing your research, reading labels, and making informed choices. It means understanding the source of your superfoods, the methods used in their cultivation, and the ethics behind their production. It's about aligning your nutritional choices with your values, ensuring that the superfoods you consume are not just beneficial for you but also for the planet.

The Holistic Approach: Superfoods as a Pillar of Well-Being

As we set the stage for a deeper exploration of superfoods, it's important to remember that they are not a magic bullet or a quick fix. They are a pillar in the holistic temple of well-being, supporting other pillars like exercise, sleep, and mental health. Incorporating superfoods into your life is not about replacing your existing diet or lifestyle; it's about enhancing it, enriching it, and elevating it to a level of health and harmony that you never thought possible.

As we conclude this introductory phase, consider this the beginning of your personal odyssey into the world of superfoods—an odyssey that promises adventure, discovery, and transformation. So fasten your seatbelt, open your mind, and prepare your palate, for you are about to embark on a journey that will not just change the way you eat but also the way you live, think, and feel.

Welcome to the transformative world of superfoods. The journey has just begun, and the best is yet to come.

Unveiling the Benefits of Superfoods

Imagine a symphony where each instrument plays a note so pure, so perfectly tuned, that the collective sound transcends music itself, becoming an ethereal experience. Superfoods offer a similar symphony of nutrients—vitamins, minerals, antioxidants, and phytonutrients—each playing its part in the grand orchestra of your health. The benefits are not just additive; they are synergistic. This means that the collective impact of these nutrients is greater than the sum of their individual effects, offering a holistic approach to well-being.

The Cellular Rejuvenation: A Fountain of Youth

What if you could age vibrantly? Superfoods offer a plethora of antioxidants that combat oxidative stress, a primary factor in aging. These antioxidants rejuvenate your cells, essentially turning back the clock, or at least slowing its relentless tick. The result is not just a youthful appearance but a youthful vitality that permeates every aspect of your life.

The Immunity Fortress: Your Shield in a World of Microbial Invaders

In a world where new strains of viruses and bacteria seem to emerge every day, having a robust immune system is not just an advantage; it's a necessity. Superfoods like garlic, ginger, and various berries are rich in compounds that enhance your immune response. They act as your personal knights in shining armor, defending your castle—your body—from microbial invaders. This is not about replacing vaccines or medications but fortifying your natural defenses to make you more resilient.

The Metabolic Symphony: Tuning Your Body's Orchestra

Metabolism is your body's orchestra, a complex interplay of biochemical reactions that sustain life. Superfoods can be the conductors of this metabolic symphony, optimizing processes like digestion, nutrient absorption, and energy production. Foods like chia seeds, rich in fiber, improve digestion and nutrient absorption. Others like quinoa provide a complete protein source, essential for tissue repair and growth. The result is a body that functions not just adequately but optimally, a well-tuned orchestra playing a harmonious metabolic symphony.

The Cognitive Revolution: Nourishing the Seat of Consciousness

Your brain is the seat of your consciousness, the epicenter of your thoughts, emotions, and memories. Nourishing it is not just about preventing cognitive decline; it's about enhancing cognitive prowess. Superfoods like walnuts and blueberries are rich in omega-3 fatty acids and antioxidants that improve brain function. They are the fuel for your mental engine, enhancing everything from memory and focus to creativity and emotional stability.

The Emotional Landscape: Food for the Soul

While the connection between diet and physical health is well-established, the link between diet and emotional well-being is often overlooked. Foods like dark chocolate and various fruits not only nourish your body but also elevate your mood. They are rich in compounds that stimulate the release of endorphins, the body's natural feel-good chemicals. This is not about replacing therapy or medications but complementing them, creating a holistic approach to emotional well-being.

The Energetic Matrix: Fueling the Fire Within

Energy is the currency of life, the fuel that powers every cellular process, every thought, every action. Superfoods like spirulina and goji berries are energy powerhouses, rich in nutrients that optimize cellular energy production. They are the high-octane fuel for your biological engine, enhancing not just your physical stamina but also your mental clarity and emotional resilience.

The Hormonal Harmony: The Unsung Heroes of Health

Superfoods like flaxseeds and broccoli are rich in compounds that balance your hormones, optimizing everything from your metabolic rate and muscle growth to your mood and reproductive health.

The Sensory Experience: A Feast for the Senses

Finally, let's not forget the sensory experience that superfoods offer. The vibrant colors, the diverse textures, and the rich flavors make every meal a feast for the senses. This is not just about nourishing your body but also about enriching your life, turning every meal into a sensory celebration, a moment of mindfulness and joy.

As we navigate through the labyrinth of life, let superfoods be your guide, your ally, and your inspiration. They offer a holistic approach to health that transcends the physical, touching the emotional, the mental, and even the spiritual dimensions of your being. So, as you incorporate these miraculous foods into your daily life, know that you are not just eating; you are evolving, transforming, and transcending. Welcome to the heart of the superfood revolution.

The Culmination: Making Superfoods a Lifestyle, not a Trend

As we've journeyed through the myriad benefits of superfoods, it's essential to recognize that knowledge alone isn't power; it's the application of knowledge that empowers us. The real magic happens when these nutrient-dense foods become a seamless part of your daily routine. It's not about a radical overhaul of your diet overnight; it's about making incremental changes that are sustainable in the long run. Start by replacing one meal or even just a snack with a superfood alternative. The key is consistency, not intensity. Over time, these small changes accumulate into a transformative experience that elevates your health to new heights.

In a world inundated with marketing gimmicks and flashy labels, it's easy to get swayed by the latest "superfood" trend. However, it's crucial to be a mindful consumer. Not all superfoods are created equal, and their nutritional value can vary based on factors like soil quality, harvesting methods, and processing techniques. So, when you're shopping, opt for organic, non-GMO, and locally sourced products whenever possible. This not only ensures that you're getting the highest nutritional bang for your buck but also supports sustainable farming practices.

One of the most common misconceptions about superfoods is that they're not as tasty as their less nutritious counterparts. This couldn't be further from the truth. The world of superfoods is a culinary playground, offering a diverse palette of flavors, textures, and aromas. With a little creativity and experimentation, you can create dishes that are as delicious as they are nutritious. For instance, a smoothie bowl can become a canvas for a colorful array of fruits, nuts, and seeds. A simple salad can be elevated with the addition of superfood herbs and spices. The possibilities are endless, limited only by your imagination.

The Family Affair: Making Health a Collective Endeavor

Health is not an individual pursuit; it's a collective endeavor. When you make the transition to a superfood-rich diet, involve your family in the journey. Make it a fun and educational experience for your kids by letting them pick a new superfood to try each week. Engage your partner in the cooking process, turning it into a bonding activity rather than a chore. When health becomes a family affair, it creates a supportive environment that makes it easier to stick to your new lifestyle.

One of the biggest challenges people face in incorporating superfoods into their daily life is time—or the perceived lack thereof. The good news is that superfoods can be incredibly time-efficient. Many of them, like chia seeds or goji berries, require no preparation and can be easily added to your meals. Others, like quinoa or kale, can be batch-cooked and used in multiple meals throughout the week. With a little planning, you can make superfoods a convenient and effortless part of your busy life.

Another concern people often have is the cost associated with superfoods. While it's true that some superfoods can be more expensive than conventional foods, it's essential to view this as an investment in your health. The long-term benefits—reduced medical bills, increased productivity, and enhanced quality of life—far outweigh the short-term costs. Moreover, many superfoods are incredibly nutrient-dense, meaning you need less quantity to get the same nutritional value, making them cost-effective in the long run.

The Holistic Approach: Beyond the Plate

While the focus of this chapter is on superfoods, it's essential to recognize that they are just one piece of the puzzle. A holistic approach to health incorporates not just diet but also exercise, stress management, and emotional well-being. As you make superfoods a part of your daily life, also explore other avenues of holistic health. Perhaps it's taking up a mindfulness practice, engaging in regular physical activity, or simply spending more time in nature. Each of these elements complements the benefits of superfoods, creating a synergistic effect that amplifies your overall well-being.

As we conclude this chapter, let's remember that health is not a destination but a journey—a lifelong journey. Incorporating superfoods into your daily life is not a temporary fix but a long-term commitment to yourself. It's about creating a life that you don't need a vacation from, a life where each day is imbued with vitality, clarity, and a profound sense of well-being. So, as you step into this new chapter of your life, do so with intention, with curiosity, and most importantly, with love for yourself. Welcome to your new life, a life supercharged by the incredible power of superfoods.

Supplements: Navigating the Good and the Bad

The Complex World of Supplements: A Compass for Navigating the Good and the Bad

In a society that often seeks instant gratification, the allure of dietary supplements is understandable. The promise of better health, more energy, and an enhanced quality of life—all neatly packaged in a pill or a powder—can be hard to resist. But as we venture into the complex world of supplements, it's crucial to approach it with a discerning eye and an informed mind. This chapter aims to serve as your compass, guiding you through the labyrinth of choices, claims, and controversies that surround the supplement industry.

The Double-Edged Sword: The Power and Pitfalls of Supplements

Supplements can be a double-edged sword. On one hand, they offer the potential to fill nutritional gaps, enhance performance, and even mitigate the effects of chronic conditions. On the other hand, they can also be a source of unnecessary expense, false hope, and in some cases, significant health risks. The key to harnessing the benefits while avoiding the pitfalls lies in understanding the nuances that dictate the efficacy and safety of these products.

One of the most significant challenges in navigating the supplement market is the lack of stringent regulation. Unlike pharmaceuticals, which undergo rigorous testing for safety and efficacy, supplements are not held to the same standards. This lack of oversight opens the door for a wide range of quality and potency, making it essential for consumers to be proactive in their research and selection process.

The supplement industry is rife with hyperbolic claims and sensationalized marketing. From "miracle cures" for weight loss to "revolutionary formulas" for anti-aging, the buzzwords are endless. But how much of this is rooted in science, and how much is pure hype? As we delve deeper into this chapter, we'll explore the scientific evidence—or lack thereof—behind some of the most popular supplements on the market. This will equip you with the knowledge to make informed decisions, allowing you to separate the wheat from the chaff in a crowded and often confusing marketplace.

The Role of Individuality: Why One Size Doesn't Fit All

Another critical aspect to consider is the role of individuality in the effectiveness of supplements. Factors such as age, gender, lifestyle, and pre-existing health conditions can significantly influence how your body responds to a particular supplement. This underscores the importance of personalized nutrition and the need for professional guidance. Consulting with healthcare providers who are well-versed in the field of supplements can provide invaluable insights into what might work best for you.

As conscious consumers, it's also important to consider the ethical implications of our choices. Where do the ingredients come from? Are they sustainably sourced? What are the labor practices of the companies we're supporting? These questions may seem peripheral to the primary goal of improving health, but they are intrinsically linked. The choices we make have ripple effects that extend beyond our individual lives, impacting communities and ecosystems around the world.

The Holistic Perspective: Supplements as a Complement, Not a Substitute

As we navigate the intricate landscape of supplements, it's vital to remember that they are meant to complement a balanced diet and healthy lifestyle, not replace them. Relying solely on supplements while neglecting other aspects of well-being is akin to putting a band-aid on a gaping wound. True health is a holistic endeavor, encompassing not just what we ingest, but also how we move, think, and interact with the world around us.

As we embark on this exploratory journey through the world of supplements, let's do so with an open mind but also a healthy dose of skepticism. Let's be students of our bodies, keen observers of how we respond to different interventions. Let's be discerning consumers, not swayed by flashy marketing or lofty promises, but guided by evidence, ethics, and intuition. And most importantly, let's remember that supplements are just one tool in a much larger toolkit for health and well-being. The ultimate goal is not to find a magic pill but to create a harmonious symphony of lifestyle choices that empower us to live our best lives. Welcome to the nuanced, complex, but infinitely fascinating world of supplements.

The Spectrum of Supplements: From Essential Nutrients to Exotic Extracts

As we delve into the core of the supplement world, it's essential to recognize the vast spectrum of products available. From essential vitamins and minerals to exotic plant extracts and amino acids, the range is as diverse as it is expansive. This diversity can be both a blessing and a curse. While it offers a plethora of options to address various health concerns, it also creates a maze that can be difficult to navigate. Understanding the different categories of supplements and their intended uses is the first step in making sense of this complex landscape.

One of the most overlooked aspects of supplements is bioavailability—the extent and rate at which the active ingredients are absorbed and utilized by the body. Many factors can influence bioavailability, including the form of the supplement, its source, and even the time of day it's taken. For instance, fat-soluble vitamins like A, D, and E are better absorbed when taken with a meal that includes fats. Being aware of these nuances can significantly impact the effectiveness of your supplement regimen.

The Interplay with Medications: A Cautionary Tale

For those who are already on prescription medications, the interaction between drugs and supplements is a critical concern. Certain supplements can either potentiate or negate the effects of medications. For example, vitamin K can interfere with blood thinners, while some minerals like calcium can inhibit the absorption of certain antibiotics. Consulting a healthcare provider for a comprehensive review of your medications and supplements is not just advisable—it's imperative.

In recent years, the line between food and supplements has started to blur with the rise of functional foods. These are foods enriched with additional nutrients or bioactive compounds to provide health benefits beyond basic nutrition. While functional foods offer a more natural way to obtain the benefits commonly sought from supplements, they also introduce another layer of complexity. Is it better to get your omega-3s from fortified eggs or a fish oil capsule? The answer may not be straightforward and often depends on individual preferences and needs.

As we become more conscious consumers, the ethical considerations of supplement sourcing come into play. Many popular supplements are derived from plants and animals that are endangered or harvested using unsustainable practices. The booming demand for exotic herbs like Ashwagandha and Rho Diola is putting a strain on native populations and ecosystems. Being mindful of the sourcing practices of the supplements you choose is an ethical responsibility we all share.

The psychological aspects of supplementation cannot be ignored. The placebo effect, where believing in the efficacy of a treatment enhances its actual effectiveness, is a well-documented phenomenon in medicine. While this doesn't negate the genuine benefits that many supplements offer, it does raise questions about how our beliefs and expectations can influence our physiological responses.

Supplements can be expensive, and the costs can quickly add up, especially if you're taking multiple products. It's essential to weigh the financial investment against the potential health benefits. Sometimes, lifestyle changes like improved diet and increased physical activity can offer similar benefits at a fraction of the cost. However, for those with specific nutrient deficiencies or medical conditions, supplements may provide a necessary and invaluable solution.

The Quest for Quality: Beyond the Label

Finally, the quality of supplements is a paramount concern. With lax regulations, the market is rife with subpar products that may not contain what their labels claim. Independent third-party testing, certifications from reputable organizations, and transparent sourcing practices are markers of high-quality products. Your health is too important to compromise on quality.

As we navigate through the intricate world of supplements, the key takeaway is to approach it with a balanced perspective. Supplements offer incredible potential to enhance our well-being, but they are not a panacea. They should be viewed as one component of a holistic approach to health, complementing rather than replacing a balanced diet, regular exercise, and a healthy lifestyle. Armed with knowledge, discernment, and a dash of skepticism, you're well-equipped to make informed choices in this ever-evolving field.

The Final Word: Making Informed Choices in the World of Supplements

As we reach the culmination of our exploration into the world of supplements, it's crucial to emphasize the importance of personalization. The one-size-fits-all approach is a relic of the past. We are all unique, with individual health needs, lifestyle factors, and even genetic predispositions that can influence how our bodies respond to supplements. The future of supplementation is not just about what's on the store shelves; it's about what's right for you.

While the internet is a treasure trove of information, it can also be a minefield of misinformation. The role of healthcare providers in guiding your supplement choices cannot be overstated. A qualified healthcare provider can offer diagnostic tests to identify any deficiencies or imbalances, provide evidence-based recommendations, and even tailor a supplement regimen to your specific needs. This collaborative approach ensures that you're not just taking supplements, but taking the right ones for you.

Beyond the physiological benefits, there's an emotional aspect to consider. Knowing that you're taking steps to improve your health can offer a significant psychological boost. This sense of empowerment can be a catalyst for broader lifestyle changes, from adopting a more balanced diet to engaging in regular physical activity. However, it's essential to keep this in perspective. Supplements can enhance your well-being, but they're not a substitute for a holistic approach to health.

As conscious consumers, we have the power to influence the market. By choosing supplements that are sustainably sourced, ethically produced, and transparently labeled, we're voting with our wallets for a more responsible industry. This collective action can drive change, pushing companies to adopt more ethical practices and encouraging innovation in product quality and transparency.

The Long Game: Supplements as a Lifelong Commitment

For many, supplementation is not a quick fix but a long-term commitment. As our bodies age, our nutritional needs change, and what worked for us in our 30s may not be sufficient in our 40s or beyond. Regular check-ups and adjustments to your supplement regimen can ensure that you're meeting your body's evolving needs. This long-term view is not just about maintaining good health; it's about enhancing your quality of life at every stage.

The Skeptic's Corner: Questioning and Validating

Skepticism is healthy, especially in a field rife with bold claims and marketing hype. Always question the sources of your information, the credibility of the claims made, and the science—or lack thereof—behind a product. This critical mindset will serve you well, helping you separate the wheat from the chaff in a crowded and often confusing marketplace.

While the journey into supplementation is deeply personal, there's value in community. Online forums, social media groups, and even local community events offer platforms to share experiences, seek advice, and learn from others. These communal spaces can be invaluable, but remember to apply your critical thinking skills here too. What works for one person may not work for you.

The Final Takeaway: An Empowered Consumer is a Healthy Consumer

In conclusion, navigating the world of supplements is a complex but rewarding endeavor. The key to success lies in being an informed, skeptical, and empowered consumer. Supplements offer a potent tool in your health arsenal, but they are most effective when used as part of a broader, more holistic approach to well-being. Your journey doesn't end when you swallow that pill or capsule; it's an ongoing process of learning, adapting, and striving for a healthier, happier you.

By taking a nuanced, balanced, and informed approach, you're not just enhancing your physical health; you're enriching your emotional and ethical well-being too. In a world where we're constantly bombarded with information and choices, taking control of your health through informed decisions is perhaps the most empowering step you can take. And that, ultimately, is the essence of navigating the good and the bad in the world of supplements.

Book 6: Mind, Body, and Spiritual Alignment

The Psychological Benefits of an Alkaline Lifestyle

A Journey into the Mind's Well-Being

When we think about an alkaline lifestyle, our minds often gravitate towards the physical benefits: increased energy, better digestion, and a stronger immune system, to name a few. However, the impact of alkalinity extends far beyond the corporeal realm. It reaches into the depths of our psychological well-being, offering a sanctuary for the mind in a world that often feels chaotic and overwhelming.

Adopting an alkaline lifestyle is not merely a dietary change; it's a paradigm shift that affects every facet of your life, including your mental health. This shift is not just about what you consume but how you perceive the world around you. The alkaline mindset is one of balance, harmony, and mindfulness. It's a worldview that encourages you to be present, to be grateful, and to be intentional in your choices, whether they relate to food, relationships, or your inner thoughts.

In our fast-paced society, stress is often an unwelcome companion. It lurks in the corners of our minds, affecting our sleep, our relationships, and even our self-esteem. Here's where the alkaline lifestyle shines as a buffer against stress. Foods rich in alkaline properties are known to reduce inflammation, a key contributor to stress. But it's not just about the food. The very principles of an alkaline lifestyle—mindfulness, balance, and harmony—act as psychological tools to manage and mitigate stress.

Emotional Resilience: The Alkaline Advantage

Life is a rollercoaster of emotions. We all experience highs and lows, joys and sorrows. Emotional resilience is the ability to navigate these ups and downs with grace and poise. An alkaline lifestyle fosters this resilience by nourishing not just the body but the mind. The focus on mindfulness and balance equips you with the emotional tools to face life's challenges head-on, without being overwhelmed.

One of the cornerstones of an alkaline lifestyle is mindfulness, the practice of being fully present and engaged in the moment. Mindfulness is not just a trendy buzzword; it's a mental skill that has been shown to reduce symptoms of anxiety and depression. When you're mindful, you're not worrying about the future or regretting the past; you're enjoying the richness of the present moment. This focus on the "now" is a natural extension of the alkaline philosophy, which emphasizes balance and harmony in all things, including your mental state.

The psychological benefits of an alkaline lifestyle don't stop at the individual level; they ripple out into the community. When you're mentally balanced and emotionally resilient, it positively impacts your interactions with others. You become a source of positivity and strength, a beacon for those who may be struggling with their own mental health. In this way, the alkaline lifestyle serves as a catalyst for communal well-being, fostering a sense of unity and mutual support.

The Power of Choice: Taking Control of Your Mental Health

Perhaps the most empowering aspect of an alkaline lifestyle is the power of choice. You choose what to eat, how to think, and how to live. These choices, in turn, shape your mental health. When you opt for alkaline foods, engage in mindful practices, and cultivate emotional resilience, you're making a conscious choice to prioritize your psychological well-being.

The Journey Ahead: A Lifelong Commitment to Mental Wellness

As we delve deeper into the intricacies of the alkaline lifestyle and its psychological benefits, it's important to remember that this is a lifelong journey. Mental wellness is not a destination but a continuous process of growth, adaptation, and self-discovery. The alkaline lifestyle offers a roadmap for this journey, providing the tools and principles to navigate the complexities of the human mind.

In conclusion, the psychological benefits of an alkaline lifestyle are manifold and deeply interconnected with the core principles of balance, harmony, and mindfulness. As we move forward, we'll explore these facets in greater detail, offering practical tips and insights to enrich your mental landscape. But for now, let's revel in the empowering realization that an alkaline lifestyle is not just a pathway to physical health but a gateway to mental freedom.

The Alkaline Mind: A Sanctuary for Mental Health

As we delve deeper into the core of the psychological benefits of an alkaline lifestyle, it's essential to understand that the mind is a sanctuary, a sacred space that needs nurturing and care. Just as an alkaline diet nourishes the body, an alkaline mindset nourishes the mind. This mindset is not a fleeting thought or a temporary state; it's a way of life. It's a commitment to mental clarity, emotional stability, and an unwavering sense of purpose.

While the alkaline lifestyle is often associated with a balanced pH level in the body, it's equally crucial to consider its impact on the brain's neurochemistry. Neurotransmitters like serotonin, dopamine, and norepinephrine play pivotal roles in regulating mood, focus, and stress response. An alkaline lifestyle, rich in nutrient-dense foods and mindful practices, can help maintain a balanced neurochemical environment. This balance is not just a biochemical phenomenon; it's a psychological asset that enhances cognitive function, emotional well-being, and overall mental health.

Emotional Intelligence: The Alkaline Way

Emotional intelligence is the ability to understand, manage, and effectively express one's own emotions, as well as engage and navigate successfully with the emotions of others. The alkaline lifestyle, with its emphasis on mindfulness and balance, naturally cultivates emotional intelligence. When you're in tune with your body, you become more aware of your emotional state, making it easier to manage your reactions to life's challenges. This heightened emotional intelligence is a valuable asset in personal relationships, professional settings, and even in the inner dialogue you have with yourself.

Cognitive function encompasses various mental abilities, including memory, attention, problem-solving, and language skills. A balanced, alkaline lifestyle can significantly impact these abilities. For example, the antioxidants found in alkaline foods can combat oxidative stress, a known contributor to cognitive decline. Moreover, the alkaline lifestyle's focus on mindfulness can improve attention span and problem-solving skills. The result is a sharper, more agile mind capable of navigating the complexities of modern life.

Self-compassion is often overlooked in discussions about mental health, yet it's a cornerstone of psychological well-being. An alkaline lifestyle encourages self-compassion by promoting mindfulness and emotional balance. When you're mindful, you're more likely to recognize negative self-talk and replace it with affirming thoughts. This shift towards self-compassion has a ripple effect, enhancing not just your relationship with yourself but also your interactions with others.

The Alkaline Lifestyle: A Catalyst for Positive Change

The alkaline lifestyle serves as a catalyst for positive change, not just in your diet but in your overall approach to life. It's a holistic transformation that transcends the boundaries of physical health to enrich your mental and emotional well-being. This transformation is not a solitary journey; it's a communal experience that fosters a sense of belonging and interconnectedness. When you adopt an alkaline lifestyle, you're not just improving your life; you're contributing to a collective upliftment, a communal journey towards holistic health and happiness.

Resilience is the ability to bounce back from adversity, to adapt and thrive in the face of challenges. The alkaline lifestyle, with its emphasis on mental clarity and emotional balance, naturally fosters resilience. When you're resilient, life's inevitable ups and downs become manageable, even surmountable. This resilience is not a passive trait but an active skill, honed and refined through the principles and practices of an alkaline lifestyle.

As we navigate the intricacies of the alkaline lifestyle and its psychological benefits, it's important to remember that this is not a quick fix or a temporary solution. It's a lifelong commitment to mental wellness, a continuous journey of self-discovery and growth. The alkaline lifestyle offers a roadmap for this journey, providing the tools and principles to navigate the complexities of the human mind.

The psychological benefits of an alkaline lifestyle are multi-faceted and deeply interconnected with the core principles of balance, harmony, and mindfulness. It's a holistic approach that addresses the mind, body, and spirit, offering a comprehensive pathway to mental wellness.

The Alkaline Lifestyle as a Pillar of Mental Wellness

As we draw this section to a close, it's worth emphasizing that an alkaline lifestyle is not just a dietary choice; it's a pillar of mental wellness. It's a holistic approach that transcends the physical realm to deeply impact your psychological state. The alkaline lifestyle is not a fad or a trend; it's a timeless wisdom that has the power to transform your mental landscape, offering you the tools to navigate the complexities of modern life with grace and resilience.

The alkaline lifestyle is a journey, not a destination. It's a continuous process of self-discovery and growth. It's about embracing the present moment, being mindful of your choices, and taking responsibility for your mental well-being. This journey is not a solitary endeavor; it's a collective experience that fosters a sense of community and interconnectedness. When you embark on this journey, you're not just improving your life; you're contributing to a larger movement, a global shift towards holistic health and happiness.

Mindfulness is the art of being fully present, aware of where we are and what we're doing, without being overly reactive or overwhelmed by what's happening around us. The alkaline lifestyle naturally cultivates mindfulness by promoting mental clarity and emotional balance. When you're mindful, you're more attuned to your emotional state, making it easier to manage stress, anxiety, and depression. This heightened sense of mindfulness is a valuable asset in personal relationships, professional settings, and even in the inner dialogue you have with yourself.

The Alkaline Lifestyle: A Catalyst for Positive Change

The alkaline lifestyle serves as a catalyst for positive change, not just in your diet but in your overall approach to life. It's a holistic transformation that transcends the boundaries of physical health to enrich your mental and emotional well-being. This transformation is not a solitary journey; it's a communal experience that fosters a sense of belonging and interconnectedness. When you adopt an alkaline lifestyle, you're not just improving your life; you're contributing to a collective upliftment, a communal journey towards holistic health and happiness.

The Alkaline Lifestyle and the Power of Choice

One of the most empowering aspects of the alkaline lifestyle is the power of choice. Every day, you have the opportunity to make choices that impact your mental well-being. Whether it's choosing nutrient-dense foods, engaging in mindful practices, or cultivating positive relationships, these choices have a cumulative effect on your psychological state. The power of choice is not a burden; it's a privilege, a freedom that allows you to shape your mental landscape according to your values and aspirations.

As we navigate the intricacies of the alkaline lifestyle and its psychological benefits, it's important to remember that this is not a quick fix or a temporary solution. It's a lifelong commitment to mental wellness, a continuous journey of self-discovery and growth. The alkaline lifestyle offers a roadmap for this journey, providing the tools and principles to navigate the complexities of the human mind.

The Alkaline Lifestyle and the Future of Mental Health

As we look towards the future, it's clear that the alkaline lifestyle has a significant role to play in shaping the landscape of mental health. With the increasing prevalence of mental health disorders and the growing awareness of the limitations of conventional treatments, there's a pressing need for holistic approaches that address the root causes of mental ailments. The alkaline lifestyle offers a compelling alternative, a holistic approach that addresses the mind, body, and spirit, offering a comprehensive pathway to mental wellness.

In conclusion, the psychological benefits of an alkaline lifestyle are multi-faceted and deeply interconnected with the core principles of balance, harmony, and mindfulness. It's a holistic approach that addresses the mind, body, and spirit, offering a comprehensive pathway to mental wellness. As we move forward, let's celebrate the empowering realization that an alkaline lifestyle is not just a pathway to physical health but a gateway to mental freedom. It's a transformative journey that offers the promise of a brighter, happier, and more fulfilling life. So, as you turn the page, remember that the alkaline lifestyle is not just a chapter in a book; it's a chapter in your life, a story that's still being written, a journey that's just beginning.

Meditation, Mindfulness, and Alkalinity:

The Symbiotic Trio for Holistic Health

As we delve into this transformative chapter, let's first acknowledge the profound convergence of ancient wisdom and modern science. Meditation, mindfulness, and alkalinity—these are not just buzzwords or trends. They are timeless principles that have been practiced and revered for centuries, now backed by scientific research. They form a symbiotic trio that can profoundly impact not just your physical well-being but your mental and spiritual health as well.

Meditation is often misunderstood as a complex spiritual practice reserved for monks or spiritual gurus. In reality, it's a simple yet powerful tool accessible to everyone. At its core, meditation is the art of focused attention. It's about quieting the mind to connect with the present moment. But how does this relate to an alkaline lifestyle? The answer lies in the body's pH balance. A calm, focused mind contributes to homeostasis—the body's natural state of balance. Stress, on the other hand, triggers the release of cortisol, a hormone that can make your body more acidic. Meditation, therefore, serves as a natural antidote to acidity, aligning perfectly with the principles of an alkaline lifestyle.

Mindfulness: The Bridge Between Thought and Action

Mindfulness takes the principles of meditation a step further. While meditation teaches you to control your thoughts, mindfulness equips you with the skills to translate that mental clarity into daily actions. Every choice you make, from the foods you eat to the words you speak, impacts your body's pH levels. Mindfulness ensures that these choices align with the principles of alkalinity. It's not just about eating the right foods; it's about consuming them mindfully. It's not just about physical exercise; it's about being present in every movement. Mindfulness, therefore, serves as the bridge between your thoughts and actions, ensuring that your lifestyle remains alkaline not just in theory but in practice.

Alkalinity: The Foundation for Mental Clarity

Alkalinity is often discussed in the context of physical health, but its impact on mental well-being is equally significant. An alkaline body is a well-oxygenated body, and a well-oxygenated body is a well-functioning brain. The clarity of thought that comes from an alkaline lifestyle is not a mere coincidence; it's a direct result of the body's optimal functioning. This mental clarity serves as the foundation for both meditation and mindfulness, making alkalinity the cornerstone of this symbiotic trio.

The beauty of integrating meditation, mindfulness, and alkalinity into your lifestyle lies in their interconnectedness. Each practice reinforces the other, creating a virtuous cycle of well-being. Meditation enhances your mental clarity, making it easier to make alkaline choices. Those alkaline choices, in turn, improve your physical health, making it easier to meditate. And mindfulness serves as the glue that holds it all together, ensuring that these practices are not isolated events but integrated parts of your daily life.

As we navigate the complexities of modern life, filled with stress, distractions, and conflicting priorities, the principles of meditation, mindfulness, and alkalinity offer a sanctuary. They provide a holistic framework for not just surviving but thriving in the modern world. Whether you're a busy professional juggling multiple responsibilities or someone seeking deeper spiritual connection, these practices offer practical solutions. They equip you with the tools to manage stress, improve focus, and make choices that align with your highest well-being.

As we embark on this enlightening journey through the chapter, let's remember that adopting meditation, mindfulness, and an alkaline lifestyle is not a one-time event but a lifelong commitment. It's a commitment to your highest well-being, a pledge to honor the sanctity of your mind, body, and spirit. And as you'll discover in the pages that follow, this commitment is not a burden but a liberating journey—a journey towards holistic health, lasting happiness, and profound spiritual awakening.

The Alchemy of Inner Transformation: Unpacking the Core Principles

Let's begin by diving deeper into the essence of meditation. Imagine your mind as a sanctuary, a sacred space where you can retreat from the chaos of the external world. This sanctuary is not a place of escape but a realm of clarity, where you can discern the subtle energies that influence your physical and emotional state. When you meditate, you're not just closing your eyes and taking deep breaths; you're actively participating in the alchemy of inner transformation. You're shifting your internal pH balance towards alkalinity by reducing mental and emotional toxins like stress, anxiety, and negative thoughts.

Now, let's transition from the meditative mind to the mindful life. Mindfulness is not a sporadic practice you engage in when you find the time; it's a way of life. It's the art of living consciously, of making each moment an opportunity for growth and transformation. When you eat, you're not just consuming food; you're nourishing your body and soul. When you speak, you're not just communicating; you're resonating vibrations that can either uplift or deplete your energy. Mindfulness is the lens through which you view your interactions, choices, and even your thoughts. It's the conscious filter that helps you align your daily life with the principles of alkalinity.

Alkalinity is not just a dietary choice; it's a cellular symphony. Every cell in your body is a living entity, and when these cells are in harmony, you experience optimal health. An alkaline environment is conducive to this cellular harmony. It's like tuning an orchestra; each instrument (cell) must be finely tuned (alkaline) to contribute to a beautiful symphony (optimal health). When your body is alkaline, your cells can perform their functions efficiently, leading to better nutrient absorption, more effective toxin elimination, and a natural resilience against diseases.

The Symbiosis: How Meditation, Mindfulness, and Alkalinity Interact

It's crucial to understand how these three pillars—meditation, mindfulness, and alkalinity—interact in a symbiotic relationship. Meditation serves as the foundation, providing you with the mental clarity and emotional balance that make mindful living possible. Mindfulness is the active application of this clarity in your daily choices, ensuring that you maintain an alkaline state. Alkalinity, in turn, enhances your mental and emotional well-being, making both meditation and mindfulness more effective. It's a self-reinforcing cycle, a virtuous circle that leads to holistic well-being.

The benefits of integrating meditation, mindfulness, and alkalinity into your life extend beyond personal well-being. They have a ripple effect that influences your relationships, your work, and your contribution to society. When you're in a state of holistic health, you're not just a better version of yourself; you're a catalyst for positive change. You inspire those around you to embark on their own journeys of self-discovery and transformation. You contribute to a collective shift towards a more conscious, compassionate, and harmonious world.

The Practicalities: Making It Work in a Busy Life

Let's address the elephant in the room: How do you integrate these practices into a busy, demanding life? The answer is simpler than you might think. It's not about carving out hours for meditation or drastically altering your diet overnight. It's about small, sustainable changes. It's about taking five minutes during your lunch break to practice mindful breathing. It's about choosing a glass of alkaline water over a soda. It's about pausing before reacting in a stressful situation to choose a more balanced response. These small choices accumulate, leading to a profound transformation over time.

As we navigate the complexities of this chapter, let's remember that this is a lifelong journey. There are no quick fixes or magic pills. The path to holistic health through meditation, mindfulness, and alkalinity is a winding road filled with challenges, discoveries, and moments of profound insight. It requires patience, commitment, and a willingness to embrace the process, knowing that each step brings you closer to your truest self.

In summary, the core principles of meditation, mindfulness, and alkalinity offer a comprehensive framework for holistic health. They are interconnected practices that reinforce each other, creating a virtuous cycle of physical, emotional, and spiritual well-being.

The Last Mile: Sealing the Covenant of Holistic Health

As we approach the end of this transformative chapter, it's essential to recognize that the journey towards holistic health is not a linear path but a spiral. You circle around the core principles of meditation, mindfulness, and alkalinity, each time gaining a deeper understanding and a more nuanced application. This is the unseen bridge that connects these seemingly disparate elements into a cohesive, life-altering philosophy.

The concept of an alkaline mind is a groundbreaking paradigm shift. We often focus on the body when discussing alkalinity, but the mind is equally susceptible to acidic thoughts that can disrupt our mental equilibrium. Just as we strive to maintain an alkaline body for optimal health, cultivating an alkaline mind through meditation and mindfulness is crucial. This state of mind is not just about positive thinking; it's about clarity, focus, and emotional resilience. It's about being so rooted in your inner sanctuary that external circumstances lose their power to disrupt your peace.

The mind and body are not separate entities but part of a harmonious existence. When you meditate, you're not just calming the mind; you're also creating an alkaline environment in the body. When you practice mindfulness, you're not just making conscious choices; you're also influencing your cellular health. This is the mind-body symphony, a harmonious existence where each component is in tune with the other, creating a melodious flow of life energy that nourishes your entire being.

The transformation doesn't stop with you. When you embody the principles of meditation, mindfulness, and alkalinity, you become a beacon of light in a world clouded by confusion and suffering. Your transformation has a ripple effect that extends from your immediate circle to society at large. You inspire change, not by preaching, but by living your truth. You show people that it's possible to live a life of balance, health, and inner peace, even in the midst of chaos.

In this journey, you become an everyday alchemist, transforming the mundane into the sacred. Your daily activities, whether it's eating, working, or even resting, become rituals of self-care and expressions of your highest self. You learn to find the extraordinary in the ordinary, the sacred in the mundane, and the transformative power in the everyday choices you make. This is the essence of living a life aligned with the principles of meditation, mindfulness, and alkalinity.

The Legacy: Passing the Torch

As you walk this path, you're not just improving your life; you're contributing to a legacy. You're part of a lineage of seekers, healers, and visionaries who have dared to step outside the conventional paradigms of health and wellness to explore something more profound, more holistic, and more empowering. By embracing these principles, you're passing the torch to the next generation, empowering them to live healthier, more conscious lives.

As we reach the final note of this chapter, understand that this is not a conclusion but an invitation—an invitation to continue exploring, questioning, and evolving. The principles of meditation, mindfulness, and alkalinity are not static doctrines but living philosophies that grow and evolve as you do. They are your companions in this lifelong journey towards holistic health, offering you tools, insights, and perspectives that enrich your life in ways you can't even begin to imagine.

In closing, the integration of meditation, mindfulness, and alkalinity is not just a health regimen; it's a life philosophy. It's a holistic approach to well-being that transcends diet, exercise, and stress management, touching the core of who you are and how you interact with the world. It's a transformative journey that begins with the individual but has the power to change the world, one conscious choice at a time.

Yoga, Physical Activity, and Their Role in Alkaline Living

The Alchemy of Movement: A New Perspective

As we delve into this transformative chapter, let's first acknowledge that the body is not just a vessel to carry us through life; it's an intricate, intelligent system that communicates with us in ways we often overlook. The way we move, breathe, and engage with the world has a profound impact on our internal environment, including our body's pH levels. This is where the alchemy of movement comes into play, transforming not just our physical state but also our mental and spiritual well-being.

When most people think of yoga, they envision a serene setting with individuals contorted into various poses. While this imagery captures the essence of the practice, yoga is much more than a series of postures. It's a holistic system that integrates mind, body, and spirit, aligning perfectly with the principles of alkaline living. Yoga is not just about flexibility; it's about creating a harmonious flow of energy that helps to balance your body's pH levels. When you engage in yoga, you're not just stretching muscles; you're also stretching your consciousness, expanding your awareness, and elevating your vibrational frequency.

Physical activity is often touted for its benefits in weight management and cardiovascular health. However, its role in maintaining an alkaline state is seldom discussed. Exercise helps to oxygenate the blood, remove toxins, and enhance metabolic processes, all of which contribute to a more alkaline environment. The beauty of this is that you don't have to be an athlete to reap these benefits. Whether it's a brisk walk, a swim, or a dance class, the key is to find activities that you enjoy and that make you feel alive. This is the physicality of alkalinity—a symbiotic relationship where movement enhances your alkaline state, and your alkaline state, in turn, enhances your capacity for movement.

The Mindful Mover: Intentionality in Action

One of the most overlooked aspects of physical activity is the role of intentionality. When you move with awareness, when you're fully present in the activity, you're practicing mindfulness. This state of being mindful while moving is a potent form of meditation that can significantly impact your alkaline levels. It's not just about going through the motions but about feeling each movement, understanding its purpose, and appreciating its impact on your body. This is the essence of being a mindful mover, and it's a practice that can be incorporated into any form of physical activity, from yoga to weightlifting to running.

In the realm of yoga and physical activity, there's an interplay between masculine and feminine energies, often referred to as 'Yang' and 'Yin' in Eastern philosophies. Yang activities are dynamic, intense, and heat-generating, like power yoga or high-intensity interval training (HIIT). Yin activities are more passive, gentle, and cooling, like restorative yoga or leisurely swimming. Both are essential for creating a balanced, alkaline state. The key is to recognize when your body needs the fiery intensity of Yang or the soothing calmness of Yin and to incorporate both into your routine.

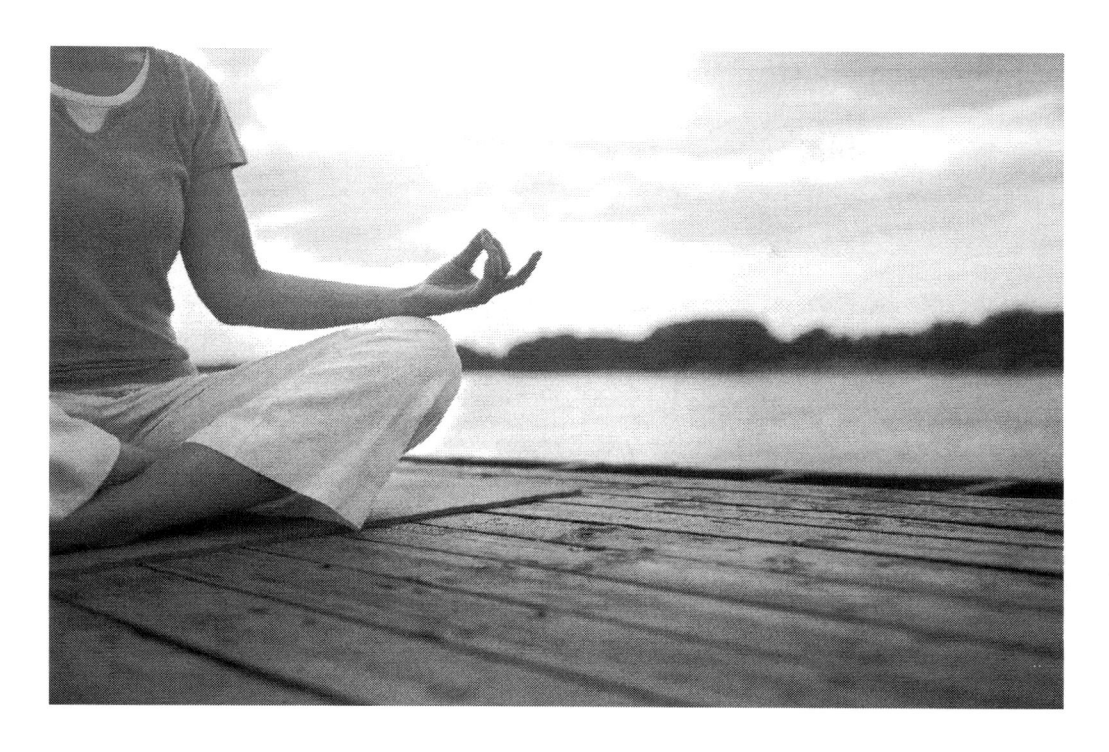

The Sacred Geometry of the Body: Alignment and Integrity

In yoga, much emphasis is placed on alignment—not just the alignment of your limbs but also the alignment of your intentions, your breath, and your focus. This concept of alignment extends to alkaline living. When your actions, thoughts, and lifestyle choices are in alignment with the principles of alkalinity, you create a state of integrity that permeates every cell in your body. This is the sacred geometry of the body, a state where everything is in its right place, functioning optimally, and resonating with the universal laws of health and well-being.

As we wrap up this introductory exploration, let's remember that the journey towards an alkaline lifestyle is not just an external endeavor; it's a journey within. It's about tuning into your body's wisdom, listening to its subtle cues, and responding in ways that honor its innate intelligence. Yoga and physical activity are not just tools for physical transformation; they're gateways to a deeper, more meaningful relationship with yourself.

In the following sections, we'll delve deeper into the nuances of yoga and physical activity, exploring their multifaceted roles in alkaline living. But for now, let this serve as a prelude to transformation, an invitation to engage with your body in a more conscious, intentional, and loving manner.

The Breath of Life: Pranayama and Alkalinity

As we journey deeper into the core of this topic, let's begin by exploring the breath, often referred to as "Prana" in yogic philosophy. Pranayama, the art of breath control, is a cornerstone of yoga that has profound implications for alkaline living. When you breathe deeply, you're not merely filling your lungs with air; you're also infusing your cells with oxygen, which aids in maintaining an alkaline state. The breath is a bridge between the mind and body, and mastering it can be a transformative experience that elevates your alkaline lifestyle to new heights.

The Energetic Body: Chakras and Alkalinity

In yoga, the concept of chakras, or energy centers, is pivotal. These chakras are not just metaphysical constructs; they have physiological counterparts that influence various systems in the body. For instance, the solar plexus chakra, located near the stomach, is often linked to digestion—a key factor in maintaining alkalinity. By engaging in specific yoga poses that target these energy centers, you can enhance your body's ability to sustain an alkaline state. This is the energetic body in action, a subtle yet powerful aspect of your being that plays a crucial role in your overall wellness.

The Rhythm of Movement: Flow and Fluidity

In physical activities like dance or martial arts, there's an inherent rhythm, a flow that participants tap into. This flow state is not just a psychological peak experience; it's also a physiological one. When you're in the flow, your body operates more efficiently, your metabolic processes are optimized, and your system naturally leans towards alkalinity. The rhythm of movement, therefore, is not just an aesthetic quality but a functional one that has tangible benefits for your alkaline lifestyle.

The Mind-Muscle Connection: Beyond Physicality

In any form of physical activity, the mind-muscle connection is vital. This is the ability to focus your mental energy on your movements, to be fully present in the activity. When you achieve this level of concentration, you're not just exercising your body; you're also exercising your mind. This dual engagement has a synergistic effect, enhancing your body's alkaline balance while also sharpening your mental clarity. It's a holistic approach that transcends the boundaries of physicality, entering the realm of conscious living.

While high-intensity activities have their place, it's essential to balance them with restorative practices like Yin Yoga or Tai Chi. These activities are not just 'cool-down' sessions; they're integral components of an alkaline lifestyle. They help to reduce inflammation, improve circulation, and facilitate detoxification—all key factors in maintaining an alkaline state. The healing touch of these restorative practices is like a balm for the soul, a nurturing embrace that brings you back to your center.

Whether you're practicing yoga or engaging in any other physical activity, there's a multisensory experience happening. The feel of the ground beneath your feet, the rhythm of your breath, the sensation of your muscles contracting and expanding—these are all part of a symphony of senses that you can tune into. When you become mindful of these sensations, you're practicing what can be termed as 'mindfulness in motion.' This practice enhances your awareness, deepens your connection to your body, and contributes to a balanced, alkaline state.

For those who are more athletically inclined, the concept of being an 'Alkaline Athlete' may resonate. This is not about how fast you can run or how much weight you can lift; it's about how well you can maintain an alkaline state while pushing your physical limits. It's a new paradigm that challenges conventional notions of athleticism, placing equal emphasis on internal balance and external performance.

The Art of Balance: Harmonizing Extremes

In the quest for an alkaline lifestyle, balance is key. Too much of anything, even a good thing, can tip the scales towards acidity. This is where the art of balance comes into play. It's about harmonizing the extremes, integrating the Yin and Yang aspects of your lifestyle to create a harmonious, alkaline state. Whether it's balancing intense workouts with restorative practices or integrating mindfulness into your daily activities, the art of balance is a skill that can be honed over time.

As we transition to the concluding segment of this chapter, let's carry forward this newfound understanding of the intricate relationship between yoga, physical activity, and alkaline living. It's a relationship that's not just theoretical but deeply experiential, one that you can explore, experience, and embody as you continue on your journey towards holistic wellness.

The Culmination: Embodying the Essence of Yoga, Physical Activity, and Alkaline Living

As we draw this chapter to a close, it's essential to recognize that the journey towards an alkaline lifestyle is not a sprint but a marathon. It's a lifelong commitment that requires a holistic approach, one that harmonizes the mind, body, and spirit. The alchemy of transformation is a subtle process, and it's in this subtlety that the magic happens. When you engage in yoga and physical activity with a conscious intention to support your alkaline lifestyle, you're not just changing your habits; you're transforming your life.

Think of your body as a living canvas, a work of art that you're continually creating and recreating. Every yoga pose you strike, every lap you swim, every mountain you climb—these are the brushstrokes that define your masterpiece. But remember, a true work of art is not just about aesthetics; it's about the essence, the soul of the creation. Similarly, your body is not just a physical entity; it's a living, breathing manifestation of your inner world. When you treat it as such, you're not just living an alkaline lifestyle; you're embodying it.

In the realm of metaphysics, it's often said that everything is energy, and energy vibrates at different frequencies. When you're living an alkaline lifestyle, supported by yoga and physical activity, you're essentially vibrating at a higher frequency. This is not just a poetic metaphor; it's a scientific fact. The molecular structure of an alkaline body is different, more harmonious, and this harmony resonates at a cellular level. It's the resonance of being, a state of existence where you're not just surviving; you're thriving.

Life is a symphony, a complex interplay of various elements that come together to create a harmonious existence. Yoga and physical activity are the instruments in this symphony, and alkalinity is the melody that ties it all together. When you strike the right chords, when you find that perfect balance, you're not just making music; you're making magic. It's the symphony of the soul, a harmonious existence that transcends the mundane and touches the divine.

The practices of yoga and physical activity are not new; they're ancient wisdom passed down through generations. What's new is the context, the modern world in which we're applying these timeless truths. In a world that's increasingly chaotic and stressful, the need for an alkaline lifestyle is more critical than ever. It's not just about combating diseases or enhancing physical performance; it's about finding peace in a restless world. It's the wisdom of the ancients, applied in a modern context, for a future that's yet to be written.

The Dance of Life: Choreographing Your Destiny

Life is a dance, a delicate balance between various elements that define our existence. Yoga and physical activity are the steps in this dance, and alkalinity is the rhythm that guides us. When you master this dance, you're not just moving through life; you're choreographing your destiny. You're taking control of the narrative, rewriting the script, and becoming the hero of your own epic saga.

In the hustle and bustle of modern life, it's easy to lose touch with our inner world. Yoga and physical activity serve as gateways to this sacred space, a sanctuary where we can retreat and recharge. When this space is alkaline, it's not just a refuge; it's a fortress, a stronghold that protects us from the onslaught of external stressors. Cultivating this inner sanctity is not a luxury; it's a necessity, a vital aspect of holistic wellness that's often overlooked but never undervalued.

As we take the final bow, let's give a standing ovation to our higher selves, the part of us that aspires for greatness, that yearns for enlightenment, that strives for an alkaline lifestyle. It's this higher self that guides us through the labyrinth of life, that whispers words of wisdom in our moments of doubt, that celebrates our victories, no matter how small. It's the unsung hero of our journey, the silent partner in our quest for holistic wellness.

In conclusion, the integration of yoga and physical activity into an alkaline lifestyle is not just a strategy; it's a philosophy, a way of life that honors the sacredness of our existence. It's a holistic approach that nurtures the mind, nourishes the body, and nurtures the soul. It's the path less traveled, but it's the only path worth taking. So take that step, strike that pose, climb that mountain, and as you do, know that you're not just living; you're thriving, you're flourishing, you're becoming the best version of yourself. And in that becoming, you'll find that you're not just surviving; you're truly, deeply, authentically alive.

Book 7: Alkaline Gourmet – A Recipe Book

Breakfast: Energizing Alkaline Starters

The Dawn of a New Day: Breakfast, The Alkaline Way

As the first rays of sunlight filter through your curtains, a new day beckons. The choices you make in these early hours set the tone for the rest of your day. Breakfast, often dubbed the most important meal, is not merely a ritual of refueling. It's a sacred act of self-care, a moment where you can nourish not just your body but also your soul. In this chapter, we delve into the transformative power of starting your day with energizing alkaline starters.

Imagine waking up to a symphony of flavors, a culinary overture that not only tantalizes your taste buds but also invigorates your spirit. This is what an alkaline breakfast aims to achieve. It's not about bland smoothies or uninspiring oatmeal; it's about creating a feast that celebrates the richness of natural, alkaline-forming ingredients. From vibrant fruit bowls to nutrient-packed green smoothies, the options are as diverse as they are delicious.

The beauty of an alkaline breakfast lies in the alchemy of its ingredients. Each element, carefully chosen, serves a purpose. The fruits bring in a burst of antioxidants, the nuts provide the much-needed healthy fats, and the seeds offer a sprinkle of fiber. It's a carefully orchestrated dance of nutrients, where each player shines but also contributes to the ensemble. This is not just food; it's medicine, it's therapy, it's love in its purest form.

In our fast-paced lives, breakfast often becomes a rushed affair, a quick bite before we dive into the chaos of the day. An alkaline breakfast invites you to slow down, to savor each bite, to relish the textures and flavors that dance on your palate. It's an exercise in mindfulness, a meditative experience that grounds you, centers you, and prepares you for the challenges that lie ahead.

Let's talk about energy, that elusive force that powers our lives. A conventional breakfast, laden with sugars and processed foods, offers a quick burst of energy, followed by an inevitable crash. An alkaline breakfast, on the other hand, provides sustained energy, fueling your fire without burning you out. It's the kind of energy that doesn't just get you through the day; it elevates your day, transforming mundane tasks into opportunities for joy and fulfillment.

The benefits of an alkaline breakfast extend beyond the physical realm. When you nourish your body with alkaline-forming foods, you're also nourishing your mind. You're enhancing your mental clarity, boosting your mood, and setting a positive emotional tone for the day. It's a holistic approach to wellness, one that recognizes the intricate connection between the body and the mind, the tangible and the intangible.

The Art of Crafting: Your Personal Masterpiece

Creating an alkaline breakfast is not just a culinary task; it's an artistic endeavor. It's about crafting a meal that reflects your individuality, your preferences, your needs. Whether you're a smoothie aficionado or a chia pudding enthusiast, the canvas is yours to paint. And the best part? There are no rules, only guidelines. You're the artist, the chef, the alchemist, and this is your personal masterpiece.

As you take the last sip of your alkaline tea or the final bite of your avocado toast, know that the impact of this meal extends far beyond the breakfast table. It's a ripple effect that influences your choices for the rest of the day, inspiring you to make healthier decisions, to live more consciously, to be more present. It's not just a meal; it's a movement, a philosophy, a way of life.

So, as you embark on this culinary adventure, remember, you're not just feeding your body; you're feeding your soul. And in that sacred act of nourishment, you'll find the energy, the vitality, the zest to not just live another day, but to truly make it count.

Crafting Your Alkaline Breakfast Experience

The kitchen is more than a room with appliances; it's a sanctuary where the alchemy of wellness begins. As you step into this sacred space each morning, you're not just a cook; you're a wellness architect. The ingredients you select, the recipes you choose, and the techniques you employ are the building blocks of your health. In the alkaline kitchen, every ingredient has a purpose, and every dish is a testament to your commitment to holistic well-being.

One of the most enriching aspects of an alkaline breakfast is its alignment with the seasons. Nature, in its infinite wisdom, provides us with fruits and vegetables that are not just delicious but also perfectly suited for our nutritional needs at different times of the year. A summer breakfast might feature a smoothie bowl adorned with fresh berries, while a winter morning could be warmed by a hot quinoa porridge spiced with cinnamon. This seasonal approach not only adds variety to your meals but also ensures that you're getting a diverse range of nutrients throughout the year.

The Nutritional Choreography: A Dance of Elements

An alkaline breakfast isn't a random assortment of foods; it's a carefully choreographed dance of nutritional elements. Proteins, fats, and carbohydrates are balanced in a way that maximizes energy and minimizes digestive stress. For instance, a chia seed pudding made with almond milk provides a harmonious blend of protein, healthy fats, and fiber, ensuring that you're satiated but not sluggish. This nutritional choreography is the secret sauce that makes an alkaline breakfast not just a meal but a wellness experience.

Spices and herbs are the unsung heroes of the alkaline kitchen. They do more than just add flavor; they bring a bouquet of health benefits to the table. Turmeric, with its anti-inflammatory properties, can be a golden addition to your morning smoothie. Fresh mint leaves can elevate a simple fruit salad while aiding digestion. The use of spices and herbs is an art form, a way to paint your breakfast canvas with strokes of flavor and wellness.

The Mind-Gut Connection: Emotional Nutrition

We often overlook the emotional aspect of eating, especially during the morning rush. However, the act of consuming an alkaline breakfast can be a form of emotional nutrition. The colors, textures, and flavors can uplift your mood, setting a positive emotional tone for the day. When you take the time to appreciate the sensory experience of your meal, you're not just nourishing your body; you're also feeding your soul.

In a world obsessed with convenience, preparing an alkaline breakfast might seem like a luxury. But let's reframe this narrative. Investing time in crafting a nourishing meal is an investment in your health, productivity, and overall well-being. It's an act of self-respect, a declaration that you're worth the effort. And the returns on this investment are exponential, manifesting as enhanced focus, sustained energy, and a fortified immune system.

The Ritual of Preparation: A Meditative Practice

The process of preparing an alkaline breakfast can be a meditative practice in itself. The act of washing fruits, chopping vegetables, or stirring a pot of oatmeal can be grounding experiences. They offer a momentary pause, a break from the digital noise and mental clutter. As you engage in these simple acts, you're not just preparing food; you're cultivating mindfulness, anchoring yourself in the present moment.

While an alkaline breakfast is a deeply personal experience, its joy multiplies when shared. Whether it's a weekend brunch with family or a quick weekday breakfast with a loved one, these shared meals become more than just social events; they're communal wellness rituals. They offer an opportunity to spread the alkaline love, to inspire and be inspired, to create a collective momentum towards holistic health.

In the grand tapestry of alkaline living, breakfast holds a place of honor. It's not just the first meal of the day; it's the first chapter in your daily wellness story. As you navigate through the myriad options and opportunities that alkaline breakfasts offer, remember that each choice is a brushstroke in the masterpiece that is your health. So, embrace the journey, savor the experience, and let the energizing alkaline starters illuminate the path to your best self.

The Culmination of Morning Alchemy: The Lasting Impact of Energizing Alkaline Starters

The choices you make in the morning reverberate throughout the day. An alkaline breakfast is not a one-time event but a catalyst for sustained wellness. It sets the rhythm for your metabolic orchestra, harmonizing energy levels, mood, and cognitive function. The morning meal is a promise to your body—a pledge of nourishment and care. When you honor this commitment, you're not just fueling your body; you're fortifying your spirit.

The act of preparing and consuming an alkaline breakfast can be elevated to a daily ritual. It's a moment of pause, a sanctuary of calm in a world that often feels chaotic. This ritual is a form of self-care, a daily affirmation that says, "I am worth the time. I am worth the effort." It's a meditative space where the act of chopping fruits, blending smoothies, or brewing herbal teas becomes a form of mindfulness. This ritualistic approach transforms the mundane into the sacred, making each breakfast a spiritual experience.

An alkaline breakfast is a symphony of nutrients, each playing its part in the grand composition of your health. The proteins lay the foundation, the healthy fats add depth, and the complex carbohydrates bring in the melodies. This nutrient symphony is not just music to your taste buds but a lasting overture for your body. It sets the stage for optimal digestion, efficient energy utilization, and effective detoxification. The nutrients in your alkaline breakfast are the unsung heroes, working behind the scenes to ensure that the rest of the day unfolds in wellness.

The emotional benefits of an alkaline breakfast extend far beyond the morning hours. The vibrant colors of fruits, the rich textures of nuts and seeds, and the aromatic spices create a sensory experience that uplifts your mood. This emotional echo can be a powerful ally in managing stress and enhancing mental well-being. When you start the day on a positive note, you're more resilient in the face of challenges, more focused in your tasks, and more compassionate in your interactions.

Your commitment to an alkaline breakfast can inspire those around you. Whether it's your family adopting healthier eating habits or your colleagues showing interest in your green smoothies, your choices create a social ripple effect. You become a living testament to the transformative power of alkaline living, a beacon that lights the way for others. This social impact amplifies the personal benefits, creating a cycle of collective wellness.

The alkaline diet emphasizes plant-based, organic, and seasonal foods, which have a lower environmental impact compared to processed and animal-based foods. By choosing an alkaline breakfast, you're making a conscious choice to minimize your environmental footprint. It's a small but significant step towards sustainable living, a way to align your personal wellness with the well-being of the planet.

The Legacy of Morning Wellness: A Lifelong Journey

An alkaline breakfast is not an end but a beginning—a stepping stone in your lifelong journey towards holistic health. It's a legacy you leave for yourself, a daily investment in your future well-being. As you age, this legacy becomes increasingly valuable, offering you the resilience to navigate life's challenges and the vitality to enjoy its blessings.

As we conclude this exploration of energizing alkaline starters, let's make a pact—a commitment to excellence in our morning choices. Let's vow to honor the sanctity of our bodies, to celebrate the richness of nature's bounty, and to cherish the emotional and spiritual dimensions of eating. Let's promise to make each breakfast not just a meal but a masterpiece—a work of art that nourishes the body, nurtures the soul, and nourishes the spirit.

In the grand narrative of your life, let the story of each day begin with an alkaline breakfast. Let it be the prologue to a day lived in harmony, a day imbued with vitality, and a day that echoes the timeless wisdom of alkaline living. Here's to mornings that energize, to breakfasts that empower, and to a life that embodies the essence of alkaline excellence.

Lunch: Nutrient-Packed Midday Meals

The Midday Metamorphosis: Unveiling the Power of Nutrient-Packed Alkaline Lunches

Lunch is often relegated to a mere pit stop in our daily race against time. We scarf down whatever is convenient, giving little thought to the nutritional value or the impact on our well-being. But what if we reframe this midday meal as a milestone, a pivotal moment that can either propel us forward or hold us back? In the realm of alkaline living, lunch is not just a break from work; it's a transformative experience that can redefine your relationship with food and, by extension, with yourself.

The beauty of an alkaline lunch lies in its simplicity and its complexity—simple because it relies on whole, unprocessed foods, and complex because each ingredient brings a unique nutrient profile to the table. Imagine a salad where leafy greens provide a rich source of iron and calcium, avocados offer healthy fats, and a sprinkle of chia seeds adds a protein punch. This is not just a meal; it's a carefully orchestrated symphony of nutrients, each playing its part to nourish your body and soul.

The Mindful Midday: A Pause for Reflection and Rejuvenation

In the hustle and bustle of modern life, lunch often becomes a rushed affair, consumed in front of a computer screen or on the go. An alkaline lunch invites you to pause, to step away from the chaos and engage in mindful eating. It's a moment to savor the flavors, to appreciate the textures, and to listen to your body's cues. This act of mindfulness extends beyond the meal itself; it becomes a form of meditation, a daily practice that enhances your emotional well-being and mental clarity.

The foods you choose for lunch have a direct impact on your energy levels for the rest of the day. A meal high in processed carbs and sugars may give you a quick energy boost, but it's often followed by a crash that leaves you feeling lethargic and unfocused. An alkaline lunch, on the other hand, provides sustained energy, thanks to its balance of complex carbs, proteins, and healthy fats. It's the kind of fuel that empowers you to tackle your afternoon tasks with vigor, whether it's a high-stakes meeting or a creative project.

The Social Fabric: Lunch as a Community Experience

Lunch is often a social affair, a time to connect with colleagues, friends, or family. An alkaline lunch can serve as a conversation starter, an opportunity to share your journey towards holistic health and perhaps inspire others to make healthier choices. It's a subtle form of advocacy, a way to spread the message of alkaline living without preaching or judging. Your lunch becomes a testament to your values, a tangible expression of your commitment to wellness and sustainability.

Preparing an alkaline lunch is not just a culinary task; it's a creative endeavor. It's an opportunity to experiment with flavors, to play with colors, and to arrange your ingredients in a visually appealing manner. This creative process is not just for aesthetic pleasure; it's a form of self-expression, a way to infuse your personality into your meals. And let's not forget the joy of discovery—the thrill of stumbling upon a new ingredient or a novel combination that takes your taste buds on an unexpected journey.

The Holistic Harmony: Aligning Body, Mind, and Spirit

An alkaline lunch is not an isolated event; it's part of a holistic approach to wellness that encompasses physical health, emotional balance, and spiritual growth. When you choose foods that are in harmony with your body's natural pH levels, you're also choosing foods that nourish your mind and uplift your spirit. It's a form of self-care that goes beyond calories and nutrients; it's a celebration of your innate potential for healing, transformation, and transcendence.

As we embark on this exploration of nutrient-packed alkaline lunches, let's approach it with an open heart and a curious mind. Let's view each meal as an opportunity for growth, each ingredient as a stepping stone on our path to holistic health. Let's embrace the diversity of flavors, the richness of textures, and the depth of nutrients that an alkaline lunch has to offer.

In the grand tapestry of alkaline living, lunch occupies a central panel, a vibrant tableau that reflects our daily struggles and triumphs. It's a narrative woven with threads of choice and consequence, a story that unfolds one meal at a time. So, let's make each lunch count. Let's make it a masterpiece of nourishment, a testament to our resilience, and a tribute to the transformative power of alkaline living.

The Art of Balance: Harmonizing Flavors and Nutrients

When it comes to crafting an alkaline lunch that's both delicious and nourishing, balance is key. Think of your plate as a canvas, where each ingredient contributes not just to the overall flavor profile but also to a balanced nutrient intake. The sweetness of a ripe tomato, the earthiness of quinoa, the zest of a lemon—all these elements come together in a harmonious blend that satisfies the palate and fuels the body. This is not just cooking; it's culinary alchemy, a transformative process that turns simple ingredients into nutrient-packed masterpieces.

One of the most enriching aspects of alkaline cooking is its alignment with the natural cycles of the Earth. Seasonal eating is not just a trend; it's a way to connect with the rhythms of nature, to celebrate the diversity of flavors that each season brings. Imagine the joy of biting into a sun-ripened peach in the summer or savoring a bowl of hearty squash soup in the fall. These are not just meals; they are sensory experiences that ground us in the present moment, reminding us of the beauty and abundance that surround us.

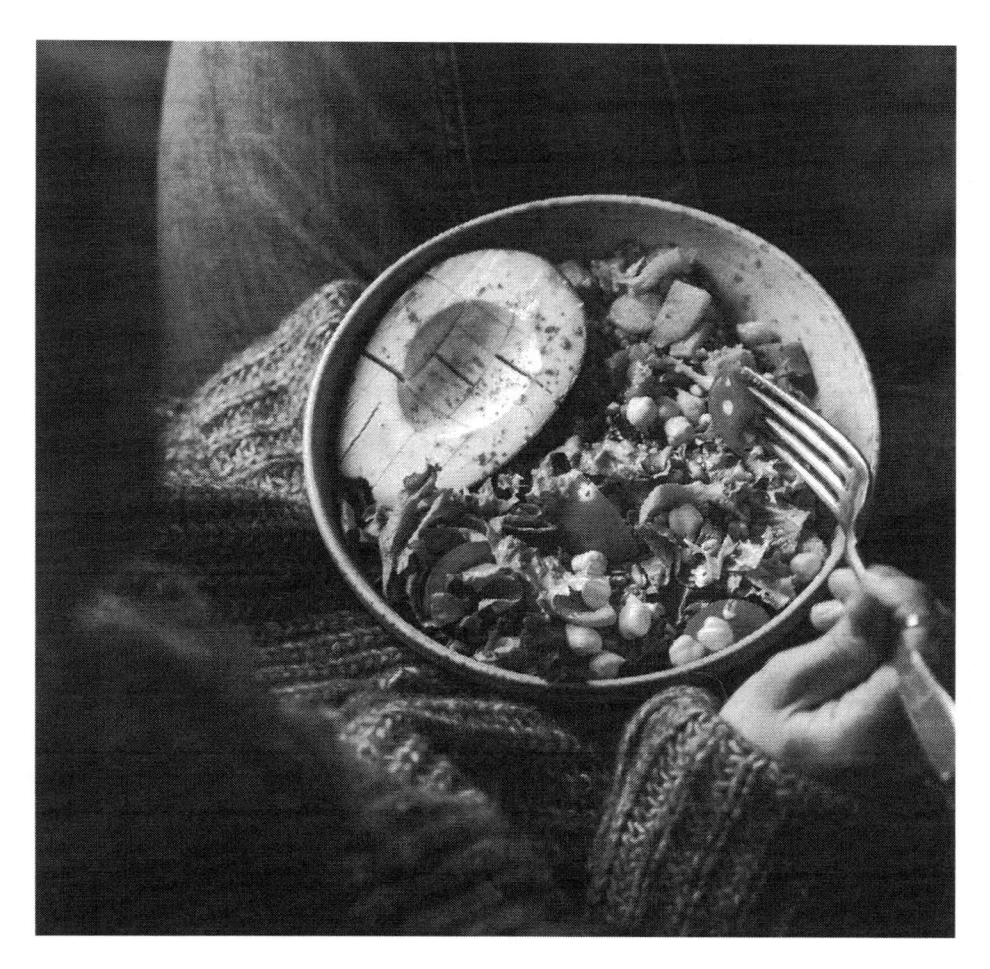

The Global Fusion: A Culinary Journey Across Cultures

Alkaline cooking is not confined to any particular cuisine; it's a global movement that transcends geographical and cultural boundaries. Whether it's a Mediterranean-inspired chickpea salad or an Asian-style stir-fry with alkaline-friendly vegetables, the possibilities are endless. This global fusion is not just about variety; it's about inclusivity, about embracing the culinary traditions of diverse communities and adapting them to fit an alkaline lifestyle. It's a celebration of our shared humanity, a testament to the universal appeal of wholesome, nourishing food.

In our fast-paced world, time is often the biggest obstacle to healthy eating. The good news is that an alkaline lunch can be as quick and easy or as slow and savory as you like. From 15-minute salads to slow-cooked stews, there's a wide range of options to suit your lifestyle and schedule. The key is planning and preparation. A well-stocked pantry and a weekly meal plan can go a long way in making your midday meals both convenient and nutritious.

When we talk about nutrient-packed lunches, we often focus on macronutrients like proteins, fats, and carbs, or micronutrients like vitamins and minerals. But an alkaline lunch offers something more—a unique combination of phytonutrients, enzymes, and antioxidants that work in synergy to promote optimal health. These bioactive compounds are the unsung heroes of alkaline cooking, the secret ingredients that elevate your meals from merely nutritious to truly transformative.

The Emotional Resonance: Food as Mood Enhancer

Let's not underestimate the emotional impact of a well-crafted alkaline lunch. Food is not just fuel; it's a mood enhancer, a comfort provider, and sometimes even a source of emotional healing. The act of eating can be a form of self-care, a way to nurture your emotional well-being in the midst of a hectic day. Whether it's the comforting warmth of a homemade soup or the invigorating freshness of a crisp salad, each meal has the potential to lift your spirits and brighten your mood.

An alkaline lunch is not just about personal health; it's also about the health of our planet. By choosing organic, locally-sourced ingredients, you're making a conscious choice to reduce your carbon footprint and support sustainable farming practices. It's a small but significant step towards a more ethical and responsible way of living, a way to align your dietary choices with your values and beliefs.

The Aesthetic Appeal: Presentation Matters

Finally, let's not forget the aesthetic aspect of a nutrient-packed alkaline lunch. The colors, the textures, the presentation—all these elements contribute to the overall dining experience. A beautifully arranged plate is not just visually pleasing; it's also more appetizing, which in turn enhances nutrient absorption and digestion. So take a few extra minutes to garnish your dish, to arrange your ingredients in a visually appealing manner. It's the final touch that completes your culinary masterpiece, the icing on the cake that makes your alkaline lunch truly unforgettable.

In the grand scheme of alkaline living, lunch is not just a meal; it's an experience, a daily ritual that nourishes your body, enriches your soul, and elevates your consciousness. It's a multi-dimensional feast that engages all your senses, a culinary journey that takes you from the familiar to the exotic, from the simple to the sublime. So, let's savor this journey, one bite at a time, as we delve deeper into the art and science of nutrient-packed midday meals.

The Lasting Impact of Nutrient-Packed Midday Meals

As we draw the curtain on our exploration of nutrient-packed midday meals, it's essential to recognize that the impact of these lunches extends far beyond the plate. Each bite you take is not just a momentary indulgence but a long-term investment in your well-being. The nutrients you absorb, the flavors you savor, and the textures you experience are all part of a larger narrative—a narrative that shapes your relationship with food, your body, and ultimately, your life.

The foods you consume at lunchtime don't just fuel your body; they also nourish your mind. The alkaline ingredients, rich in essential nutrients, play a vital role in cognitive function. They help to sharpen your focus, elevate your mood, and enhance your mental clarity. This is particularly crucial in the middle of a busy day when your energy levels are waning, and your mind is cluttered with the chaos of life's demands. A nutrient-packed lunch acts as a reset button, aligning your mind and body in a state of harmonious coexistence.

In many cultures, lunch is more than just a meal; it's a social event, a time for family, friends, and colleagues to come together in a shared experience of nourishment and connection. The act of sharing a meal can strengthen bonds, foster a sense of community, and create lasting memories. In this context, a nutrient-packed alkaline lunch becomes a catalyst for meaningful interactions, a way to enrich not just your own life but also the lives of those around you.

In our fast-paced society, meals are often rushed, consumed in a state of distraction or stress. But a nutrient-packed lunch invites you to slow down, to practice the art of mindful eating. It encourages you to savor each bite, to appreciate the complexity of flavors and the richness of textures. This is not just about enhancing your culinary experience; it's about cultivating a mindset of mindfulness that permeates all aspects of your life—from your eating habits to your emotional well-being.

The choices you make at lunchtime have a cumulative effect on your long-term health. Consistently opting for nutrient-packed meals can help to prevent chronic diseases, boost your immune system, and enhance your metabolic function. It's a proactive approach to healthcare, a way to take control of your destiny rather than leaving it to chance or circumstance. And the benefits are not just physical;

they're also psychological, contributing to a sense of empowerment and self-efficacy that can transform your outlook on life.

The Environmental Footprint: A Conscious Consumer

Your lunch choices also have an ecological impact. By opting for organic, locally-sourced ingredients, you're contributing to a more sustainable food system, one that respects the integrity of the Earth and its natural resources. It's a form of environmental stewardship, a way to align your personal values with your actions, to be a conscious consumer in a world of mindless consumption.

There's an undeniable joy in crafting a beautiful, nutrient-packed lunch—a sense of accomplishment, a burst of creative energy. It's a form of self-expression, a way to channel your creativity into something tangible and nourishing. And the rewards are immediate, both in the pleasure of the eating experience and the long-term benefits to your health.

As we conclude this section, let's remember that the journey towards nutrient-packed midday meals is not a destination but a continuous process—a lifelong commitment to your health, your happiness, and your holistic well-being. It's a journey that invites you to explore, to experiment, and to evolve, to be an active participant in the grand adventure of life.

So, as you close this book and step back into the hustle and bustle of your daily routine, take a moment to reflect on the profound impact that a simple lunch can have on your life. Let it be a source of inspiration, a touchstone for mindful living, and a catalyst for positive change. And may each bite you take be a step towards a healthier, happier, and more harmonious existence.

Dinner: Hearty Alkaline Delights
The evening's prelude: The meaning of dinner

As the sun dips below the horizon, casting its golden farewell in the sky, the atmosphere changes palpably. The hustle and bustle of the day is winding down, and the evening heralds itself with the promise of rest and rejuvenation. It is at this time of transition that dinner takes center stage: a meal that has the power to elevate or diminish the quality of the night ahead. In the context of an alkaline lifestyle, dinner becomes more than just a meal: it is a celebration of life, a nourishing ritual that aligns body, mind and soul.

Imagine a plate filled with vibrant colors: deep greens, radiant reds, and sun-kissed yellows. These are not just shades, but visual representations of the nutrients that make up an alkaline, hearty dinner. The ingredients chosen are the building blocks of this meal, each providing a unique blend of vitamins, minerals and antioxidants. From leafy green vegetables to protein-rich legumes, the components of an alkaline dinner are carefully curated to provide a balanced spectrum of nutrients designed to nourish you from the inside out.

Creating a hearty alkaline dinner is like composing a symphony. Each element, whether a spice, herb, or vegetable, plays its part in a larger whole, contributing its unique note to the overall melody. The interplay of flavors and textures is a rhythmic dance that tantalizes the palate, making each bite an experience to savor. The crispness of a freshly picked vegetable, the smoothness of a well-crafted sauce, the flavor explosion of a sprinkling of herbs-these are the nuances that turn a meal into a culinary masterpiece.

Connecting the soul: Dinner as a time for reflection and connection

In the rush of modern life, dinner often becomes a hurried affair, consumed in front of a screen or on the go. But a hearty alkaline dinner invites one to pause, sit at the table and participate in the ancient ritual of breaking bread. It is a time for reflection, sharing the day's experiences and connecting with loved ones. This meal becomes a sacred space, a momentary refuge from the chaos of the world, where to nourish not only the body but also the soul.

The benefits of a hearty alkaline dinner go far beyond immediate sensory pleasure. This meal serves as the day's nutritional encore, providing the essential nutrients that support cellular repair, immune function, and metabolic balance during sleep. It is the final act of the day's nutritional performance, setting the stage for a restful night's rest and preparing the body to face the challenges of the next day.

The act of eating a hearty alkaline dinner becomes a form of culinary mindfulness, a practice that encourages you to be fully present in the experience. From the aroma wafting through the air during meal preparation to the sensation of the first bite on the tongue, every moment is an opportunity to engage the senses and immerse yourself in the joy of nourishment.

The beauty of a hearty alkaline dinner lies in its versatility. Whether you crave the spiciness of a Mexican chili or the comforting warmth of an Italian stew, the principles of alkaline cooking can be adapted to a wide range of culinary traditions. It is a global palette that invites you to explore the world through your taste buds while remaining true to the principles of alkaline living.

As we embark on this exploration of hearty alkaline dinners, remember that this is only the opening act of a lifelong journey of culinary discovery. Each meal is an opportunity to experiment, learn and grow, to deepen our understanding of the intricate relationship between food and wellness. So as you flip through the pages of this chapter, let your imagination run wild, your taste buds dance, and your soul be nourished by the transformative power of a rich alkaline dinner. Each meal is a celebration of life, a testament to the healing power of food and a stepping stone on the path to holistic wellness.

Crafting Your Hearty Alkaline Dinner

As you stand in your kitchen, the evening's blank canvas awaits your culinary artistry. The ingredients are your colors, the utensils your brushes, and the plate your frame. But unlike a traditional artist, your masterpiece is not just to be admired; it's to be devoured, to nourish, to heal. In the realm of alkaline cooking, the dinner hour is where you can truly let your creativity shine. It's where you can experiment with flavors, textures, and ingredients that not only please the palate but also fuel the body in the most holistic way possible.

In the world of alkaline cuisine, the concept of a "hearty" dinner transcends the mere filling of the stomach. It's about creating a harmonious blend of nutrients that serve multiple functions—energizing the body, aiding digestion, promoting cellular repair, and preparing the system for a night of restful sleep. It's a symphony where each nutrient plays its part, contributing to the overall well-being of the individual. For instance, incorporating leafy greens like kale and spinach provides a rich source of magnesium, which not only aids in digestion but also acts as a natural relaxant, setting the stage for a peaceful night.

Spices are the unsung heroes of alkaline cooking. They do more than just add flavor; they elevate the entire dining experience. Take turmeric, for example. This golden-hued spice is not only a staple in alkaline cooking but also a powerful anti-inflammatory agent. When incorporated into a hearty dinner, it serves a dual purpose—enhancing taste while promoting health. Similarly, herbs like basil and oregano not only add a burst of flavor but also contain potent antioxidants that combat oxidative stress, making your dinner not just a meal but a medicinal experience.

The Ritual of Cooking: A Mindful Practice

The act of preparing a hearty alkaline dinner is not just about the end result; it's about the journey. It's a meditative practice that invites you to be fully present, to engage with each ingredient as if it were a sacred object, to treat each step of the cooking process as a ritual of self-care. As you chop, sauté, and simmer, you're not just cooking; you're crafting a nourishing experience for both body and soul. It's an opportunity to disconnect from the digital world and connect with the tactile, sensory experience of creating something from scratch.

Dinner, especially a hearty alkaline one, is best enjoyed in the company of loved ones. It's a communal experience that goes beyond the mere act of eating. It's about sharing stories, creating memories, and building bonds. It's a time to put away the screens and engage in meaningful conversations, to laugh, to debate, to celebrate the simple joy of being together. And what better way to do this than over a meal that not only satisfies the taste buds but also nourishes the body and soul?

The Versatility Factor: Adapting to Individual Needs

One of the most beautiful aspects of alkaline cooking is its versatility. Whether you're a busy professional looking for a quick yet nutritious meal, a parent trying to please picky eaters, or someone managing specific health issues, a hearty alkaline dinner can be adapted to meet individual needs without compromising on taste or nutritional value. From one-pot wonders to elaborate multi-course meals, the possibilities are endless.

As you delve deeper into the world of alkaline cooking, you'll find that it's not just about personal health; it's also about the health of the planet. Opting for organic, locally-sourced ingredients is not just a lifestyle choice but an ethical stance. It's a commitment to sustainability, to reducing your carbon footprint, and to supporting local farmers and communities. Every choice you make, from the vegetables you pick to the spices you use, has a ripple effect, making your hearty alkaline dinner an act of conscious living.

The Culmination: A Symphony of Sensory Delights

As you sit down to enjoy your hearty alkaline dinner, take a moment to savor the experience. Smell the aroma, admire the colors, taste the flavors, and feel the textures. Let it be a sensory symphony that not only pleases the palate but also nourishes the soul. Let it be a testament to the transformative power of mindful eating, of conscious living, and of the endless possibilities that await you in this journey toward holistic well-being.

In this central part of our exploration, we've delved into the multifaceted experience that is a hearty alkaline dinner. It's a meal that serves as a mirror, reflecting your values, your creativity, and your commitment to a life well-lived. So, as you continue on this culinary adventure, let each dinner be a stepping stone, a learning experience, and most importantly, a hearty celebration of the beautiful complexity that is life.

Desserts: Guilt-Free Alkaline Treats

The Last Bite: Savoring the Essence of Hearty Alkaline Delights

As you take the last bite of your hearty alkaline dinner, a sense of satisfaction washes over you. It's not just the physical fullness you feel; it's a deeper, more profound sense of fulfillment. You've not only nourished your body but also fed your soul. This is the moment to pause and reflect, to savor the afterglow of a meal that was so much more than a mere assembly of ingredients. It was a culinary journey, a narrative woven through flavors, textures, and aromas, each element carefully chosen to contribute to your holistic well-being.

As you lean back in your chair, your body begins the intricate process of digestion. It's a symphony of enzymes, acids, and gut flora working in harmony to extract the nutrients from the food you've consumed. But because you've chosen an alkaline meal, this process is smoother, more efficient. The alkaline nature of the ingredient's aids in quicker digestion, reducing the chances of bloating or discomfort. It's as if your body is thanking you, acknowledging the care you've taken in selecting foods that are not just delicious but also deeply nourishing.

The Evening Ritual: Completing the Circle

The act of cleaning up after dinner is often seen as a chore, but in the context of a hearty alkaline meal, it becomes part of the ritual. As you wash the dishes, store the leftovers, and wipe down the counters, you're completing the circle. You're putting to rest the culinary adventure you embarked upon, making space—both physical and metaphorical—for new experiences. It's a moment to appreciate the transient nature of life, the ebb and flow of moments that make up our days.

The benefits of a hearty alkaline dinner extend beyond the dinner table. As you transition into the evening, you'll find that the choices you made during the meal prep have a direct impact on the quality of your sleep. The magnesium-rich leafy greens, the anti-inflammatory spices, and the balanced combination of proteins and healthy fats all contribute to a state of relaxation, setting the stage for a night of restorative sleep. It's holistic health in action, a testament to the interconnectedness of diet, lifestyle, and well-being.

The Emotional Resonance: Food as Love Language

For many, food is a love language, a way to express care, affection, and even creativity. When you invest time and effort into preparing a hearty alkaline dinner, you're sending a message—not just to yourself but also to those you share the meal with. You're saying, "I care about you. I value your health. I honor your presence in my life." It's a message that resonates on an emotional level, strengthening bonds and deepening relationships.

No culinary adventure is without its learning curves, and the world of alkaline cooking is no exception. Perhaps the quinoa was a tad overcooked, or the seasoning not quite right. These are not failures; they're stepping stones, opportunities to refine your skills, to experiment, to grow. Each meal is a chapter in your ongoing journey toward holistic health, a journey that is as much about the process as it is about the destination.

Your choice to embrace alkaline cooking has a ripple effect that goes beyond your personal health. It's a statement, a declaration of your commitment to a more sustainable, ethical way of living. It's a vote for local farmers, for organic produce, for ethical sourcing. It's a contribution, however small, to a larger movement that seeks to harmonize human health with planetary well-being.

The Final Note: A Symphony's End, A New Beginning

As the evening winds down, take a moment to appreciate the full scope of what you've accomplished. You've not just prepared a meal; you've orchestrated an experience that nourished body, mind, and soul. And as you lay your head down for the night, know that this is not the end but a new beginning. Tomorrow offers another opportunity to explore, to create, to nourish. But for now, rest easy, knowing that you've done your part in crafting a life that is not just lived but savored, one hearty alkaline dinner at a time.

In closing, the essence of a hearty alkaline dinner lies not just in the food on the plate but in the experience, it offers—a holistic journey that nourishes the body, enriches the soul, and contributes to a more sustainable, ethical way of living. It's a celebration of life's simple joys and complex flavors, a testament to the transformative power of mindful eating.

The Sweet Spot: The Art and Science of Guilt-Free Alkaline Treats

When it comes to desserts, the word "guilt-free" often seems like an oxymoron. But in the realm of alkaline gourmet, it's a reality. Imagine a canvas of flavors where every brushstroke is deliberate, every hue a calculated choice. Crafting the perfect alkaline dessert is akin to alchemy, a blend of science and artistry. It's about understanding the chemistry of ingredients, how coconut oil melds with cacao, how the tartness of berries can be balanced by the natural sweetness of agave nectar. It's a culinary dance, each step choreographed to create a harmonious finale.

The Emotional Connection: Desserts as Soul Food

Let's face it; desserts are often tied to our emotions. They're the comfort we seek after a long day, the joy we share at celebrations, the love we offer to friends and family. But traditional desserts, laden with sugar and unhealthy fats, often leave us with a sense of guilt. Alkaline desserts change this narrative. They allow us to indulge without compromising our health, to savor flavors without the accompanying emotional baggage. It's like having your cake and eating it too, quite literally.

In mainstream desserts, the focus is often on taste, with little regard for nutritional value. Alkaline desserts flip this script. Each ingredient is a powerhouse of nutrients, carefully selected not just for its flavor but also for its health benefits. Take, for instance, the humble chia seed, often used as a binding agent in alkaline desserts. It's a source of Omega-3 fatty acids, fiber, and antioxidants. Or consider cacao, the unprocessed form of cocoa, rich in flavonoids and essential minerals. In alkaline desserts, every bite is a step toward better health.

Eating an alkaline dessert is not just a gustatory experience; it's a feast for all the senses. The vibrant colors of fruit-based desserts catch your eye, the aroma of spices like cinnamon and nutmeg fill the air, the texture of nut-based crusts add a tactile dimension, and the symphony of flavors dance on your palate. It's a multi-sensory experience designed to delight and satisfy, to make each moment of indulgence a memorable one.

The Versatility: A Dessert for Every Occasion

One of the most remarkable aspects of alkaline desserts is their versatility. Whether it's a casual weekday dinner or a grand holiday feast, there's an alkaline dessert that fits the bill. From simple fruit salads drizzled with alkaline-friendly sweeteners to elaborate raw cakes adorned with edible flowers, the options are endless. It's a testament to the creativity and innovation that alkaline cooking brings to the table, challenging the conventional wisdom that healthy eating is boring or restrictive.

In our fast-paced lives, eating often becomes a mindless activity, done in a rush or while multitasking. Alkaline desserts invite us to slow down, to savor each bite, to be present in the moment. It's an exercise in mindfulness, a chance to connect with our food and, by extension, with ourselves. As you take that bite of a coconut-cacao truffle or a slice of avocado-lime pie, you're not just eating; you're engaging in a form of self-care, a momentary pause in the hustle and bustle of life.

Alkaline desserts are not confined to any one cuisine or culture. They draw inspiration from culinary traditions around the world, from the tropical flavors of the Caribbean to the exotic spices of the East. It's a global tapestry of tastes, a culinary journey that transcends geographical boundaries. It's also an opportunity to explore new ingredients, to expand your culinary repertoire, and to embrace the diversity that our world has to offer.

In a world grappling with issues like climate change and ethical consumerism, our food choices matter. Alkaline desserts offer an ethical alternative, a way to indulge without contributing to environmental degradation. By opting for organic, locally-sourced ingredients, you're making a statement, casting a vote for a more sustainable, ethical way of life.

In essence, alkaline desserts are not just a category of recipes; they're a philosophy, a holistic approach to indulgence that aligns with the principles of health, sustainability, and ethical living. They challenge the status quo, offering a new paradigm for what desserts can and should be. It's a culinary revolution, one that invites you to partake not just with your taste buds but with your heart and soul. So, as you explore the world of guilt-free alkaline treats, remember that each dessert is more than just a sweet ending; it's a celebration of life's complexities, a tribute to the beauty of mindful living.

The Final Word: A Sweet Farewell

As we reach the end of this exploration into the world of guilt-free alkaline desserts, it's essential to reflect on the lasting impact these culinary creations can have on our lives. Unlike traditional desserts that offer fleeting pleasure followed by lingering guilt, alkaline desserts provide a sense of satisfaction that endures. They nourish not just the body but also the soul, serving as a testament to the transformative power of mindful eating.

The beauty of alkaline desserts lies not just in their flavors but also in their ability to change perceptions. They challenge the deeply ingrained notion that desserts are a guilty pleasure, a forbidden indulgence. By offering a healthier alternative, they empower us to make better choices, to redefine our relationship with food. And this change doesn't just stop at the individual level; it has a ripple effect, influencing family, friends, and even the broader community. It's a culinary revolution, one that starts in the kitchen but extends far beyond it.

One of the most remarkable achievements of alkaline desserts is their ability to harmonize taste and health, to create a balance that has long eluded mainstream desserts. It's a delicate equilibrium, achieved through meticulous ingredient selection, precise measurements, and expert techniques. It's the art of creating flavors that tantalize the palate while nourishing the body, of crafting desserts that are as pleasing to the eye as they are beneficial to the soul. It's a balance that elevates alkaline desserts from mere food items to culinary masterpieces.

While we've made significant strides in the world of alkaline desserts, the journey is far from over. There's still much to explore, from exotic ingredients to innovative cooking techniques. The field is ripe for experimentation, inviting culinary enthusiasts and health-conscious individuals alike to venture into uncharted territory. It's an exciting time to be part of this movement, to contribute to the growing body of knowledge, and to witness the evolution of alkaline desserts as they transition from niche delicacies to mainstream staples.

As we indulge in these guilt-free treats, it's important to recognize that we're also partaking in a legacy, a tradition that has its roots in ancient wisdom and modern science. It's a legacy that we have the privilege and the responsibility to pass down to future generations, to ensure that the principles of alkaline living continue to thrive. By sharing these recipes, by teaching our children the value of mindful eating, we're laying the foundation for a healthier, happier future.

As you close this chapter and perhaps even venture into your kitchen to try out some of these recipes, remember that you're not just a passive reader but an active participant in this alkaline revolution. Each time you choose an alkaline dessert over a sugar-laden treat, each time you share these recipes with loved ones, you're making a statement, taking a stand for a healthier way of life. It's a call to action, an invitation to be part of something bigger than yourself, to contribute to a movement that has the potential to change lives.

In conclusion, guilt-free alkaline desserts are not just a culinary trend; they're a lifestyle choice, a conscious decision to prioritize health without sacrificing pleasure. They offer a new way to experience desserts, one that aligns with the principles of holistic well-being. From the alchemy of flavors to the emotional connection, from the nutritional benefits to the sensory experience, every aspect of alkaline desserts is designed to enrich your life. So, as you take that final bite, savor not just the flavors but also the journey you've embarked on, a journey towards a more mindful, fulfilling, and healthful life.

Book 8: Liquid Nutrition – Beyond Water

The Science Behind Alkaline Water

The Elemental Elixir: Unveiling the Science Behind Alkaline Water

Water, the most basic element of life, has been with us since the dawn of time. It's the cornerstone of our existence, the medium in which life began, and the sustenance that has nurtured civilizations. But what if I told you that the water you know—the water you've been drinking all your life—could be transformed into something even more beneficial? Welcome to the world of alkaline water, a subject that has captivated scientists, health enthusiasts, and skeptics alike.

The term "pH" might evoke memories of high school chemistry, but its implications for your health are far-reaching. The pH scale measures how acidic or alkaline a substance is, ranging from 0 to 14. Neutral water has a pH of 7, but alkaline water typically has a pH of 8 or 9. This might seem like a minor difference, but it's this shift in pH that turns regular water into a liquid asset for your health.

One of the most fascinating aspects of alkaline water is its molecular structure. Unlike regular water, alkaline water contains smaller molecular clusters. These clusters are easier for your cells to absorb, making hydration more efficient. Imagine your cells as parched wanderers in a desert, and alkaline water as a more accessible oasis. The easier it is to drink from the oasis, the quicker the wanderers can continue on their journey, revitalized and renewed.

Alkaline water is not just about pH; it's also about minerals. Essential minerals like calcium, potassium, and magnesium are often found in higher concentrations in alkaline water. These minerals don't just add flavor; they play a vital role in your body's physiological processes. They're the conductors in the symphony of your body's functions, ensuring that each cellular instrument plays its part in harmony.

You've probably heard about antioxidants, those miraculous molecules that fight off the damaging effects of free radicals in your body. Alkaline water has a negative oxidation-reduction potential (ORP), making it a natural antioxidant. In the paradoxical world of antioxidants, a negative ORP is actually a positive attribute. It means the water has the ability to neutralize harmful free radicals, acting as a sort of molecular bouncer for your cells.

The Detoxification Phenomenon: A River of Renewal

Our bodies are constantly bombarded by toxins, from the air we breathe to the food we eat. Alkaline water acts as a river of renewal, flushing out these toxins and cleansing our system. It's like a spring cleaning for your insides, a detoxification process that leaves you feeling rejuvenated and revitalized.

It's natural to be skeptical about something that promises so many benefits. After all, we live in an age where misinformation is rampant, and "miracle cures" are a dime a dozen. But the science behind alkaline water is backed by numerous studies, peer-reviewed papers, and testimonials from those who've experienced its benefits firsthand. It's not a magic potion, but a scientifically supported advancement in hydration technology.

As we delve deeper into the science of alkaline water, it's crucial to consider its accessibility and sustainability. While alkaline water is becoming more widely available, it's essential to ensure that it's produced and distributed in an ethical, sustainable manner. The goal is not just better hydration for the individual but a healthier planet for all.

As we embark on this journey to explore the science behind alkaline water, I invite you to keep an open mind. We'll delve into the chemistry, the biology, and even the controversy, all while keeping our focus on what matters most: your health and well-being. So pour yourself a glass of alkaline water, and let's dive into a subject that's as refreshing as it is enlightening.

In this chapter, we'll explore the science behind this elemental elixir, breaking down complex concepts into digestible insights. We'll sift through the research, separate fact from fiction, and emerge with a clearer understanding of why alkaline water is more than just a trend—it's a transformative force in the realm of health and wellness.

The Alkaline Equation: A Deep Dive into the Science

When alkaline water enters your system, it's like a guest arriving at a party—eager to mingle, ready to make connections. But this isn't just any party; it's a biochemical ballet, and alkaline water is the prima ballerina. As it courses through your veins, it interacts with enzymes, proteins, and cellular machinery, subtly altering the biochemistry in ways that are profoundly beneficial. It's not just hydration; it's a physiological transformation.

Your body is constantly striving to maintain a delicate balance between acidity and alkalinity, known as the acid-base balance. This balance is crucial for normal cellular function. When you consume alkaline water, you're essentially giving your body a helping hand in maintaining this balance. It's like a tightrope walker using a balancing pole; the added stability makes the performance not just possible but graceful.

We often think of hydration in simple terms: water in, thirst out. But hydration is a complex process involving osmosis, ion channels, and cellular pumps. Alkaline water, with its smaller molecular clusters, revolutionizes this process. It hydrates not just faster but smarter, targeting cells that are most in need of hydration and supercharging the entire system.

Emerging research has shown that the gut is like a second brain, influencing everything from mood to cognitive function. Alkaline water, rich in beneficial minerals and negative ions, fosters a healthier gut environment. This, in turn, sends positive signals to the brain, creating a harmonious dialogue between the gut and the mind. It's a conversation that leads to better mental clarity, enhanced focus, and a sense of well-being.

The Inflammation Equation: Cooling the Fires Within

Inflammation is the body's natural response to injury or infection, but chronic inflammation can be a silent killer. Alkaline water, with its antioxidant properties, helps to neutralize the free radicals that contribute to inflammation. It's like a firefighter dousing the flames, bringing relief to inflamed tissues and organs.

Metabolism is the sum total of all the chemical reactions in your body, and it's influenced by a myriad of factors, including hydration. Alkaline water, by virtue of its superior hydrating capabilities, gives your metabolism a subtle but significant boost. It's like adding high-octane fuel to a car; the performance improves, the engine runs smoother, and you get more mileage out of every drop.

At the cellular level, alkaline water is a maestro, orchestrating a symphony of biological processes. It enhances nutrient absorption, optimizes energy production, and facilitates waste removal. Each cell becomes a finely-tuned instrument, playing its part in the grand orchestra of your body. The result is a feeling of vitality, an effervescence that permeates every aspect of your life.

The Skeptic's Reckoning: Empirical Evidence and Clinical Trials

For those who demand empirical evidence, rest assured that the benefits of alkaline water are not just anecdotal. Numerous clinical trials and scientific studies have corroborated its health benefits, from improved hydration to reduced markers of oxidative stress. It's a body of evidence that's growing by the day, converting skeptics into believers, one glass at a time.

While the existing research is promising, there's an ethical imperative for more rigorous, large-scale studies. The potential of alkaline water to improve public health is too significant to ignore. It's a call to action for scientists, healthcare providers, and policy-makers to invest in research that could transform lives on a global scale.

The Personal Paradigm Shift: Your Health, Your Choice

Ultimately, the science behind alkaline water invites you to make a personal paradigm shift. It challenges you to rethink your hydration habits, to elevate your health choices, and to experience the transformative power of intelligent hydration. It's not just a sip; it's a leap—a leap into a future where wellness flows as naturally as water itself.

In this central part of our exploration, we've delved into the intricate science that makes alkaline water a transformative force in health and wellness. We've navigated the biochemical, physiological, and even psychological terrains that this unique form of hydration impacts. As we continue this journey, let's carry with us the understanding that science is not just about data and experiments; it's about enriching lives, one drop at a time.

The Transformative Power of Alkaline Water

As we reach the conclusion of this deep dive into the science behind alkaline water, it's essential to recognize that this isn't just about quenching thirst or even just about hydration. It's about a personal revolution—a new way of living that's grounded in scientific understanding but elevated by human experience. It's about making choices that not only serve your body but also nourish your soul.

The transformative power of alkaline water doesn't stop at the individual level. Its impact ripples out, affecting families, communities, and even societies at large. Imagine a world where people are not just surviving but thriving, where healthcare costs are reduced because preventative measures are taken seriously. Alkaline water, with its myriad health benefits, could be a cornerstone in building this new reality.

In a world where access to clean water is still a challenge for many, the conversation around alkaline water takes on an ethical dimension. Health is a human right, and as we discuss the benefits of alkaline water, we must also consider how to make it accessible to all. It's not just a question of science or even of personal health; it's a matter of social justice.

As we embrace the health benefits of alkaline water, we must also consider the environmental impact. How can we ensure that the production and consumption of alkaline water are sustainable? From eco-friendly packaging to responsible sourcing, every choice we make has a ripple effect on the planet. It's a holistic approach that considers not just individual well-being but the health of the Earth.

Any revolutionary idea faces its share of skepticism, and alkaline water is no exception. However, as the scientific evidence mounts and as more people experience its benefits firsthand, a cultural shift is happening. What was once viewed with skepticism is now being embraced as a legitimate and valuable health resource. It's a shift from doubt to acceptance, from questioning to experiencing.

The Medical Community: A Call for Collaboration

The potential of alkaline water to improve public health is too significant to ignore. It's a call to action for the medical community to collaborate with researchers, holistic health practitioners, and even patients themselves. By working together, we can create a body of evidence that stands up to scrutiny and that guides people in making informed health choices.

While our focus has been on the science behind alkaline water, it's worth noting that many people experience what they describe as a spiritual benefit. They speak of a sense of harmony and balance that goes beyond the physical. While this may not be quantifiable in scientific terms, it's an essential part of the human experience and deserves acknowledgment.

The Final Toast: To Your Health and Well-Being

As we wrap up this exploration, let's raise a glass—a glass of alkaline water, of course—to your health and well-being. May you be inspired to delve deeper, to question freely, and to experience fully. May you find in alkaline water not just a means of hydration but a catalyst for transformation.

This is not the end but merely a milestone on your journey toward optimal health and well-being. Consider this an invitation to continue exploring, questioning, and experiencing. The science behind alkaline water offers a foundation, but your personal experience will build the house—a house of health, happiness, and holistic well-being.

In closing, let's ponder the legacy we wish to leave. A world where science and experience harmonize, where health is not a privilege but a right, and where each choice we make contributes to a healthier, happier world. Alkaline water, with its scientific backing and transformative potential, is more than a trend; it's a testament to what's possible when we marry science with the human spirit.

In this final section, we've journeyed from the personal to the global, touching on the ethical, environmental, and even spiritual dimensions of alkaline water. We've considered its potential to transform not just individual lives but the very fabric of our society. And as we take this last sip, let's carry with us the profound understanding that the science behind alkaline water is not just about molecules and pH levels; it's about the alchemy of turning knowledge into action, science into experience, and experience into a life well-lived. Cheers to that.

Crafting Nutrient-Packed Smoothies

The Smoothie Revolution: More Than a Trend

Welcome to the world of nutrient-packed smoothies, a universe where the blender is your canvas, fruits and vegetables are your palette, and your body is the ultimate beneficiary. This is not just about mixing some fruits and veggies; it's about crafting a liquid symphony that nourishes your body, delights your taste buds, and elevates your spirit.

Smoothies have become a cultural phenomenon, but let's be clear: this is not a fad. This is a revolution in how we approach nutrition, wellness, and even the art of eating. It's a shift from processed foods laden with artificial ingredients to whole, natural foods that come from the Earth. It's about reclaiming our health without sacrificing pleasure or convenience.

When we talk about crafting nutrient-packed smoothies, we're talking about a holistic approach to nutrition. It's not just about protein, carbs, and fats; it's about vitamins, minerals, antioxidants, and phytonutrients. It's about understanding the synergistic relationships between different ingredients and how they can enhance each other's nutritional value. For example, pairing vitamin C-rich fruits with iron-rich greens can enhance iron absorption, turning your smoothie into a nutritional powerhouse.

One of the most beautiful aspects of smoothies is the ability to tailor them to your specific needs. Whether you're an athlete looking for a post-workout recovery drink, a busy parent seeking a quick but nutritious breakfast, or someone dealing with specific health issues like inflammation or digestive problems, there's a smoothie recipe for you. It's personalized nutrition at its finest.

Crafting nutrient-packed smoothies is also a culinary adventure. It's an opportunity to experiment with flavors, textures, and colors. It's a chance to discover new ingredients, like exotic fruits, superfood powders, or even edible flowers. And let's not forget the visual appeal—a beautifully crafted smoothie can be a feast for the eyes, making the experience even more enjoyable.

Let's not underestimate the psychological benefits of this smoothie journey. The act of selecting fresh ingredients, blending them into a delicious concoction, and savoring the result is a form of self-care. It's a moment to pause, to nourish yourself, and to celebrate the simple joys of life. It's mindfulness in a glass.

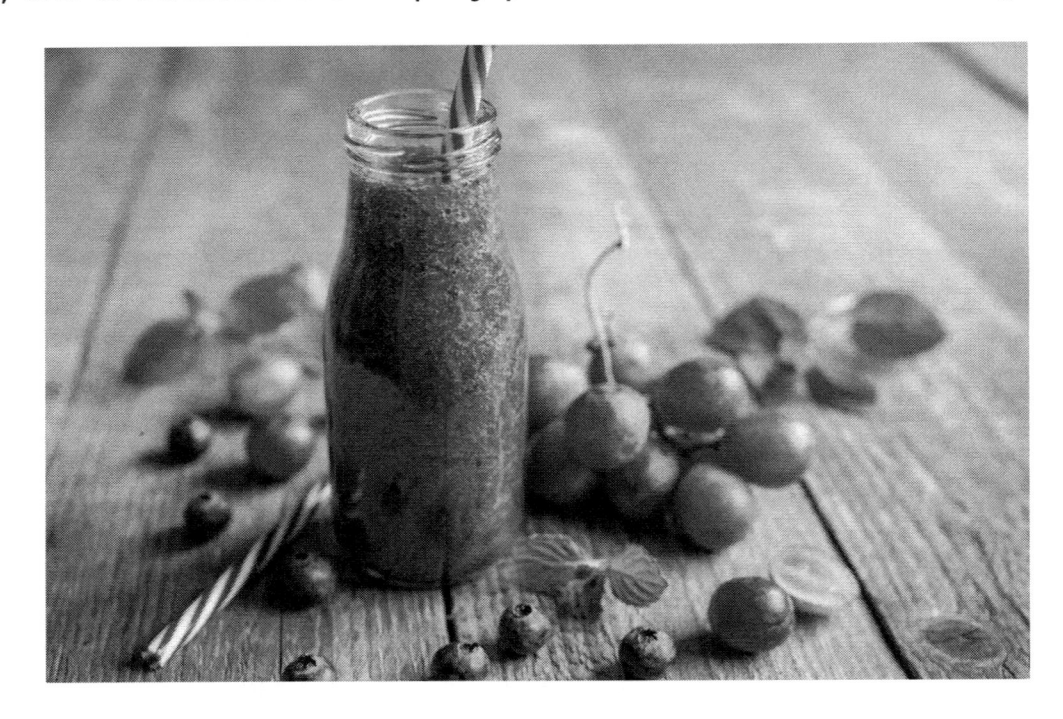

In our fast-paced world, one of the biggest challenges is finding the time to eat healthily. Smoothies offer a convenient solution without compromising on nutrition. A well-crafted smoothie can be a complete meal, providing all the essential nutrients your body needs. And the best part? You can take it with you wherever you go.

The Sustainability Angle: Good for You, Good for the Planet

As we embrace the health benefits of smoothies, let's also consider the environmental impact. By choosing organic, locally-sourced ingredients, we're not just nourishing ourselves but also supporting sustainable farming practices. It's a win-win situation for both our health and the planet.

Smoothies are not just a solitary pleasure; they're also a way to connect with others. Whether it's sharing a recipe, enjoying a smoothie with a loved one, or even hosting a smoothie party, it's an experience that brings people together. It's a celebration of health, taste, and community.

As we embark on this journey of crafting nutrient-packed smoothies, let's take a moment to savor the possibilities. Imagine the burst of flavors, the rainbow of colors, and the surge of vitality you'll feel with each sip. This is not just a drink; it's a lifestyle choice, a statement of intent, and a step towards a healthier, happier you.

In this initial exploration, we've touched upon the multifaceted dimensions of smoothies—from their nutritional prowess to their role in personal and planetary well-being. As we delve deeper into the specifics, let's carry with us this holistic perspective. After all, a smoothie is more than the sum of its ingredients; it's a microcosm of our approach to life and health. So, grab your blender, unleash your creativity, and let's craft some liquid magic. Cheers to a nourishing journey ahead!

The Nutritional Choreography: The Dance of Macronutrients and Micronutrients

Crafting a nutrient-packed smoothie is akin to composing a symphony. Each ingredient plays a specific role, contributing to the overall harmony of flavors and nutrients. The sweetness of a ripe banana, the tartness of fresh berries, the earthiness of spinach, and the zing of ginger—when blended together, these elements create a balanced, satisfying experience that goes beyond mere sustenance. It's a culinary masterpiece that speaks to your senses while nourishing your body.

In the realm of smoothies, the interplay between macronutrients—proteins, fats, and carbohydrates—and micronutrients—vitamins and minerals—is a dance that requires finesse. It's not just about throwing in a handful of kale or a scoop of protein powder; it's about understanding how these elements work together to fuel your body. For instance, the healthy fats in avocado can help your body absorb the fat-soluble vitamins in leafy greens, making your smoothie not just delicious but also more effective as a nutritional source.

Texture plays a crucial but often overlooked role in the enjoyment of smoothies. The creaminess of yogurt, the smoothness of almond milk, or the crunch of chia seeds can transform your smoothie from a mere drink to an indulgent treat. It's this tactile experience that makes each sip a moment to savor, elevating your smoothie from a quick meal replacement to a culinary event.

The seasons offer a rotating palette of flavors and nutrients, and embracing this natural cycle can add a layer of richness to your smoothie-crafting journey. Imagine the sweetness of summer peaches, the tartness of autumn apples, or the earthy goodness of winter root vegetables. Each season brings its own set of nutrient-dense ingredients that not only taste better but are also more in tune with your body's seasonal needs.

Smoothies can be more than just a meal; they can be a form of medicine. Ingredients like turmeric, known for its anti-inflammatory properties, or spirulina, rich in antioxidants, can turn your smoothie into a healing elixir. It's not about replacing medical treatment but enhancing your body's natural ability to heal and thrive. This is where the wisdom of ancient herbal remedies meets the convenience of modern nutrition.

While a smoothie may seem like a simple concoction, the art lies in the layering of flavors, textures, and nutrients. It's about starting with a solid base, adding complexity with a variety of fruits and vegetables, enhancing flavor with herbs and spices, and finally, elevating the nutritional profile with superfoods or supplements. Each layer serves a purpose, and when done right, the result is a complex, satisfying, and incredibly nutritious beverage.

The Mindful Sip: The Ritual of Enjoyment

The act of drinking a smoothie can be a form of mindfulness, a moment to pause and appreciate the richness of the experience. Feel the coolness as you take the first sip, notice the interplay of flavors as they unfold on your palate, and sense the surge of energy as the nutrients are absorbed into your system. It's a holistic experience that engages all your senses, reminding you to be present in the moment.

As we craft these nutrient-packed smoothies, let's also be mindful of the ethical choices we make. Opting for organic, sustainably-sourced ingredients is not just a personal health choice but a statement of our values. It's about being conscious consumers who understand the impact of our choices on the environment and the community.

It's a microcosm of our approach to health and wellness—a blend of science, art, ethics, and mindfulness. It's a testament to our ability to take control of our nutrition, to make conscious choices, and to find joy in the simple act of nourishing ourselves.

So, as you stand before your blender, ingredients in hand, remember that you're not just making a smoothie; you're crafting a nutrient-packed masterpiece that embodies your commitment to health, wellness, and conscious living. Cheers to your health and the delicious journey that awaits!

The Personal Touch: Your Unique Nutritional Blueprint

As we reach the crescendo of our exploration into crafting nutrient-packed smoothies, let's not forget the most crucial element: you. Your body, your taste preferences, and your nutritional needs are as unique as your fingerprint. The beauty of smoothies lies in their adaptability. They can be tailored to fit your specific requirements, whether you're an athlete needing a protein boost, a busy parent looking for quick nutrition, or someone dealing with specific health issues. The smoothie becomes not just a drink but a personalized nutritional blueprint.

The concept of intuitive eating has been gaining traction, and it's something that can be beautifully applied to the world of smoothies. It's about listening to your body, understanding what it needs, and then crafting a smoothie that aligns with those needs. Some days, you might crave the refreshing zing of citrus fruits, signaling a need for Vitamin C. Other days, you might lean towards leafy greens, perhaps indicating a need for iron or calcium. This intuitive approach turns the act of smoothie-making into a form of self-care, a daily ritual where you check in with yourself.

The act of crafting a nutrient-packed smoothie has implications that ripple out beyond your kitchen. It's a commitment to a certain quality of life, a pledge to treat your body with respect. This simple act can be a catalyst for broader changes in your lifestyle. It can inspire you to make healthier choices in other areas, be it exercise, sleep, or stress management. The smoothie becomes a symbol of your broader commitment to holistic well-being.

We often underestimate the impact of nutrition on our emotional well-being. The ingredients you choose for your smoothies can have a profound effect on your mood and mental clarity. Foods rich in omega-3 fatty acids, such as flaxseeds or chia seeds, can improve brain function. Ingredients like dark chocolate or blueberries have antioxidants that can uplift your mood. By being mindful of these aspects, your smoothie can become a tool for emotional as well as physical nourishment.

As you master the art of crafting nutrient-packed smoothies, consider this a form of wisdom that can be passed down. Whether it's teaching your children about the benefits of different ingredients or sharing recipes with friends, this knowledge becomes a generational gift. It's a way to empower your loved ones to take control of their nutrition, to make informed choices, and to live a healthier life.

In a world grappling with environmental challenges, the choices we make in our kitchen have far-reaching consequences. By opting for locally sourced, organic ingredients, you're making an ethical choice that benefits not just you but the planet. It's a small but significant step towards a more sustainable lifestyle, adding another layer of meaning to your daily smoothie ritual.

The Toast to Your Health: A Culminating Moment

So here's to you, the artist and the consumer of this liquid nutrition. As you take that final sip, savor it. Let it be a moment of gratitude, not just for the nourishment you've provided your body but for the journey you've undertaken to reach this point. It's a journey of self-discovery, of tuning into your body's needs, of making ethical choices, and of embracing a holistic approach to health and well-being.

In this simple act of crafting a smoothie, you've done something extraordinary. You've taken disparate elements—fruits, vegetables, liquids, and supplements—and blended them into a harmonious whole. But more importantly, you've taken steps towards integrating the disparate elements of your life—nutrition, emotional well-being, ethical choices, and personal growth—into a harmonious whole.

As you rinse out your blender, ready to start anew tomorrow, carry with you the lessons and the joys of today. Your smoothie is more than just a drink; it's a testament to the life you're choosing to live, one sip at a time. Cheers to your health, your wisdom, and your ever-evolving journey in the world of liquid nutrition.

Herbal Teas: Benefits, Brewing, and Best Practices

The Alchemy of Herbal Teas: A Journey into Liquid Gold

Picture this: a steaming cup of herbal tea, its aroma wafting through the air, inviting you to take a sip. The experience is almost poetic, a momentary pause in the hustle and bustle of life, offering not just comfort but also a treasure trove of health benefits. Welcome to the world of herbal teas, a realm where the ancient wisdom of natural healing meets the modern quest for a balanced life.

Herbal teas are not merely a substitute for your regular cup of coffee or black tea; they are a lifestyle choice. Unlike traditional teas, which are brewed from the leaves of the Camellia sinensis plant, herbal teas are made from a variety of herbs, flowers, roots, and even bark. This opens up a universe of flavors and health benefits, each blend offering its unique bouquet of healing properties.

The first sip of an herbal tea is like the opening note in a symphony, setting the tone for what's to come. Whether it's the calming essence of chamomile, the invigorating zest of peppermint, or the earthy richness of rooibos, each herbal tea offers a distinct sensory experience. This is not just about taste; it's about how the tea makes you feel. The warmth that spreads through your body, the clarity that descends upon your mind, and the sense of peace that envelops your soul—these are the intangible benefits that elevate herbal teas from a mere beverage to a holistic experience.

The Healing Whisper: The Underlying Benefits

Herbal teas are often touted for their health benefits, and rightly so. From aiding digestion to reducing inflammation, boosting immunity, and even combating anxiety, the range of therapeutic effects is vast. But what often goes unnoticed is the subtler form of healing that takes place. It's the kind of healing that doesn't show up in lab tests or medical reports but manifests in quieter ways: better sleep, increased energy levels, improved focus, and a general sense of well-being.

Brewing herbal tea is not just a means to an end; it's a ritual, an act of self-care. The few minutes you spend steeping the herbs in hot water are an opportunity for mindfulness, a break from the incessant chatter of daily life. The act of brewing becomes a meditative practice, allowing you to be present in the moment, attuned to the subtle changes in color and aroma as the herbs release their essence into the water.

The Essence of Herbal Teas: More Than Just a Beverage

One of the most empowering aspects of herbal teas is the ability to create your own blends. While pre-packaged teas are convenient, there's something incredibly satisfying about mixing your own herbs, tailoring the blend to your specific needs and preferences. Whether you're looking to unwind after a stressful day, boost your immune system during flu season, or simply enjoy a flavorful cup of tea, the possibilities are endless.

In a world where consumer choices have far-reaching implications, opting for sustainably sourced, organic herbal teas is a statement of your values. It reflects a commitment to not just personal well-being but also ecological balance. By choosing ethical brands, you're contributing to a larger movement that values environmental stewardship and social responsibility.

The Communal Experience: Sharing the Elixir

Herbal teas have a communal aspect, often enjoyed in the company of loved ones. Whether it's a tea ceremony that honors ancient traditions or a simple tea break with friends, the act of sharing a cup of herbal tea is a celebration of community and connection. It's a reminder that well-being is not just an individual pursuit but a collective endeavor.

As we delve deeper into the fascinating world of herbal teas, we'll explore the nuances that make each blend unique, the ancient wisdom that underpins their healing properties, and the modern practices that allow us to enjoy these benefits today. So, as you take that first, soul-warming sip, know that you're embarking on a journey that transcends the boundaries of time and culture, a journey into the heart of nature's own pharmacy. Welcome to the alchemy of herbal teas.

The Heart of the Brew: Unveiling the Secrets of Herbal Teas

When you steep a blend of herbs in hot water, you're essentially performing a form of alchemy. The water acts as a solvent, extracting the essential oils, flavors, and medicinal compounds from the herbs. What you end up with is a liquid that's far more than the sum of its parts—a concoction that can soothe, heal, energize, or detoxify. The beauty of this process is that it's both an art and a science, a balance between intuition and knowledge.

Herbal teas offer a wide range of health benefits that cater to the diverse needs of modern life. For instance, teas like chamomile and lavender are renowned for their calming effects, making them ideal for stress management and better sleep. On the other hand, ginger and peppermint teas are excellent for digestive health. Then there are teas like echinacea and elderberry, known for boosting the immune system. The list goes on, addressing everything from hormonal balance to cognitive function.

While the health benefits of herbal teas are often the main attraction, the flavor experience is equally compelling. The rich tapestry of tastes and aromas that these teas offer is a culinary adventure in itself. From the spicy kick of ginger to the floral notes of chamomile, each sip is a journey that tantalizes the palate while nourishing the body. And let's not forget the sheer joy of discovering a new blend that resonates with your taste buds—a pleasure that's both simple and profound.

The act of drinking herbal tea can be a form of mindfulness, a way to connect with the present moment. As you hold the warm cup in your hands and take that first sip, you're not just consuming a beverage; you're engaging in a ritual that grounds you, that brings you back to yourself. This is particularly important in a world where we're constantly bombarded with information and distractions. The tea becomes a tool for mental clarity, a liquid form of meditation that you can integrate into your daily routine.

The Seasonal Symphony: Aligning Teas with Natural Cycles

One of the most enriching ways to enjoy herbal teas is to align your choices with the seasons. In winter, for example, warming spices like cinnamon and cloves can add both flavor and heat, while in summer, cooling herbs like mint and lemongrass offer a refreshing respite. This seasonal approach not only enhances the sensory experience but also aligns with the body's natural rhythms, optimizing the health benefits you receive.

In recent years, there's been a surge in artisanal tea makers who are elevating the craft to new heights. These are individuals and small businesses that source high-quality, often organic, ingredients to create blends that are both innovative and traditional. This movement is not just about better-tasting teas; it's about ethical sourcing, sustainability, and a deeper connection between the grower, the maker, and the consumer.

The Spectrum of Benefits: A Panacea for Modern Ailments

Herbal teas are incredibly versatile, and their use extends beyond the teacup. For instance, they can be used as a base for smoothies, offering an extra layer of flavor and nutrition. They can also be incorporated into cooking, used in everything from marinades to desserts. Some people even use herbal teas in their skincare routines, harnessing their antioxidant and anti-inflammatory properties.

Herbal teas are a global phenomenon, enjoyed by cultures around the world. Each region has its own traditional blends and rituals, from the Moroccan mint tea ceremonies to the Ayurvedic teas of India. This global tapestry adds another layer of richness to the herbal tea experience, allowing us to explore different cultures and traditions one cup at a time.

The Last Sip: A Final Word on Herbal Teas

As we've journeyed through the world of herbal teas, it's crucial to remember that the ultimate tea experience is deeply personal. The herbs that resonate with you may not have the same effect on someone else. It's a relationship between you and the plant, a dialogue that evolves over time. You'll find that certain teas become your go-to for specific situations, whether it's a cup of chamomile to wind down after a long day or a peppermint blend to kickstart your morning. This personalization is not just about preference; it's about listening to your body and understanding what it needs.

In a world where consumer choices have far-reaching impacts, opting for sustainable and ethically sourced teas is more than a trend; it's a responsibility. Many tea brands are now offering organic, fair-trade options that ensure the farmers are paid fairly and the environment is not harmed in the process. This ethical approach aligns perfectly with the holistic philosophy that herbal teas embody. When you sip such a cup, you're not just nourishing yourself; you're contributing to a chain of goodness that benefits the planet and its inhabitants.

There's a meditative quality to the act of brewing and drinking tea. From boiling the water to steeping the herbs and finally savoring each sip, each step can be a mindful act. You can elevate this daily habit into a personal ritual by adding elements that make it special. Maybe it's a particular teacup that you use only for this purpose, or perhaps it's a series of affirmations you recite as the tea steeps. This ritualistic element adds a layer of spiritual nourishment to the physical benefits the tea provides.

The Community Aspect: Sharing the Brew

Tea has always been a social beverage, a means of connecting with others. Whether it's a tea party with friends or a quiet cup with a loved one, the act of sharing tea amplifies its benefits. It becomes a medium for conversation, for sharing stories and experiences. In a way, each cup becomes a small but significant celebration of community and connection.

The world of herbal teas is vast and ever-expanding. New blends and herbs are continually being discovered, each with its unique set of benefits and flavors. This means that your tea journey is not a static experience but a dynamic one that evolves with you. As you grow and change, you'll find new teas that resonate with your current state of being. It's a lifelong journey of discovery that promises endless opportunities for both healing and pleasure.

The Healing Cup: A Holistic Approach to Well-being

In the grand tapestry of holistic health, herbal teas hold a special place. They offer a form of nourishment that is both gentle and powerful, addressing not just physical ailments but emotional and spiritual imbalances as well. When integrated into a broader wellness strategy, they serve as a valuable tool for achieving and maintaining optimal health.

As we move forward, the role of herbal teas in health and wellness is likely to grow. With ongoing research into the medicinal properties of herbs, we can expect even more targeted blends designed for specific health issues. At the same time, the rise of virtual tea communities and online platforms will make it easier for tea enthusiasts to share knowledge and recommendations.

As we come to the end of this exploration, consider this your personal invitation to dive deeper into the world of herbal teas. Start experimenting with different blends, pay attention to how they make you feel, and most importantly, enjoy the process. Remember, each cup is an opportunity for healing, for mindfulness, and for simple, unadulterated joy. So go ahead, put the kettle on, and pour yourself a cup of wellness. Your body, mind, and soul will thank you.

In the end, herbal teas are not just a topic to be studied but an experience to be lived. They encapsulate a philosophy that recognizes the interconnectedness of all things, the delicate balance between body, mind, and spirit. As you sip your way through life, may each cup bring you closer to that harmonious state of being. Cheers to your health, your well-being, and the many cups of herbal bliss that await you.

Book 9: Women's Health – An Alkaline Approach

Nutrition Across Different Life Stages

The Dance of Life

As we delve into the intricate tapestry of women's health through an alkaline lens, we arrive at a pivotal chapter—Nutrition Across Different Life Stages. This chapter is not just a guide; it's an ode to the ever-changing, ever-evolving journey of womanhood. From the first blush of adolescence to the wisdom-filled years of maturity, a woman's nutritional needs are as dynamic as the life she leads. And in this dance of life, nutrition serves as the music that orchestrates our well-being.

Before we explore the specific nutritional needs at various life stages, let's establish why an alkaline approach is particularly beneficial for women. The alkaline diet, rich in plant-based foods and low in processed items, naturally aligns with a woman's physiological needs. It offers a balanced array of nutrients while promoting a healthy pH level in the body. This balance is crucial because it lays the foundation for optimal hormonal health, which, as we'll see, plays a significant role at every stage of a woman's life.

The Maiden Voyage: Adolescence and Nutrition

The adolescent years are a whirlwind of change, not just emotionally and mentally, but also physically. It's a time when nutritional choices can have long-lasting impacts. An alkaline diet rich in fruits, vegetables, and whole grains can provide the essential nutrients for bone development, cognitive function, and emotional well-being. It's not just about avoiding the pitfalls of junk food; it's about embracing a lifestyle that sets the stage for a lifetime of health.

The Fertile Crescent: Nutrition in the Childbearing Years

As women transition into their childbearing years, the role of nutrition takes on new dimensions. Now, it's not just about individual well-being; it's about the potential for nurturing new life. An alkaline diet can be particularly beneficial during this stage. Foods rich in folic acid, calcium, and iron are not just menu items; they're building blocks for both mother and child. And let's not forget the hormonal fluctuations that accompany menstrual cycles, pregnancy, and breastfeeding. An alkaline diet can help regulate these hormonal shifts, making this life stage not just manageable but truly vibrant.

The Season of Wisdom: Menopause and Beyond

Menopause is often viewed through a lens of decline, a fading away of fertility and youth. But what if we reframe it as a season of wisdom, a time when a woman comes into her full power? Nutrition plays a crucial role in this reframing. The alkaline diet, rich in phytoestrogens found in foods like flaxseeds and soy, can help manage menopausal symptoms. Moreover, the high mineral content in alkaline foods supports bone health, a significant concern for post-menopausal women.

The Emotional Landscape: Nutrition as Emotional Well-being

We often focus solely on the physical aspects of nutrition, overlooking its profound impact on our emotional and mental health. Women, often being the emotional anchors of their families, can benefit immensely from the mood-regulating effects of an alkaline diet. Foods rich in Omega-3 fatty acids, magnesium, and antioxidants are not just nutrients; they're emotional balancers, stress relievers, and mental clarity enhancers.

As we navigate through the different stages of life, it's essential to remember that nutrition is not a static concept; it's a dynamic, evolving practice. Your needs today may not be your needs a decade from now, and that's perfectly okay. The key is to remain attuned to your body, to listen to its subtle signals, and to adjust your nutritional choices accordingly.

As we continue to explore the role of alkaline nutrition in women's health, we stand on the cusp of exciting new discoveries. Ongoing research is shedding light on the intricate connections between diet, hormonal health, and overall well-being. As we move forward, we can expect even more personalized nutritional guidelines tailored to each life stage, offering women a roadmap for a lifetime of vibrant health.

In this section, we've set the stage for a deep dive into the specific nutritional needs that accompany the various stages of a woman's life. We've looked at the overarching principles that make an alkaline approach particularly beneficial for women, and we've touched upon the emotional and mental aspects that are often overlooked in nutritional discourse. As we delve deeper into each life stage in the following sections, keep in mind that this is your journey, unique to you. Your dance of life is yours to choreograph, and nutrition is the music that will guide your steps.

The Alchemy of Womanhood: The Core of Nutrition Across Life Stages

Adolescence is a time of metamorphosis, where the cocoon of childhood begins to unravel, revealing the first glimpses of the woman to come. It's a stage where the body demands a diverse array of nutrients to fuel rapid growth and hormonal changes. The alkaline diet shines here, offering a cornucopia of essential nutrients like calcium for bone density, iron for blood health, and Omega-3s for cognitive development. It's not just about what to eat but how to eat. Mindful eating practices, such as savoring each bite and being present during meals, can instill habits that last a lifetime.

The Fertility Waltz: Nutrition in the Reproductive Years

The reproductive years are a dance of their own, a waltz between womanhood and the potential for motherhood. Nutrition during this phase is like a duet between you and your body, where each step is synchronized for optimal health. An alkaline diet rich in folic acid, for instance, is not just beneficial for you; it's a gift to your future child, reducing the risk of neural tube defects. Moreover, the alkaline approach can help manage Polycystic Ovary Syndrome (PCOS), a condition that affects many women in their childbearing years. Foods like leafy greens and legumes, rich in magnesium and antioxidants, can help regulate insulin levels, a key factor in PCOS management.

Menopause is often framed as an ending, but let's reframe it as a new beginning, a different kind of music in the ongoing symphony of a woman's life. Nutrition here is about grace, about understanding the changing tempo of your body and adapting accordingly. Phytoestrogens found in flaxseeds and fermented soy products can help manage hot flashes and mood swings. Moreover, the alkaline diet's emphasis on bone health becomes crucial here, as the risk of osteoporosis increases post-menopause.

The Emotional Cadence: Nutrition for the Soul

We've talked about the body, but what about the soul? Emotional well-being is a crucial aspect of overall health, especially for women who often serve as the emotional pillars of their families. Foods rich in tryptophan, like nuts and seeds, can boost serotonin levels, acting as natural mood lifters. The alkaline diet also emphasizes hydration, and let's not underestimate the power of water. Proper hydration can alleviate symptoms of anxiety and depression, offering a sense of emotional buoyancy.

The Wisdom Years: The Grand Finale

As women move into the later stages of life, the focus often shifts from nurturing others to self-care, and rightfully so. This is the time to reap the benefits of a life well-lived and well-fed. Antioxidant-rich foods like berries and dark leafy greens can help manage age-related conditions like macular degeneration and cognitive decline. It's also a time when many women explore spirituality more deeply, and the clarity that comes from an alkaline diet can be a valuable ally on this spiritual journey.

The Universal Dance: Nutrition as a Collective Responsibility

While this chapter focuses on individual choices, it's essential to recognize that nutrition is also a collective responsibility. In a world where processed foods are often more accessible and affordable than fresh produce, advocating for systemic change is crucial. Whether it's supporting local farmers, pushing for better food labeling, or educating the next generation, your individual choices can ripple out to create broader societal transformation.

Nutrition is not a one-size-fits-all prescription; it's a lifelong journey of learning and adaptation. As new research emerges, be open to tweaking your alkaline approach. Maybe it's incorporating a newly discovered superfood or adjusting your meal timings based on your body's natural circadian rhythms. The key is to stay curious, stay engaged, and most importantly, stay attuned to your body's ever-changing needs.

In the heart of this chapter, we've navigated the intricate choreography of women's nutritional needs across different life stages. From the hormonal surges of adolescence to the wisdom-infused years of maturity, each stage offers its unique challenges and triumphs. The alkaline approach serves as a versatile, adaptable partner in this dance, providing the nutritional balance and emotional harmony to make each stage not just survivable, but truly thrive able. As we move forward, let this be your guide, your nutritional choreography, in the grand dance of life.

The Culmination: Harmonizing Nutrition Across Life's Symphony

As we've navigated the labyrinth of women's nutritional needs across different life stages, one thing becomes abundantly clear: the choices we make resonate deeply within us. Each decision to opt for an alkaline food over an acidic one, to hydrate adequately, or to engage in mindful eating is like striking a chord in the symphony of our lives. These choices are not isolated notes; they form a melody that reverberates through our physical and emotional well-being, echoing into our relationships, our work, and our sense of self.

While individual choices are pivotal, we don't make these choices in a vacuum. We are influenced by our families, our communities, and the broader culture. This is why it's crucial to recognize the role of community in shaping our nutritional habits. Whether it's a family dinner, a community potluck, or a holiday celebration, these gatherings can either reinforce alkaline choices or push us towards acidic pitfalls. The power of community can be harnessed to create a culture of health, where alkaline foods are not just an individual choice but a collective value.

Nutritional science is a dynamic field, continually evolving as new research emerges. While the core principles of the alkaline approach have stood the test of time, it's essential to stay updated with the latest findings. For instance, the role of gut health in overall well-being is a relatively new area of research that aligns beautifully with the alkaline philosophy. Probiotic-rich foods like fermented vegetables can be integrated into your alkaline regimen to support gut health, thereby enhancing nutrient absorption and emotional well-being.

As we age, our relationship with food often reaches a crescendo, a peak of wisdom where we understand not just the "what" but also the "why" behind our choices. This is the stage where many women become the nutritional gatekeepers of their families, passing down the wisdom accumulated over a lifetime. It's a profound responsibility but also a remarkable opportunity to shape the health of future generations. The alkaline approach, with its emphasis on natural, nutrient-dense foods, offers a solid foundation upon which to build this legacy.

The Encore: The Ongoing Journey of Nutritional Mastery

Life is not a one-act play; it's a series of encores, each presenting an opportunity for growth and refinement. The same is true for your nutritional journey. As you move through different life stages, your body's needs will change, and your alkaline approach will need to adapt. This adaptability is not a sign of inconsistency; it's a hallmark of mastery. Whether it's incorporating new superfoods, adjusting meal timings, or exploring novel cooking techniques, each adjustment is an encore in your lifelong performance of well-being.

It's easy to focus on the challenges, the missed notes, and the occasional dissonance in our nutritional journey. But let's not forget to celebrate the triumphs, the high notes that make the journey worthwhile. Whether it's reaching a health milestone, discovering a new favorite alkaline recipe, or simply feeling vibrant and energized, these moments deserve a standing ovation. They serve as affirmations that you're on the right path, fueling your resolve to continue this enriching journey.

The Final Bow: Acknowledging the Unseen Conductors

As we take our final bow, let's acknowledge the unseen conductors in our lives—the healthcare providers, the researchers, the farmers, and most importantly, the women who came before us. Their wisdom, labor, and sacrifices have shaped the stage upon which we perform our nutritional symphony. As we exit the stage, let's carry forward their legacy, fine-tuning our performance while setting the stage for those who will follow us.

In the grand tapestry of life, nutrition is not just a thread; it's a vibrant color that adds depth, texture, and beauty to the overall design. As women, our relationship with nutrition is not a static entity but a dynamic interplay that evolves across different life stages. The alkaline approach serves as a versatile palette, offering a spectrum of nutritional hues to paint each stage with vitality, balance, and grace. So, as the curtain falls on this topic, let it rise on a new act in your life—one where you're not just a passive spectator but an active performer, choreographing your unique dance of health and well-being.

Addressing Women's Health Concerns Naturally

The Dawn of a New Perspective

In a world where quick fixes and pharmaceutical solutions often take center stage, the idea of addressing women's health concerns naturally might seem like a step back. But is it really? The truth is, the natural approach to women's health is not a rejection of modern medicine but rather an expansion of it. It's an acknowledgment that our bodies are complex ecosystems, influenced by a myriad of factors—diet, lifestyle, environment, and yes, even our thoughts and emotions.

The alkaline approach serves as a cornerstone in this natural paradigm. It's not just about what we eat, but how what we eat affects our entire being. Alkaline foods, rich in essential nutrients and devoid of toxic elements, provide the body with the tools it needs to heal, rejuvenate, and thrive. This is particularly significant for women, who often juggle multiple roles and responsibilities, leaving them susceptible to a range of health issues from hormonal imbalances to stress-related ailments.

The Feminine Mystique: Unique Health Challenges

Women's bodies are a marvel of nature, capable of creating life, enduring immense physical changes, and adapting to various life stages. However, this complexity also makes women more susceptible to certain health concerns. Issues like menstrual irregularities, menopause symptoms, and certain types of cancers are unique to women. The natural approach, rooted in the alkaline philosophy, offers not just symptom relief but aims for holistic well-being.

One of the most overlooked aspects of women's health is the intricate connection between emotional and physical well-being. Stress, anxiety, and emotional turmoil can manifest physically, exacerbating existing health issues or even creating new ones. The alkaline approach extends beyond diet to include practices like mindfulness, meditation, and natural stress-relief techniques, recognizing that emotional balance is crucial for physical health.

We don't live in isolation. Our health is continually influenced by our environment—from the air we breathe to the products we use. Women, in particular, are exposed to a range of beauty and personal care products, many of which contain harmful chemicals. The natural approach advocates for a cleaner, more organic lifestyle, encouraging women to scrutinize not just what goes into their bodies but what goes on them.

Perhaps the most empowering aspect of the natural approach to women's health is the agency it provides. It shifts the narrative from being a passive recipient of healthcare to an active participant in your own well-being. This is not to undermine the importance of professional medical advice but to complement it. It's about making informed choices—whether it's opting for organic produce, practicing yoga, or even choosing natural menstrual products.

Women's health is not just an individual concern; it's a community issue. The choices we make, the lifestyles we adopt, and the knowledge we share have a ripple effect, influencing not just our health but that of our families and communities. The natural approach, therefore, is not just a personal journey but a collective endeavor. It's about creating a culture of health, where natural, holistic practices are not the exception but the norm.

The Journey Ahead: A Lifelong Commitment

Addressing women's health concerns naturally is not a quick fix; it's a lifelong commitment. It's about tuning into your body, understanding its signals, and responding with love and care. It's a dynamic, evolving process that requires attention, education, and sometimes even a bit of trial and error. But the rewards—physical vitality, emotional balance, and a deep sense of well-being—are well worth the effort.

As we delve deeper into this chapter, we'll explore specific health concerns that women commonly face and how the alkaline approach can offer natural, effective solutions. We'll look at real-life examples, scientific studies, and practical tips to equip you with the knowledge and tools you need to take charge of your health, naturally. So let's embark on this transformative journey together, shedding old paradigms and embracing a holistic, natural approach to women's health.

The Dawn of a New Perspective: Addressing Women's Health Concerns Naturally

In a world where quick fixes and pharmaceutical solutions often take center stage, the idea of addressing women's health concerns naturally might seem like a step back. But is it really? The truth is, the natural approach to women's health is not a rejection of modern medicine but rather an expansion of it. It's an acknowledgment that our bodies are complex ecosystems, influenced by a myriad of factors—diet, lifestyle, environment, and yes, even our thoughts and emotions.

The alkaline approach serves as a cornerstone in this natural paradigm. It's not just about what we eat, but how what we eat affects our entire being. Alkaline foods, rich in essential nutrients and devoid of toxic elements, provide the body with the tools it needs to heal, rejuvenate, and thrive. This is particularly significant for women, who often juggle multiple roles and responsibilities, leaving them susceptible to a range of health issues from hormonal imbalances to stress-related ailments.

Women's bodies are a marvel of nature, capable of creating life, enduring immense physical changes, and adapting to various life stages. However, this complexity also makes women more susceptible to certain health concerns. Issues like menstrual irregularities, menopause symptoms, and certain types of cancers are unique to women. The natural approach, rooted in the alkaline philosophy, offers not just symptom relief but aims for holistic well-being.

One of the most overlooked aspects of women's health is the intricate connection between emotional and physical well-being. Stress, anxiety, and emotional turmoil can manifest physically, exacerbating existing health issues or even creating new ones. The alkaline approach extends beyond diet to include practices like mindfulness, meditation, and natural stress-relief techniques, recognizing that emotional balance is crucial for physical health.

We don't live in isolation. Our health is continually influenced by our environment—from the air we breathe to the products we use. Women, in particular, are exposed to a range of beauty and personal care products, many of which contain harmful chemicals. The natural approach advocates for a cleaner, more organic lifestyle, encouraging women to scrutinize not just what goes into their bodies but what goes on them.

The Power of Choice: Taking Control of Your Health

Perhaps the most empowering aspect of the natural approach to women's health is the agency it provides. It shifts the narrative from being a passive recipient of healthcare to an active participant in your own well-being. This is not to undermine the importance of professional medical advice but to complement it. It's about making informed choices—whether it's opting for organic produce, practicing yoga, or even choosing natural menstrual products.

Women's health is not just an individual concern; it's a community issue. The choices we make, the lifestyles we adopt, and the knowledge we share have a ripple effect, influencing not just our health but that of our families and communities. The natural approach, therefore, is not just a personal journey but a collective endeavor. It's about creating a culture of health, where natural, holistic practices are not the exception but the norm.

Addressing women's health concerns naturally is not a quick fix; it's a lifelong commitment. It's about tuning into your body, understanding its signals, and responding with love and care. It's a dynamic, evolving process that requires attention, education, and sometimes even a bit of trial and error. But the rewards—physical vitality, emotional balance, and a deep sense of well-being—are well worth the effort.

As we delve deeper into this chapter, we'll explore specific health concerns that women commonly face and how the alkaline approach can offer natural, effective solutions. We'll look at real-life examples, scientific studies, and practical tips to equip you with the knowledge and tools you need to take charge of your health, naturally. So, let's embark on this transformative journey together, shedding old paradigms and embracing a holistic, natural approach to women's health.

Tackling women's health problems naturally

When it comes to women's health, the alkaline diet offers a plethora of benefits beyond simply managing symptoms. Rich in fruits, vegetables, and whole grains, this diet is a powerhouse of essential nutrients such as vitamins, minerals, and antioxidants. These nutrients not only nourish the body, but also help regulate hormonal imbalances, which are often the root cause of many women-specific health problems, such as polycystic ovary syndrome (PCOS), endometriosis, and menopausal symptoms.

Herbs have been used for centuries to treat various ailments, and their efficacy is not just folklore. Modern science increasingly validates the medicinal properties of herbs, many of which are integral to the alkaline approach. For example, herbs such as chasteberry, black cohosh, and evening primrose oil have shown promise for alleviating menstrual disorders and menopausal symptoms. The beauty of using herbs is that they often have fewer side effects than drugs, offering a gentler but effective treatment option.

The mindful approach: Stress, hormones and women's health

Stress is a silent killer, and its impact on women's health cannot be overstated. Chronic stress can lead to hormonal imbalances, exacerbating health problems such as irregular menstruation, weight gain, and even fertility problems.

Mindfulness techniques such as meditation and deep breathing exercises, which are an integral part of the alkaline lifestyle, can be incredibly effective in managing stress. By reducing stress, we can bring hormone levels back into balance, thereby improving various aspects of women's health.

If diet and herbs are key, physical activity is another pillar of the alkaline approach to women's health. Exercise is not just about weight management; it is a powerful tool for hormonal balance. Physical activities such as yoga and Pilates are particularly beneficial because they focus on holistic well-being, improving both physical stamina and mental clarity. In addition, exercise releases endorphins, the body's natural painkillers, which can help relieve menstrual cramps and body aches.

The environmental aspect: Detoxifying the world

The environment in which we live plays an important role in our health. From the air we breathe to the water we drink; environmental toxins can have devastating effects on our bodies. Women, who often use a variety of personal care products, are particularly at risk. Switching to natural and organic products can significantly reduce the toxin load, improving health outcomes. The alkaline approach supports this lifestyle change, emphasizing the importance of clean living.

Emotions and physical health are closely linked, especially for women. Emotional upsets can manifest as physical symptoms. Conditions such as irritable bowel syndrome (IBS) and fibromyalgia are often triggered or worsened by emotional stress. The alkaline approach recognizes this connection and incorporates emotional well-being into its holistic health model. Practices such as journaling, mindful communication, and emotional intelligence exercises can help improve emotional and physical health.

Women's health is not just an individual journey, but a collective endeavor. The wisdom of one person can serve as a lesson for many. Community support, therefore, is invaluable. Whether sharing recipes, workout tips or even personal stories, a supportive community can make the journey to natural health much more enriching. The alkaline approach encourages the creation of this community, recognizing that collective wisdom is often superior to individual knowledge.

Taking a natural approach to women's health is not a temporary solution, but a lifelong commitment. It is about making daily choices that honor your body and its unique needs. The alkaline approach, with its emphasis on natural foods, herbs and holistic practices, offers a sustainable path to long-term health and well-being.

As we move forward, we will delve into specific strategies, supported by scientific research and real-world testimonials, to naturally address common women's health problems. From dietary changes to herbal remedies and lifestyle modifications, you will be equipped with a complete toolkit to take charge of your health, naturally.

A Holistic Blueprint for Women's Health

The alkaline approach is not a one-size-fits-all solution but a framework that empowers you to listen to your body, understand its unique needs, and make informed choices. It's about reclaiming your health narrative and becoming an active participant in your well-being.

Adopting the alkaline lifestyle is not a temporary fix but a lifelong commitment to holistic well-being. It's a paradigm shift that requires you to unlearn many conventional beliefs about health and wellness. But the rewards are immeasurable. From hormonal balance to emotional well-being, the benefits permeate every aspect of your life, offering a holistic solution to a range of women's health concerns.

One of the most empowering aspects of the alkaline approach is the emphasis on informed choices. Whether it's selecting herbs for menstrual relief or choosing organic produce, every decision is an opportunity to honor your body. And the more informed you are, the better choices you'll make. This is not about following a set of rigid rules but about understanding the 'why' behind each choice, thereby making the journey towards natural health a fulfilling one.

The Role of Intuition: Listening to Your Body

In a world inundated with health advice, it's easy to overlook the most important source of guidance—your body. Your body is an incredible machine, capable of sending you signals when something is amiss. The alkaline approach encourages you to tune into these signals. Whether it's a food craving or a physical symptom, listening to your body can provide invaluable insights into your health.

We've talked about the importance of emotional well-being in women's health. But it's worth reiterating that your emotional landscape plays a crucial role in your physical health. Stress, anxiety, and emotional upheavals can manifest as physical symptoms, and addressing these emotional triggers is often the first step towards healing. Practices like mindfulness, journaling, and emotional intelligence exercises can be incredibly effective in this regard.

The journey towards natural health is not a solitary endeavor. It's a collective journey, enriched by shared experiences and wisdom. Whether it's a support group, an online forum, or even a circle of friends, a supportive community can be a powerful catalyst for change. The alkaline approach recognizes the value of collective wisdom and encourages community building as a cornerstone of holistic health.

The Future Outlook: The Evolving Landscape of Women's Health

As we look towards the future, it's clear that the landscape of women's health is evolving. With growing awareness and research, natural approaches like the alkaline diet are gaining mainstream acceptance. And as more women share their success stories, the movement towards natural health is only going to gain momentum. This is not a passing trend but a paradigm shift, one that promises a healthier, more empowered future for women everywhere.

In conclusion, addressing women's health concerns naturally is not just about symptom management but about holistic well-being. It's a multi-dimensional approach that encompasses physical, emotional, and even environmental factors. And while the journey may be challenging, the rewards are life-changing. So as you turn the page, remember that the most important step in any journey is the first one. And you've already taken it by choosing to empower yourself with knowledge and choice. Your health is your most valuable asset, and you have the tools to protect and nurture it, naturally.

Let's carry forward the spirit of empowerment and collective wisdom. Let's commit to making informed choices, listening to our bodies, and supporting each other in this journey towards optimal health. After all, the path to natural health is not a destination but a journey, one that promises a lifetime of well-being and fulfillment.

Beauty, skin care and alkaline practices

An introduction to skin care and alkaline practices

Welcome to a transformative topic that promises to redefine your understanding of beauty and skin care. We often associate beauty with external attributes, forgetting that true beauty is a reflection of our internal health. This chapter aims to bridge this gap, offering you a holistic perspective on beauty that transcends superficial treatments and delves into the heart of well-being.

The alkaline approach to beauty is not just another trend; it is a paradigm shift that challenges conventional wisdom. It is about understanding that the skin is a living, breathing organ that responds to life choices. Alkaline philosophy holds that a balanced internal environment is the basis of radiant skin and overall beauty.

Skin: The body's largest organ

Before we delve into alkaline practices that can improve your beauty regimen, let's take a moment to appreciate the skin. It is not just a protective covering, but a complex organ that performs multiple functions, from regulating temperature to eliminating toxins. The skin is a mirror that reflects internal health, and understanding this connection is the first step in taking a holistic approach to beauty.

The concept of acid-alkaline balance is central to this chapter. The body seeks to maintain a slightly alkaline pH level, and any deviation can lead to various health problems, including skin problems. An acidic environment can exacerbate conditions such as acne, eczema and premature aging. The alkaline approach aims to restore this balance, offering a natural solution to a range of skin problems.

The role of nutrition: You are what you eat

The saying "you are what you eat" has particular relevance when it comes to skin care. The alkaline diet, rich in natural fruits, vegetables and herbs, provides essential nutrients that nourish the skin from within. It is not just about eliminating harmful foods, but adopting a diet that enriches the body and, by extension, the skin.

Hydration plays a key role in maintaining skin health. But the alkaline approach takes it a step further by emphasizing the quality of the water you consume. Alkaline water, with its higher pH level, offers additional benefits such as better hydration and detoxification, contributing to clearer, brighter skin.

The mind-skin connection: Stress and complexion

You have probably noticed that stress can affect your skin. Alkaline philosophy recognizes the mind-skin connection and offers holistic solutions such as meditation and mindfulness to manage stress. These practices not only improve mental well-being, but also have a positive impact on the skin.

Throughout this chapter we will explore various alkaline practices that can be incorporated into your skin care regimen. From herbal face masks to alkaline baths, these practices offer natural alternatives to chemical-based products. Most importantly, they encourage you to consider skin care as an integral part of your overall health journey.

As you embark on this enlightening journey, remember that the alkaline approach to beauty is not a quick fix, but a lifestyle choice. It is a commitment to understanding your body, respecting its needs, and making informed choices that contribute to your overall well-being. And as you will discover, the benefits are not just skin-deep.

From practical advice to transformative practices, this chapter promises to be a treasure trove of wisdom that will enable you to reclaim your natural beauty in the most authentic way possible.

After all, beauty is not only about looking good, but also about feeling good in your own skin, literally and metaphorically. And that, dear reader, is the essence of the alkaline approach to beauty, skincare and overall well-being.

The Alkaline Approach to Beauty and Skincare: A Deeper Dive

The alkaline diet is not just about what you put in your body; it's also about what you put on your body. Your skin absorbs nutrients and minerals, and the alkaline diet provides an array of beneficial elements that can enhance your skin's health. Foods rich in antioxidants like berries, leafy greens, and nuts can combat free radicals, which are a leading cause of skin aging. The alkaline diet also emphasizes hydration, which is crucial for maintaining skin elasticity and preventing dryness.

Herbs have been used for centuries to treat various ailments, and their application in skincare is equally potent. Plants like aloe vera, chamomile, and lavender have natural anti-inflammatory properties that can soothe irritated skin. Herbs like turmeric and ginger are rich in antioxidants and can be used in face masks to rejuvenate your skin. The alkaline approach encourages the use of these natural remedies over chemical-laden products, aligning your skincare routine with your overall health goals.

The Detoxification Process: Clearing the Canvas

Detoxification is a buzzword in the beauty industry, but in the alkaline context, it takes on a more profound meaning. The alkaline diet is inherently detoxifying, helping to eliminate toxins that can lead to skin issues like acne and eczema. Alkaline water, with its higher pH, can flush out toxins more effectively than regular water. This detoxification process is not just about clear skin; it's about setting the stage for your body to absorb nutrients more efficiently, which in turn enhances your skin's natural glow.

Mindfulness and Beauty: The Inner-Outer Connection

The alkaline approach recognizes that your mental state has a direct impact on your physical appearance. Stress can trigger hormone imbalances that may lead to skin problems. Mindfulness techniques, such as meditation and deep-breathing exercises, can help manage stress levels. When you are mentally balanced, it reflects on your skin—reducing redness, improving complexion, and even slowing down the aging process.

The Role of Physical Activity: Sweat It Out

Exercise is another pillar of the alkaline lifestyle that has direct benefits for your skin. Physical activity increases blood flow, which helps nourish skin cells and keep them vital. Sweat removes toxins, and the increased heart rate improves circulation, giving your skin a youthful, radiant appearance. Whether it's yoga, jogging, or even a brisk walk, incorporating physical activity into your routine can be a game-changer for your skin.

The Importance of Sleep: Beauty Rest Defined

We've all heard of beauty sleep, but few realize how crucial it is. During sleep, your body goes into repair mode, producing new skin cells and boosting collagen production. The alkaline approach emphasizes the importance of quality sleep, recommending practices like winding down before bed and keeping electronic devices away to ensure a restful night. The result? You wake up with refreshed, glowing skin, ready to face the day.

Customizing Your Alkaline Skincare Routine: Tailoring to Your Needs

The beauty of the alkaline approach is its adaptability. While the principles remain constant, you can tailor your skincare routine to suit your specific needs. For instance, if you have dry skin, you might focus more on hydration and use herbs that offer intense moisturization. If you're prone to acne, your routine might include more detoxifying elements. The key is to listen to your body and adjust accordingly.

Lastly, it's worth noting that the alkaline approach to beauty is inherently sustainable. By opting for natural, organic products, you're not just doing your skin a favor; you're also contributing to a healthier planet. Many alkaline skincare products come in eco-friendly packaging, and the focus on local, organic ingredients reduces your carbon footprint.

The alkaline approach to beauty and skincare is revolutionary because it doesn't treat these aspects as isolated from your overall health. It integrates them into a holistic lifestyle that benefits not just your appearance but your entire well-being. It's a comprehensive, sustainable, and most importantly, effective way to achieve the radiant skin and natural beauty we all desire. And as you'll find, when you look good, you feel good, and when you feel good, you look absolutely stunning. That's the alkaline way—a holistic path to beauty, inside and out.

The Alkaline Journey to Lasting Beauty: A Final Reflection

The alkaline lifestyle is not a quick fix or a fad; it's a commitment to holistic well-being that naturally extends to beauty and skincare. When you embrace this lifestyle, you're not just opting for a healthier diet or a more mindful way of living; you're choosing a path that harmonizes your internal and external selves. This harmony manifests in clearer skin, a radiant complexion, and an overall sense of vitality that no cosmetic product can replicate.

In a world of instant gratification, the alkaline approach teaches us the value of consistency. Just as one unhealthy meal won't ruin your health, a single alkaline facial won't transform your skin overnight. It's the daily commitment to alkaline practices—be it your diet, skincare routine, or stress management techniques—that yields visible and lasting results. Over time, you'll notice not just superficial changes, but a deep-rooted sense of well-being that radiates from the inside out.

Let's talk about the emotional transformation that accompanies the physical one. When you look good, you feel good, and this newfound confidence has a ripple effect on every aspect of your life. You become more open to new experiences, more comfortable in your own skin, and more in tune with your body's needs. This isn't vanity; it's self-love, and it's a crucial aspect of mental health that we often overlook.

Embarking on an alkaline journey doesn't mean walking the path alone. There's a burgeoning community of alkaline enthusiasts who share tips, recipes, and words of encouragement. This sense of community not only makes the journey more enjoyable but also holds you accountable. It's easier to stick to a skincare routine or a diet plan when you know there's a community cheering you on, sharing in your challenges and celebrating your victories.

The Ethical Dimension: Beauty Without Cruelty

One of the most compelling aspects of the alkaline approach to beauty and skincare is its ethical dimension. By opting for natural, cruelty-free products, you're making a statement about the kind of world you want to live in—one where beauty doesn't come at the expense of our furry friends or our planet. This ethical commitment amplifies the joy you derive from your beauty routine, making each scrub, mask, or moisturizer not just an act of self-care, but also an act of global responsibility.

Let's address the elephant in the room: cost. Many people shy away from natural products, assuming they're more expensive. While the initial cost may be higher, the long-term financial benefits are significant. Natural products are generally more concentrated and last longer, and their effectiveness reduces the need for multiple skincare items. Moreover, the health benefits of an alkaline lifestyle can save you a fortune in medical bills down the line.

The Time Factor: Integrating Alkaline Practices into a Busy Life

For those juggling a hectic lifestyle, the thought of incorporating an alkaline skincare routine may seem daunting. But it's all about smart planning. Many alkaline practices can be seamlessly integrated into your daily life. For instance, making a nutrient-packed alkaline smoothie takes no longer than pouring a bowl of sugary cereal. Similarly, natural face masks can be applied while you're answering emails or doing household chores. It's not about finding extra time; it's about optimizing the time you already have.

In conclusion, the alkaline approach to beauty and skincare is not a trend; it's a lifestyle choice that offers lifelong benefits. It's a holistic model that recognizes the interconnectedness of our physical, emotional, and ethical well-being. It's a journey of self-discovery, where each day brings you closer to the best version of yourself. And as you navigate the complexities of modern life—from stress and pollution to the inevitable aging process—you'll find that the principles of alkalinity serve as a steady guide, helping you maintain not just your beauty, but your grace, your dignity, and your zest for life.

So, as you close this chapter and perhaps ponder the steps you'll take to integrate these practices into your life, remember: beauty isn't skin deep; it's soul deep. And the alkaline way is your roadmap to a soulful, radiant beauty that stands the test of time.

Book 10: Men's Health – Strength and Vitality

Unique Nutritional Needs for Men

In today's fast-paced society, the focus on health often leans towards quick fixes and one-size-fits-all solutions. This is especially true for men, who are often expected to embody strength and vitality at all times. The societal norms surrounding masculinity can sometimes act as barriers, preventing men from addressing their unique health needs. But let's be clear: strength isn't about ignoring your needs; it's about understanding and nurturing them. That's where the alkaline approach comes into play, offering a tailored pathway to men's health that goes beyond the superficial.

It's not just societal roles that differentiate men from women; biology plays a significant part too. Men generally have higher muscle mass, different hormonal profiles, and distinct metabolic rates compared to women. These biological factors necessitate a unique approach to nutrition, one that fuels the body's specific needs for optimal functioning. The alkaline lifestyle offers a nuanced understanding of these needs, providing men with the tools to achieve not just physical strength but also mental clarity and emotional balance.

The alkaline approach is not just another diet plan or a set of rigid rules. It's a holistic lifestyle that takes into account the interconnectedness of physical health, mental well-being, and emotional stability. For men, this means a diet rich in alkaline foods that support muscle growth, enhance cognitive function, and balance hormonal levels. But it doesn't stop there; the alkaline lifestyle also incorporates stress management techniques and physical activities that are tailored to men's unique physiological makeup.

The Misconceptions: Debunking the Protein Myth

One of the most pervasive myths in men's nutrition is the overemphasis on protein, particularly animal protein. While protein is undoubtedly essential for muscle repair and growth, the source and type of protein matter immensely. The alkaline approach shifts the focus from animal-based proteins, which are often acidic, to plant-based options that are not only alkaline but also rich in other essential nutrients. This shift is not just beneficial for your body's pH levels; it also has a positive impact on your cardiovascular health, digestive system, and even your mental well-being.

We often overlook the impact of nutrition on mental health, especially for men, who are less likely to discuss emotional or psychological issues openly. The alkaline lifestyle recognizes the profound impact that your diet can have on your mental state. Foods rich in omega-3 fatty acids, antioxidants, and essential vitamins play a crucial role in enhancing mood, improving focus, and reducing stress. By adopting an alkaline diet, men can naturally boost their mental health, which in turn improves their overall quality of life.

The Lifestyle Factor: Balancing a Hectic Routine

Let's face it; modern life is hectic. Between work commitments, family responsibilities, and social engagements, finding time for health can be challenging. The beauty of the alkaline approach is its adaptability. It's not about spending hours in the kitchen or the gym; it's about making smarter choices that fit into your busy schedule. Simple swaps like choosing alkaline water over soda or opting for a plant-based snack instead of a sugary treat can make a significant difference over time.

The Journey Ahead: A Lifelong Commitment

As we delve deeper into the unique nutritional needs for men, it's essential to remember that this is a lifelong journey. It's not about quick fixes or temporary changes; it's about a sustained commitment to your well-being. The alkaline lifestyle offers a comprehensive roadmap for this journey, providing men with the nutritional guidance, emotional support, and mental clarity they need to navigate the complexities of modern life.

In the topic that follow, we will explore the intricacies of fitness, muscle building, and addressing common male health concerns through the alkaline lens. But for now, let's celebrate the first step in acknowledging and embracing the unique nutritional needs that define men's health. Because true strength lies in understanding, and the path to vitality is paved with knowledge and self-care.

The Nutritional Building Blocks: Macronutrients and Micronutrients

When it comes to men's health, the conversation often starts and ends with protein. While protein is a crucial macronutrient, especially for muscle building, it's not the only one. Carbohydrates and fats also play vital roles in energy production and hormonal balance. The alkaline approach emphasizes the importance of all three macronutrients, sourced from plant-based, alkaline-rich foods.

But let's not forget about micronutrients—vitamins and minerals that are essential for a plethora of physiological functions. For instance, zinc is crucial for testosterone production, while magnesium aids in muscle relaxation and stress reduction. The beauty of an alkaline diet is that it naturally incorporates a wide range of micronutrients, eliminating the need for synthetic supplements.

The Hormonal Equation: Testosterone and Its Role

Testosterone is often dubbed the "male hormone," responsible for many of the biological differences between men and women. It plays a role in muscle growth, fat distribution, and even mood regulation. However, modern lifestyle factors, including stress and poor diet, can lead to hormonal imbalances. The alkaline lifestyle offers a natural way to balance testosterone levels through nutrient-rich foods and stress management techniques. Foods like pumpkin seeds, leafy greens, and alkaline grains are not only testosterone-friendly but also contribute to overall hormonal balance.

The Energy Conundrum: Sustaining Vitality Throughout the Day

Men often face the challenge of maintaining consistent energy levels, especially those leading active, demanding lives. The typical solution? Caffeine and sugar-laden energy drinks. While these may offer a quick fix, they lead to energy crashes and contribute to long-term health issues. The alkaline approach focuses on sustained energy through balanced meals that include complex carbohydrates, healthy fats, and plant-based proteins. These foods provide a slow, steady release of energy, keeping you active and focused throughout the day.

The Stress Factor: Nutrition's Impact on Mental Well-being

Stress is an unavoidable aspect of modern life, but how we manage it can make all the difference. For men, stress can manifest in various ways, including fatigue, irritability, and even reduced libido. Nutrition plays a significant role in stress management. Alkaline foods rich in antioxidants and anti-inflammatory properties can naturally lower cortisol levels, the body's primary stress hormone. Incorporating foods like berries, nuts, and avocados into your diet can make a tangible difference in how you handle stress.

The Digestive Link: Gut Health and Its Systemic Effects

Recent research has highlighted the gut's role as the "second brain," affecting everything from mood to immune function. For men, optimal gut health is crucial for nutrient absorption, especially when it comes to protein and essential minerals. Alkaline foods are naturally high in fiber, promoting healthy gut flora and aiding in digestion. A well-functioning digestive system not only improves nutrient absorption but also contributes to better mental health through the gut-brain axis.

The Cardiovascular Connection: Heart Health Matters

Men are often at higher risk for cardiovascular issues, making heart health a priority. The alkaline diet is naturally low in sodium and high in potassium, helping to regulate blood pressure and improve cardiovascular function. Foods like bananas, sweet potatoes, and spinach are alkaline staples that support heart health. Moreover, the emphasis on plant-based fats ensures a healthy lipid profile, reducing the risk of atherosclerosis and other heart-related conditions.

As men age, the focus shifts towards longevity and preventive care. The alkaline lifestyle is inherently aligned with these goals. Rich in antioxidants, alkaline foods combat oxidative stress, one of the primary factors in aging. Additionally, the anti-inflammatory nature of the diet helps prevent chronic conditions that are more prevalent in older age, such as arthritis and diabetes.

The Athletic Angle: Performance and Recovery

For those engaged in athletic pursuits or intense physical work, nutrition is the cornerstone of performance and recovery. The alkaline diet provides a balanced array of nutrients that aid in muscle repair, reduce inflammation, and improve endurance. It's not just about what you eat before or after a workout; it's about consistently fueling your body with the right nutrients to perform at its best.

In summary, the unique nutritional needs of men are multi-faceted, influenced by biological factors, lifestyle choices, and even societal expectations. The alkaline approach offers a holistic, adaptable framework that addresses these needs comprehensively, setting the stage for a life of strength, vitality, and well-being.

The Legacy of Well-Being: Passing It On

As we've explored the various facets of men's unique nutritional needs, it's crucial to remember that each man's journey is his own. The alkaline lifestyle isn't a one-size-fits-all solution but rather a framework that can be adapted to meet individual needs. The first step in this journey is self-discovery. Understanding your body's specific requirements is essential for tailoring an alkaline diet that works for you. This involves not just a keen awareness of your physical state but also an emotional and mental inventory. Are you stressed? Do you feel fatigued? These are signs that your body is telling you something, and the alkaline lifestyle offers tools to listen and act.

One of the most empowering aspects of adopting an alkaline lifestyle is the power of choice it affords. Every meal becomes an opportunity to nourish your body and mind. When you choose alkaline-rich foods, you're not just eating; you're making a conscious decision to improve your health. This sense of agency is particularly important for men, who often face societal pressures to conform to certain dietary norms, like excessive meat consumption. The alkaline diet liberates you from these constraints, allowing you to make choices that align with your unique nutritional needs and ethical values.

While the primary focus of this chapter has been on nutrition, it's essential to recognize that the benefits of an alkaline lifestyle extend far beyond physical well-being. The foods you eat have a direct impact on your mental and emotional health. As you nourish your body with alkaline foods, you'll likely notice an improvement in your mental clarity, emotional stability, and overall mood. This is not a coincidence; it's a testament to the interconnectedness of human health. When you take care of one aspect of your well-being, the effects ripple out, enhancing every facet of your life.

Embarking on an alkaline lifestyle doesn't have to be a solitary endeavor. In fact, one of the most enriching aspects of this journey is the community you build along the way. Whether it's sharing recipes, discussing challenges, or celebrating milestones, the collective wisdom and support of a like-minded community can be invaluable. For men, who often find it difficult to discuss health issues openly, this sense of community can be particularly empowering. It creates a safe space to share, learn, and grow, breaking down the barriers that often hinder men from taking proactive steps in their health.

The Final Word: Your Health, Your Responsibility

Adopting an alkaline lifestyle is not a temporary fix but a lifelong commitment. As you age, your nutritional needs will evolve, and the beauty of the alkaline diet is its adaptability. Whether you're an athlete looking to optimize performance or entering the golden years and focusing on longevity, the principles of alkaline living can be adapted to meet your changing needs. This adaptability makes it a sustainable choice, one that you can commit to for the long haul.

Your journey towards optimal health doesn't just benefit you; it also sets a precedent for those around you. Whether it's your family, friends, or even your community, your choices can inspire others to take control of their health. For men, this is an opportunity to redefine what it means to be strong. Strength isn't just physical prowess; it's also the courage to make choices that defy societal norms but enrich your life in meaningful ways. By embracing the alkaline lifestyle, you're not just improving your health; you're also contributing to a broader cultural shift towards holistic well-being.

In conclusion, the unique nutritional needs of men are complex, influenced by a myriad of factors from biology to lifestyle to societal expectations. However, the alkaline approach offers a holistic, adaptable, and deeply empowering pathway to address these needs. It's a lifestyle that respects the individuality of each man, offering the tools to create a personalized health plan. But ultimately, the responsibility lies with you. Your health is your most valuable asset, and the choices you make today will shape your quality of life for years to come. So take that step, embrace the alkaline lifestyle, and embark on a journey towards a healthier, happier, and more fulfilling life.

Fitness and Muscle Building in Alkalinity

The Quest for Physical Excellence: A Universal Desire

The pursuit of physical fitness is as old as humanity itself. From the ancient Greeks' admiration of the athletic form to our modern-day obsession with gyms and fitness influencers, the quest for physical excellence remains a universal desire. Yet, in this age of information overload, the path to achieving this excellence has become increasingly muddled. Diets, workout plans, and supplements abound, each promising miraculous result. But what if the secret to optimal fitness isn't found in a protein shake or an intricate workout routine? What if it's found in the very foundation of our biological makeup—our body's pH level? Welcome to the transformative world of fitness and muscle building in alkalinity.

The concept of alkalinity isn't new, but its application in the realm of physical fitness is groundbreaking. The alkaline lifestyle, rooted in maintaining a balanced body pH, offers a fresh perspective on achieving and sustaining physical excellence. Unlike conventional fitness approaches that focus solely on external factors like exercise and diet, the alkaline approach delves deeper. It considers the internal environment of the body, aiming to create a physiological state where optimal fitness isn't just possible; it's inevitable.

The Body as a Temple: Respecting Its Natural Balance

Think of your body as a finely tuned machine or, if you prefer, a sacred temple. Either way, it operates best when it's in a state of equilibrium. An alkaline body is a balanced body, and a balanced body is more receptive to the benefits of physical exercise. It's a body where muscle recovery is expedited, energy levels are consistently high, and the risk of injury is minimized. In essence, when you align your fitness goals with the principles of alkalinity, you're not just building muscle; you're building a resilient, efficient, and harmonious system.

Fitness isn't merely a physical endeavor; it's a mental one as well. The alkaline lifestyle recognizes this intricate mind-muscle connection. When your body is in an alkaline state, your mind experiences greater clarity, focus, and resilience. These mental attributes are invaluable when it comes to physical training. They enable you to push through barriers, whether it's lifting heavier weights, running longer distances, or mastering complex yoga poses. The alkaline approach, therefore, offers a holistic path to fitness—one that harmonizes the mind and body, propelling you towards your peak physical potential.

The relationship between alkalinity and fitness is symbiotic. Just as an alkaline body enhances your fitness efforts, regular exercise contributes to maintaining an alkaline state. Physical activity encourages the efficient elimination of acidic waste products, further stabilizing your body's pH levels. This creates a virtuous cycle where your fitness activities and your alkaline lifestyle mutually reinforce each other, leading to sustainable and long-lasting results.

Adopting an alkaline approach to fitness requires a lifestyle shift, a commitment to a new way of living that goes beyond the gym. It's about making conscious choices every day—what you eat, how you manage stress, even how you breathe. These choices collectively contribute to either an acidic or an alkaline state. By consistently choosing alkalinity, you're laying a robust foundation upon which your fitness goals can flourish.

The Journey Ahead: A Path Less Traveled

As we delve deeper into this chapter, we'll explore the practical aspects of integrating alkalinity into your fitness regimen. From alkaline-rich foods that fuel your workouts to the types of exercise that complement an alkaline lifestyle, we'll provide a comprehensive guide to this revolutionary approach to fitness.

In conclusion, fitness and muscle building in alkalinity offer a holistic, sustainable, and deeply empowering pathway to physical excellence. It's a path less traveled but one that promises not just a well-sculpted body but a balanced, vibrant, and harmonious life. So, are you ready to embark on this transformative journey? The road to your best self-starts here.

The Physiology of Alkalinity: A Catalyst for Change

The human body is a complex biochemical machine, and like any machine, it has optimal operating conditions. One of these conditions is the body's pH level, a measure of its acidity or alkalinity. When we talk about fitness and muscle building in the context of alkalinity, we're essentially discussing the body's internal environment. A balanced pH level enhances cellular function, improves nutrient absorption, and optimizes energy production. These are the building blocks of physical fitness, and they set the stage for a more effective and efficient workout regimen.

The Alkaline Diet: Fueling the Fire Within

Nutrition is the cornerstone of any fitness journey, and it takes on a whole new dimension in an alkaline lifestyle. The alkaline diet emphasizes foods that are rich in minerals like potassium, magnesium, and calcium, which help to neutralize excess acidity in the body. These are the foods that not only nourish you but also prepare your body for the rigors of physical exercise. Think leafy greens, fresh fruits, nuts, and legumes—natural foods that are high in nutritional value and low in acidic residue. When your diet aligns with your body's natural state, you're not just eating; you're fueling your very life force, your vitality.

Exercise Selection: The Alkaline Way

Not all exercises are created equal, especially when viewed through the lens of alkalinity. Aerobic exercises like running, swimming, and cycling are excellent for cardiovascular health, but they also produce lactic acid, which can tip the body's pH balance toward acidity. On the other hand, resistance training, particularly weightlifting, has been shown to have a less acidic impact on the body. The key is balance. A well-rounded fitness routine that incorporates both aerobic and anaerobic exercises is ideal for maintaining an alkaline state. It's not about avoiding certain activities; it's about creating a harmonious blend that serves your body's needs.

The Recovery Equation: Rest, Rejuvenate, Rebuild

In the world of fitness, recovery is often the unsung hero. It's during these periods of rest that your muscles repair themselves, growing stronger in the process. An alkaline body expedites this recovery process. When your internal environment is balanced, inflammation is reduced, and nutrient absorption is optimized, creating the perfect conditions for muscle growth and repair. This is where the alkaline lifestyle shines, turning what is often a sore, sluggish post-workout phase into a period of rejuvenation and growth.

Stress Management: The Missing Link

Stress is an unavoidable aspect of modern life, and it has a tangible impact on your body's pH levels. Stress triggers the release of cortisol, a hormone that, among other things, can lead to a more acidic internal environment. Managing stress, therefore, is crucial for maintaining an alkaline state and, by extension, optimizing your fitness results. Techniques like mindfulness, deep-breathing exercises, and even short meditative breaks can go a long way in mitigating the effects of stress, keeping you on track in your alkaline fitness journey.

The Mindset Shift: From Routine to Ritual

One of the most transformative aspects of integrating alkalinity into your fitness regimen is the shift in mindset it necessitates. This isn't just about changing your diet or tweaking your workout routine; it's about adopting a new way of life. Your exercise sessions are no longer just routines; they become rituals—sacred practices that nourish not just your body but also your soul. This holistic approach transcends the physical, touching every aspect of your being and elevating your fitness journey into a quest for overall well-being.

While the alkaline lifestyle is a deeply personal journey, it doesn't have to be a solitary one. There's immense value in community—a collective of like-minded individuals who share your goals, understand your challenges, and celebrate your victories. Whether it's a local alkaline-focused fitness group or an online forum, finding your tribe can provide that extra layer of motivation and accountability that turns good habits into lifelong practices.

Fitness is not a destination; it's a journey, a lifelong commitment to self-improvement. The beauty of an alkaline approach to fitness is its sustainability. This isn't a quick fix or a seasonal diet; it's a way of life. And like any meaningful journey, it evolves. As you delve deeper into the nuances of alkaline living, you'll discover new foods, exercises, and stress-management techniques that resonate with you, allowing your fitness regimen to grow and evolve with you.

In sum, the concept of fitness and muscle building in alkalinity offers a holistic, multi-dimensional approach to physical well-being. It's a paradigm shift those challenges conventional wisdom, urging us to look inward, to understand our bodies at a cellular level, and to align our fitness goals with our body's natural state. The result is a more balanced, harmonious, and ultimately, a more effective path to physical excellence.

In Conclusion: The Future is Alkaline

As we've journeyed through the intricate relationship between alkalinity and fitness, we've discovered that this isn't just another health fad. It's a revolutionary approach that combines ancient wisdom with modern science. We've explored how an alkaline diet fuels your body's natural vitality, how exercise selection can be optimized for alkalinity, and how stress management and community support play pivotal roles in this holistic lifestyle. Now, let's bring it all together and look at the bigger picture.

The benefits of an alkaline approach to fitness and muscle building extend far beyond the gym. When your body is in a state of alkalinity, you're not just physically stronger; you're also mentally sharper and emotionally more resilient. This has a ripple effect on every aspect of your life. You'll find that you're more focused at work, more present in your relationships, and more engaged with the world around you. You'll discover a newfound sense of vitality that permeates through your daily life, turning mundane tasks into opportunities for growth and self-improvement.

One of the most profound aspects of adopting an alkaline lifestyle is the journey of self-discovery it initiates. As you delve deeper into this way of life, you'll start to uncover layers of yourself that you never knew existed. You'll begin to understand your body's unique needs and rhythms, and how to nourish them in a way that aligns with your natural state. This is not just a physical transformation; it's a spiritual awakening. It's about reconnecting with your true self and rediscovering what it means to live a life of purpose and meaning.

The Ethical Dimension: A Commitment to a Better World

An often-overlooked aspect of the alkaline lifestyle is its ethical dimension. By choosing natural, organic foods and sustainable practices, you're not just improving your own health; you're also contributing to a more ethical and sustainable world. It's a win-win situation where your personal gains are also gains for the planet. This adds an extra layer of fulfillment to your fitness journey, knowing that your actions are aligned with a greater good.

As you experience the transformative power of an alkaline approach to fitness, you'll naturally feel compelled to share it with others. Whether it's through social media, community workshops, or simply word of mouth, spreading the word is an integral part of this journey. You become a torchbearer, passing on the knowledge and wisdom you've gained to help others embark on their own journeys of self-discovery and transformation. In doing so, you're not just leaving a legacy; you're creating a movement.

The Road Ahead: A Lifelong Commitment

It's important to remember that fitness is not a destination; it's a lifelong journey. And like any journey, there will be ups and downs, challenges and triumphs. But what sets the alkaline lifestyle apart is its sustainability. It's not a quick fix or a temporary solution; it's a long-term commitment to your well-being. As you continue to evolve and grow, so will your understanding of what it means to live an alkaline life. It's a dynamic, ever-evolving process that keeps you engaged, inspired, and most importantly, empowered.

As we close this chapter on fitness and muscle building in alkalinity, let's take a moment to envision the future. Imagine a world where the principles of alkalinity are not just an alternative but the norm. A world where people are not just surviving but thriving, living their fullest lives in complete harmony with their natural state. This is not a utopian dream; it's a very achievable reality. And it starts with you. By embracing the alkaline lifestyle, you're taking the first step toward creating a healthier, happier, and more harmonious world for all.

So, as you step out of this chapter and into the world, carry with you the wisdom, insights, and inspirations you've gained. Let them guide you, empower you, and most importantly, let them transform you. Because the future is not just alkaline; the future is you.

Addressing Common Male Health Concerns

The Masculine Paradox: Strength vs. Vulnerability

In a society that often equates masculinity with stoicism, the subject of men's health has long been shrouded in silence. This silence is not just a social construct; it's a crisis. It's a crisis that affects fathers, brothers, and sons, often leaving them to navigate the complex landscape of health concerns alone. But here, in this sanctuary of wisdom and understanding, we break that silence. We delve into the common health concerns that plague men, not as an academic exercise, but as a crucial, life-altering dialogue.

The notion of masculinity is often tied to images of strength and invincibility. While these traits are admirable, they can also be a double-edged sword. On one hand, they inspire men to be protectors and providers, roles that are deeply ingrained in our cultural psyche. On the other hand, they create an internal conflict when men face health issues that make them feel vulnerable. This paradox often leads to avoidance, where health concerns are brushed under the rug, leading to more severe problems down the line.

The Alkaline Connection: A New Lens to View Men's Health

As we've explored in previous chapters, the alkaline lifestyle offers a holistic approach to well-being. But what does it specifically offer to men grappling with health issues? The answer lies in the interconnectedness of our bodily systems. An alkaline body is like a well-oiled machine, where each part functions in harmony with the others. This is particularly beneficial for men, who often face health concerns that are systemic rather than isolated. Conditions like heart disease, prostate issues, and high blood pressure are not just 'part' problems; they are 'whole' problems that require a holistic solution.

You've probably heard the term "mind-body connection" thrown around in wellness circles. While it may sound like a trendy catchphrase, its implications are profound, especially for men. Stress, anxiety, and depression are not just mental health issues; they manifest physically in the form of high blood pressure, digestive issues, and even chronic pain. The alkaline lifestyle, with its focus on mental clarity and emotional balance, offers men a way to address these interconnected issues in a unified manner.

The Social Dimension: Why Community Matters

Men are often conditioned to be lone wolves, to solve their problems independently. But health is not a solitary journey; it's a communal one. The support of a like-minded community can be a game-changer in addressing common male health concerns. Whether it's sharing experiences, offering advice, or simply providing a listening ear, the value of a supportive community cannot be overstated. It's not just about physical health; it's about emotional well-being, which is equally crucial in the grand scheme of men's health.

When men take proactive steps to address their health concerns, the impact reverberates through generations. It sets a precedent for younger men and boys in the family, teaching them the importance of health awareness and preventive care. This is not just a gift to oneself but a legacy of wellness for future generations. It's about changing the narrative from one of neglect to one of proactive care, from silence to dialogue, from crisis to prevention.

In Summary: A Call to Action

Addressing common male health concerns requires courage. It requires the courage to challenge societal norms, to confront one's vulnerabilities, and to take proactive steps towards better health. But this courage does not have to be a solitary endeavor. With the guidance of the alkaline lifestyle and the support of a community, men can navigate this road less traveled with confidence and resilience. As we embark on this enlightening journey through the labyrinth of men's health, let this chapter serve as a call to action. A call to break the silence, to challenge the stereotypes, and to embrace a holistic approach to well-being. It's not just about adding years to your life; it's about adding life to your years. It's about living not just as the men that society expects us to be, but as the men we are destined to be—healthy, balanced, and vibrantly alive.

So, let's take this journey together, step by step, with open minds and compassionate hearts. Let's redefine what it means to be strong, not just in body, but in spirit. Because true strength lies not in silence, but in the courage to speak, to act, and to heal.

The Cardiovascular Conundrum: More Than Just a Pump

When we talk about men's health, the conversation often gravitates towards cardiovascular issues. It's not just about the heart as an organ, but the heart as a metaphorical representation of a man's overall health. The cardiovascular system is like the highway of the body, and when there's a roadblock, everything comes to a screeching halt. High blood pressure, cholesterol, and arterial plaque are not merely numbers on a medical chart; they are signposts pointing to deeper, systemic issues. The alkaline lifestyle, rich in plant-based foods and low in processed items, offers a way to keep this highway clear and functional.

The Prostate Puzzle: A Silent Concern

Prostate health is often a taboo subject, discussed in hushed tones and veiled references. Yet, it's a concern that affects a significant number of men, especially as they age. The prostate is not just another gland; it's an integral part of the male reproductive system and urinary function. Issues like enlarged prostate or prostatitis can severely impact a man's quality of life. Here, the alkaline lifestyle comes to the rescue again, offering anti-inflammatory foods and herbs that can help maintain prostate health without the side effects of conventional treatments.

The Testosterone Tug-of-War: The Hormonal Balancing Act

Testosterone is often dubbed the "male hormone," responsible for everything from muscle mass to libido. But it's not just about physical attributes; testosterone plays a role in mood regulation, energy levels, and even cognitive function. A decline in testosterone can lead to a range of issues, from fatigue and weight gain to decreased sexual drive. The alkaline lifestyle, with its focus on nutrient-dense foods and natural supplements, can help balance these hormonal levels, offering men a holistic approach to managing this crucial aspect of their health.

The Weighty Issue: Obesity and Its Ripple Effects

Weight management is not just a cosmetic concern; it's a health imperative. Obesity is a ticking time bomb that sets off a chain reaction of health issues, from diabetes and heart disease to joint problems and sleep apnea. The alkaline lifestyle offers a sustainable way to manage weight, focusing on nourishment rather than deprivation. It's not about counting calories; it's about making each calorie count. It's about choosing foods that not only fill your stomach but also nourish your soul.

The Mental Maze: Stress, Anxiety, and Their Physical Manifestations

We've already touched upon the mind-body link, but it's worth reiterating how stress and anxiety can manifest physically. In men, chronic stress can lead to digestive issues, insomnia, and even sexual dysfunction. The alkaline lifestyle, with its emphasis on mindfulness and emotional balance, offers tools to manage this stress. Techniques like deep breathing, meditation, and even simple walks in nature can help reset the mental equilibrium, leading to better physical health.

The Sleep Paradox: Rest vs. Restlessness

Sleep is often the first casualty in a busy, high-stress lifestyle. Yet, it's one of the most crucial factors in maintaining optimal health. Lack of sleep can lead to a host of issues, from impaired cognitive function and mood swings to serious health conditions like heart disease and diabetes. The alkaline lifestyle encourages a balanced approach to life, including the importance of restful sleep. Foods rich in magnesium and herbal teas like chamomile can aid in better sleep, offering a natural alternative to over-the-counter sleep aids.

The Activity Equation: Movement as Medicine

Physical activity is not just about building muscles or achieving an aesthetic goal; it's about maintaining a state of overall well-being. Exercise has been shown to improve mood, boost the immune system, and even enhance cognitive function. The alkaline lifestyle doesn't prescribe a one-size-fits-all exercise regimen; it encourages movement that brings joy and vitality, whether it's a brisk walk, a yoga session, or even a dance class.

As we navigate through the intricate maze of men's health, it becomes evident that these issues are not isolated; they are interconnected. They are pieces of a larger puzzle that make up the complex entity known as 'man.' The alkaline lifestyle offers a holistic lens to view this puzzle, not as a series of disjointed pieces but as a cohesive whole. It's about understanding that the heart, the prostate, the hormones, the mind, and even the soul are part of this intricate web, and they all deserve equal attention and care.

So, as we journey deeper into the realm of men's health, let's carry this holistic perspective with us. Let's understand that addressing common male health concerns is not just about treating symptoms; it's about understanding the root causes and tackling them head-on. It's about empowering men to take charge of their health, to break free from societal norms, and to live a life that is not just long, but also deeply fulfilling.

As we reach the conclusion of this pivotal chapter on men's health, it's essential to recognize the power of choice. The choices you make today, from the foods you eat to the lifestyle you lead, have a profound impact on your future well-being. You're not just a passive recipient of healthcare; you're an active participant in shaping your health narrative. The alkaline lifestyle offers you a toolbox filled with holistic solutions, empowering you to take control of your health journey.

The Alkaline Advantage: A Sustainable Path to Wellness

The beauty of the alkaline lifestyle lies in its sustainability. It's not a quick fix or a fad diet; it's a lifelong commitment to wellness. It's about making conscious choices that align with your health goals, whether it's cardiovascular health, hormonal balance, or mental well-being. The alkaline lifestyle doesn't just offer a Band-Aid solution; it addresses the root causes of common male health concerns, providing a comprehensive approach to holistic well-being.

Your health choices don't just affect you; they have a ripple effect on your family, your community, and even society at large. When you prioritize your well-being, you're setting a positive example for those around you. You're contributing to a culture of health-consciousness, breaking the cycle of chronic illnesses that plague our society. Your individual health journey can inspire collective change, making the world a healthier place for future generations.

Throughout this chapter, we've emphasized the interconnectedness of physical and mental health. They're not separate entities but two sides of the same coin. Your mental state can influence your physical well-being, and vice versa. The alkaline lifestyle recognizes this intricate relationship, offering holistic solutions that cater to both your body and mind. It's not just about eating the right foods or doing the right exercises; it's about achieving a state of mental and emotional equilibrium that complements your physical wellness.

The Legacy of Dr. Sebi: A Testament to Natural Healing

Embarking on a health journey can be a daunting task, but you don't have to go it alone. The alkaline community offers a supportive network of like-minded individuals who share your commitment to holistic well-being. Whether it's sharing recipes, discussing herbal remedies, or offering emotional support, the community serves as a valuable resource in your health journey. Your part of a larger movement, a collective endeavor to redefine the standards of male health.

While we've focused on the practical aspects of men's health, it's crucial to acknowledge the philosophical underpinnings of the alkaline lifestyle. Dr. Sebi's teachings serve as a testament to the power of natural healing, challenging the conventional medical paradigm that often focuses on symptom management rather than root cause resolution. His legacy serves as a guiding light, illuminating the path to holistic wellness.

The Future is Now: A Call to Action

As we wrap up this chapter, let's not forget that the future starts now. Every choice you make, every step you take, shapes your health trajectory. The alkaline lifestyle offers you a roadmap, a guide to navigate the complex landscape of men's health. But ultimately, the journey is yours to make. It's a call to action, an invitation to take charge of your well-being, to redefine the narrative of male health for yourself and for generations to come.

Addressing common male health concerns is not a destination; it's an ongoing journey. It's a commitment to continuous learning, to adapting and evolving as new challenges arise. The alkaline lifestyle equips you with the knowledge and tools to navigate these challenges, to turn obstacles into opportunities for growth and transformation. So, as you close this chapter, remember that it's not the end; it's just the beginning of a lifelong journey towards holistic wellness. And in this journey, you're not just a passenger; you're the captain steering the ship towards uncharted waters, towards a future filled with health, vitality, and boundless possibilities.

Book 11: Alkaline Family – Raising the Next Generation

Introducing Children to Alkaline Foods

The Weight of Responsibility and the Lightness of Love

Welcome to a chapter that holds the future—quite literally. If you're reading this, chances are you're already well-versed in the benefits of an alkaline lifestyle for adults. But what about the youngest members of our families? How do we ensure that our children, the next generation, are set on a path of holistic well-being from the get-go? The family table is more than a place to eat; it's a classroom where lifelong habits are formed. It's where children first encounter the flavors, textures, and rituals that will shape their relationship with food for years to come.

As parents, guardians, or caregivers, the responsibility of shaping a child's palate and, consequently, their health, can feel overwhelming. But let's reframe that weight as an opportunity—an opportunity to instill values of health, vitality, and conscious living from a tender age. This isn't just about avoiding the pitfalls of a fast-food culture; it's about sowing the seeds of a lifestyle that reveres the natural, the wholesome, and the sustainable. It's about teaching our children to make choices that honor not just their bodies, but also the planet they inhabit.

Introducing children to alkaline foods is not merely a dietary choice; it's a foundational life skill. Just as we teach our kids to read, write, and calculate, we must also equip them with the nutritional literacy to navigate a world teeming with dietary landmines. The alkaline diet offers a robust framework for this education. Rich in fruits, vegetables, nuts, and legumes, it's a diet that supports not just physical growth but also cognitive development and emotional well-being.

The Taste Bud Challenge: Making Alkaline Foods Kid-Friendly

Let's address the elephant in the room: How do you make alkaline foods appealing to a demographic that's notoriously picky and often resistant to anything green on their plate? The answer lies in creativity and, yes, a bit of culinary sleight of hand. Think alkaline smoothies disguised as milkshakes, or zucchini noodles masquerading as spaghetti. The goal is not to trick children but to present alkaline foods in a way that resonates with their natural curiosity and sense of adventure.

Children thrive on routine. The predictability of a ritual—be it a bedtime story or a family meal—offers them a sense of security in a world that's constantly changing. Incorporating alkaline foods into these rituals can normalize them, making them a regular and expected part of a child's life. Whether it's a Saturday morning spent making alkaline pancakes or a Sunday afternoon dedicated to prepping veggies for the week, these rituals become the scaffolding upon which a lifetime of healthy eating habits can be built.

The Community Connection: It Takes a Village

While the family unit is the cornerstone of a child's nutritional education, the community plays a crucial role too. Schools, recreational centers, and even places of worship can be allies in your quest to raise an alkaline-friendly child. Advocacy and education are key here. The more we normalize alkaline eating within our communities, the easier it becomes for our children to make healthy choices outside the home.

Food is not just fuel; it's a language of love, care, and connection. When we introduce our children to alkaline foods, we're not just nourishing their bodies; we're also feeding their souls. We're teaching them to associate love and comfort with foods that heal rather than harm. This emotional imprinting can be as impactful as any nutritional fact or figure.

The Journey Begins: Your Role in a Generational Shift

As we delve deeper into the practicalities and strategies for introducing children to alkaline foods, remember that your part of a generational shift. You're at the forefront of a movement that's redefining health, not just for individuals but for society at large. And it starts with the smallest, most impressionable members of our community—our children.

So, as we embark on this enlightening journey, let's not underestimate the power of the family table, the impact of community, and the indelible mark of early emotional experiences. Let's commit to raising a generation that's not just well-fed but well-nourished, in body, mind, and spirit.

The Art of Subtle Introduction

The first step in introducing alkaline foods to children is to do it subtly. Kids are keen observers, and a sudden overhaul of their favorite meals might meet with resistance. Instead, consider a gradual approach. For instance, if your child loves mashed potatoes, try incorporating some cauliflower into the mash. Over time, you can adjust the ratio until it becomes a full-fledged cauliflower mash. The key is to make the transition so smooth that your child hardly notices the change.

The Importance of Choice and Autonomy

Children, like adults, want to feel in control of their lives, and that extends to their food choices. One effective strategy is to involve them in the grocery shopping process. Let them pick out a new vegetable or fruit they'd like to try. This sense of ownership can make them more open to tasting new alkaline foods. It's not just about telling them what's good for them; it's about empowering them to discover it for themselves.

The Power of Presentation

Never underestimate the power of a well-plated meal. Children are visual creatures, and an appealing presentation can make all the difference. Use vibrant colors, interesting shapes, and even fun dishware to make the alkaline foods more enticing. For example, you could use a cookie cutter to make star-shaped slices of watermelon or arrange a variety of colorful veggies into a rainbow on their plate. The goal is to make the experience of eating alkaline foods as enjoyable as possible.

The Role of Storytelling

Children love stories, and this can be a powerful tool in your alkaline introduction arsenal. Create engaging narratives around the food. Maybe the broccoli florets are trees in a magical forest, or the almond milk is a special potion that grants super strength. The more imaginative and engaging the story, the more likely your child will be to try the food.

Consider creating a "Taste Tester Club" within your family where everyone gets to try a new alkaline food each week and vote on whether it should become a regular part of your meals. This not only makes trying new foods fun but also gives everyone in the family a voice in their dietary choices.

Pairing unfamiliar alkaline foods with familiar favorites can be a winning strategy. If your child loves pasta, for example, try serving it with an alkaline-friendly tomato sauce loaded with veggies. The familiar taste of the pasta can make the unfamiliar vegetables more palatable. Over time, you can introduce alkaline-compliant pasta alternatives like chickpea pasta or spiralized zucchini.

The Value of Repetition

It's common for children to be hesitant about trying new foods. Sometimes, it takes multiple exposures to a new food before a child will accept it. Don't be discouraged if your child turns up their nose the first time, they try quinoa. Keep offering it in different preparations, and over time, their taste buds may adjust.

The Emotional Safety Net

It's important to create an emotionally safe environment around mealtime. Children should never be forced or coerced into eating something they don't want to. Instead, encourage them to take a "no-thank-you bite"—one small bite to try, and if they don't like it, that's okay. This takes the pressure off and makes them more willing to experiment.

Remember, the habits you're instilling now will serve your children for the rest of their lives. You're not just getting them to eat their greens; you're laying the foundation for a lifetime of healthy eating choices. You're teaching them to listen to their bodies, to make informed decisions, and to treat themselves with the love and respect they deserve.

As you successfully introduce alkaline foods to your children, you'll likely find that it has a ripple effect on your entire family, your community, and even your children's future families. You're not just raising a child; you're raising a future adult, a future parent, a future influencer in their own right.

In the grand tapestry of life, these threads—these daily choices and experiences—create a pattern of health, vitality, and conscious living. And it all starts with that first, brave bite of something new. So go ahead, take the plunge into the alkaline lifestyle with your children. The rewards will be richer than you can imagine.

The family table as a classroom

The family table is not just a place to eat: it is a classroom where life lessons are taught. When you introduce alkaline foods to your children, you are not only teaching them how to eat healthy, you are imparting values to them. Teach them the importance of making choices that honor not only their bodies but also the world around them. Alkaline foods are often more sustainable and environmentally friendly, so the teaching goes beyond personal well-being and includes a broader ethical stance.

Children are natural evangelizers. When they discover something, they love, they talk about it, share it and make it part of their identity. Imagine the ripple effect when your child, fueled by the energy and vitality that comes from a balanced, alkaline diet, becomes a beacon of health among his or her peers. They may inspire friends to try new foods or even influence their school's menu. The impact on the community can be profound, reversing the trend toward a more health-conscious and alkaline society.

The legacy of lifelong health

We often focus on the physical benefits of a healthy diet, but the emotional and psychological benefits are equally significant. Children who eat well are more likely to perform well in school, concentrate better, and have more stable emotional lives. The alkaline lifestyle is not only about the foods we eat, but also about creating a holistic environment in which our children can thrive emotionally, psychologically and physically.

As parents, we are not only raising children, but also future adults. The habits we inculcate in them today will shape their choices in adulthood. By introducing children to alkaline foods from an early age, we set them on the path to lifelong health. We reduce their risk of chronic disease, improve their quality of life and increase their potential lifespan. This is a legacy that will extend to their children, creating a cycle of health that will benefit generations to come.

Food is deeply linked to our sense of celebration and ritual. By incorporating alkaline foods into family celebrations, we can create new traditions that honor both our health and our sense of joy and community. Imagine a Thanksgiving feast with alkaline dishes, or a Fourth of July barbecue with alkaline options. These events become opportunities to celebrate our commitment to health, to share it with extended family and friends, and to create lasting memories anchored in wellness.

Life is unpredictable, and our ability to adapt is one of our greatest strengths. The same is true for diet. There will be times when sticking to an alkaline diet will be a challenge. Travel, social events or simply the chaos of life can upset our best laid plans. Teaching our children, the alkaline lifestyle also means teaching them how to adapt, how to make the best choices in every situation, and how to return to balance when life throws them off track.

The gift of empowerment

When we educate our children about the benefits of alkaline foods, we don't just give them a lesson in nutrition; we empower them. We provide them with the tools they need to take control of their own health, to question traditional dietary advice, and to make choices in line with their own well-being. This is empowerment in its truest form and is one of the most valuable gifts we can give our children.

Introducing alkaline foods to your children is not a one-time event, but a lifelong journey. It is a commitment to continually learn, adapt and grow. It is an invitation to your children to join you on a journey that leads not only to better health, but to a better way of living and being in the world.

As you close this point and move on to the next steps of your alkaline journey, remember that every step you take, no matter how small, is a step toward a brighter and healthier future, for you, for your children and for the generations to follow. This is the very essence of raising the next generation in an alkaline family, and the impact is immeasurable. It is a legacy of health, power and conscious living that will echo through the centuries. And it all starts with this first, simple step: introducing your children to the vital world of alkaline foods.

Crafting Family-Friendly Alkaline Meals
The Heart of a Healthy Home

The kitchen is often considered the heart of the home. It's where families gather, not just to eat, but to connect, share, and create memories. The act of preparing a meal is more than just a daily chore; it's a form of expression, a manifestation of love and care. When you bring the principles of alkaline eating into your kitchen, you're not just making a dietary change; you're transforming this central space into a sanctuary of health and well-being.

Crafting family-friendly alkaline meals is an art that goes beyond following recipes. It's about understanding the unique tastes and preferences of each family member and finding a way to incorporate alkaline foods in a manner that is both delicious and nutritious. It's about taking traditional family favorites and giving them an alkaline twist. Imagine a pizza night where the crust is made from spelt flour, the sauce is a lush blend of alkaline-friendly tomatoes and herbs, and the toppings are an array of colorful vegetables. Or envision a Sunday morning where pancakes are made from amaranth flour, sweetened with agave nectar, and served with a side of fresh fruit. The possibilities are endless, and the joy of discovery makes the journey incredibly rewarding.

One of the key aspects of crafting family-friendly alkaline meals is the principle of inclusion. It's not about taking things away; it's about adding more of what's good for you. Instead of focusing on what you can't have, focus on the abundance of delicious foods that are also incredibly good for you. This shift in perspective is crucial, especially for children who might be resistant to change. When they see a table full of colorful, delicious foods, the sense of deprivation vanishes, replaced by a sense of excitement and curiosity.

The Power of Meal Planning

Creativity is your best friend when it comes to alkaline cooking. Don't be afraid to experiment with new ingredients, flavors, and cooking methods. Use spices liberally to add flavor and depth to your dishes. Try different cooking techniques like roasting, steaming, or sautéing to bring out the natural flavors of alkaline foods. The more you experiment, the more you'll discover the incredible versatility and deliciousness of alkaline ingredients.

Meal planning plays a crucial role in successfully crafting family-friendly alkaline meals. It's the roadmap that guides your culinary journey. A well-thought-out meal plan takes into account the nutritional needs of each family member, the time constraints of your busy lifestyle, and the practical aspects of meal preparation. It's the key to making alkaline eating sustainable and enjoyable in the long run.

Cooking shouldn't be a solitary task relegated to one family member. Make it a family affair. Involve your children in the meal preparation process. Let them wash the vegetables, stir the pot, or even chop ingredients if they're old enough. This shared experience not only lightens the workload but also serves as an educational opportunity. It's a hands-on way for children to learn about nutrition, develop cooking skills, and appreciate the value of homemade meals.

Food is not just fuel; it's an emotional experience. The meals we share as a family create lasting memories and traditions. By crafting alkaline meals that are not just healthy but also delicious and visually appealing, you're creating a positive emotional association with nutritious food. This emotional connection is what will sustain your family's alkaline journey in the long run.

The First Step in a Lifelong Journey

Crafting family-friendly alkaline meals is the first step in a lifelong journey toward optimal health and well-being. It's a commitment that requires effort, creativity, and a dash of love. But the rewards are immeasurable. You're not just nourishing bodies; you're nourishing souls. You're not just changing a diet; you're transforming a lifestyle. And most importantly, you're setting the foundation for a legacy of health that will benefit your family for generations to come.

As you delve deeper into this chapter, keep in mind that the art of crafting alkaline meals is a skill that evolves over time. Each meal you prepare is a learning experience, a stepping stone on your path to mastering the art of alkaline cooking. So, roll up your sleeves, step into your kitchen sanctuary, and let the culinary adventure begin.

The Journey to Nutritional Harmony

Crafting family-friendly alkaline meals is akin to composing a symphony—a harmonious blend of flavors, textures, and colors that resonate with the soul. It's not just about throwing together a few alkaline ingredients and calling it a meal. It's about understanding the nuances of each ingredient, how they interact with each other, and how they can be orchestrated to create a culinary masterpiece that's both pleasing to the palate and beneficial to the body.

The Seasonal Approach

One of the most enriching aspects of alkaline cooking is the opportunity to embrace seasonal produce. Nature, in its infinite wisdom, provides us with fruits and vegetables that are not only abundant but also nutritionally optimal for each season. For instance, the refreshing watermelon in the summer hydrates and cools the body, while the hearty squash in the winter offers sustenance and warmth. By aligning your meal planning with the seasons, you're not just optimizing nutritional value but also supporting local farmers and reducing your carbon footprint.

Alkaline eating doesn't mean you have to give up your cultural heritage or the traditional dishes that have been passed down through generations. It's about adapting and evolving. Take, for example, a classic Italian pasta dish. You can easily substitute the regular pasta with zucchini noodles and create a sauce using alkaline-friendly tomatoes, garlic, and herbs. The essence of the dish remains, but it's now in harmony with your alkaline lifestyle.

The Nutritional Balance

When crafting alkaline meals, it's essential to consider the nutritional balance. A well-rounded meal should provide a good mix of protein, healthy fats, and complex carbohydrates. For protein, think beyond animal products. Quinoa, lentils, and chickpeas are excellent alkaline sources of protein. Healthy fats can be sourced from avocados, olive oil, and nuts. And for complex carbohydrates, look to root vegetables like sweet potatoes and alkaline grains like wild rice.

Eating is a sensory experience that goes beyond taste. The visual appeal of a dish, its aroma, and even its texture plays a crucial role in the overall dining experience. When crafting alkaline meals, take the time to garnish your dishes, play with colors, and create a visual feast that complements the flavors. The olfactory experience can be enhanced with the use of fresh herbs and spices, which not only add aroma but also pack a nutritional punch.

The Joy of Leftovers

In today's fast-paced world, time is a luxury many of us can't afford. But that shouldn't deter you from crafting nutritious alkaline meals. Many alkaline recipes can be made in under 30 minutes, and with a little bit of planning, you can also prepare meals in advance. Slow cookers and pressure cookers can be lifesavers, allowing you to prepare hearty meals with minimal hands-on time.

Don't underestimate the power of leftovers. Many alkaline dishes taste even better the next day, as the flavors have had time to meld. Leftovers can be repurposed in creative ways to make new meals. For instance, last night's vegetable stir-fry can become today's lunch wrap with the addition of some avocado and a spelt tortilla.

The Family Table

The family table is where bonds are strengthened, where conversations flow, and where love is shared. When you bring alkaline meals to this sacred space, you're not just feeding bodies; you're nourishing the soul. You're creating an environment where health and happiness coexist, where each family member feels cared for, and where the foundation for a lifetime of wellness is laid.

Crafting family-friendly alkaline meals is not a trend; it's a lifestyle choice that has far-reaching implications. You're setting a precedent, creating a legacy of health that will be passed down through generations. Your children will grow up with an innate understanding of what it means to nourish their bodies, and they, in turn, will pass this wisdom on to their children.

In essence, crafting family-friendly alkaline meals is a journey—a journey that each family embarks upon together, hand in hand, united in their quest for optimal health and well-being. It's a journey filled with discovery, joy, and above all, love. And it's a journey that promises a destination where the air is purer, the grass is greener, and the future is brighter. So, let's continue this journey, one alkaline meal at a time, savoring each moment and cherishing each bite.

The Art of Mindful Eating

As we draw the curtain on our exploration of crafting family-friendly alkaline meals, it's crucial to recognize that the essence of this journey is not just about food. It's about the alchemy of love and nutrition, a transformative process that turns simple ingredients into nourishing meals and, in turn, creates a sanctuary of health and happiness for the family. It's about the invisible threads of care and intention that weave through each dish, making it more than just a meal—it's a love letter to your family's well-being.

In a world that often feels like it's spinning out of control, the act of sitting down to a family meal can be a grounding experience. It's a moment to pause, to breathe, and to connect. Mindful eating is not just about savoring each bite; it's about appreciating the labor and love that went into the meal. It's about acknowledging the journey each ingredient has taken from the earth to your plate. This mindfulness amplifies the nutritional benefits of the alkaline meal, creating a holistic experience that nourishes the body, mind, and soul.

Crafting family-friendly alkaline meals is also about weaving a tapestry of generational wisdom. It's about taking the culinary traditions passed down through the ages and giving them a modern, alkaline twist. In doing so, you're creating a living legacy, a dynamic tradition that evolves yet remains rooted in its core values of health and well-being. This tapestry becomes a family heirloom, a source of knowledge and inspiration for future generations.

Life is unpredictable. There will be days when things don't go as planned—when work runs late, when traffic is a nightmare, or when you simply don't have the energy to cook. It's in these moments that the resilience of adaptability shines through. The beauty of alkaline cooking lies in its flexibility. With a well-stocked pantry of alkaline staples, you can easily whip up a nutritious meal in no time. Whether it's a simple avocado toast or a quick vegetable stir-fry, the possibilities are endless. The key is to not let perfection be the enemy of good. An imperfect alkaline meal is still better than a fast-food alternative.

Every family is a symphony of unique personalities, preferences, and needs. Crafting family-friendly alkaline meals is about composing a menu that resonates with this diverse ensemble. It's about finding the middle ground where health meets taste, where tradition meets innovation, and where simplicity meets sophistication. It's a delicate balancing act, but one that brings immense satisfaction when achieved.

The choices we make at the family dinner table have a ripple effect that extends far beyond the confines of our home. When you choose to craft alkaline meals, you're making a statement—a statement about the kind of world you want to live in. You're voting for sustainable farming practices, ethical treatment of animals, and responsible stewardship of the earth's resources. You're contributing to a collective shift towards a healthier, more harmonious world.

The Horizon of Lifelong Wellness

As we stand on the horizon of lifelong wellness, it's important to look back and appreciate how far we've come. The journey to crafting family-friendly alkaline meals is filled with trials and triumphs, challenges and celebrations. It's a journey that demands patience, commitment, and above all, love. But it's a journey worth taking, for the destination is a sanctuary of health and happiness.

In conclusion, crafting family-friendly alkaline meals is not a task; it's a privilege. It's an opportunity to express love in its purest form—through the nourishment of the bodies and souls of those we hold dear. It's a symphony of flavors, a tapestry of traditions, and a testament to the resilience and adaptability of the human spirit. Move forward in your alkaline journey, may your kitchen be filled with the aroma of wholesome cooking, may your table be surrounded by the faces of those you love, and may your life be enriched by the joy and wellness that comes from living in harmony with nature's wisdom.

Natural Remedies for Common Childhood Ailments

The Dawn of a Healthier Tomorrow

As we embark on this enlightening journey through the realm of natural remedies for common childhood ailments, let's pause for a moment to acknowledge the sacred trust that is parenthood. It's a role that comes with no instruction manual, yet it's the most consequential job we'll ever have. The health and well-being of our children are not just a responsibility; they are a sacred trust we hold for the future. And in this trust, we find our first and most enduring love—the love for our children.

In recent years, there's been a quiet revolution brewing in the way we approach family health. Gone are the days when a trip to the doctor's office was the first and only option for treating common childhood ailments. Today, more and more parents are turning to natural remedies as a first line of defense. This shift is not a rejection of modern medicine but rather a harmonious blending of ancient wisdom and contemporary science. It's a holistic approach that treats the child as a whole—body, mind, and spirit.

The Wisdom of Our Ancestors and the Alkaline Advantage

Long before the advent of modern medicine, our ancestors had an intimate understanding of the natural world. They knew which plants could heal and which could harm. They understood the rhythms of the body and how to bring it back into balance when it faltered. This wisdom was not just the domain of shamans and herbalists; it was common knowledge passed down through generations. Today, we stand on the shoulders of these giants as we rediscover the healing power of nature.

The alkaline lifestyle offers a unique advantage in this quest for natural remedies. By maintaining a balanced pH level in the body, we create an environment where disease struggles to take hold. This is particularly important for children, whose immune systems are still developing. An alkaline diet rich in fruits, vegetables, and herbs can act as a natural shield, protecting our little ones from common ailments like colds, allergies, and digestive issues.

The Role of Intuition

Nature offers us a symphony of elements, each with its unique properties and potentials. Take, for example, the humble ginger root. This unassuming plant is a powerhouse of anti-inflammatory and antimicrobial properties. A simple ginger tea can work wonders for a sore throat or an upset stomach. Then there's lavender, a fragrant herb known for its calming effects. A few drops of lavender oil in a diffuser can help ease the symptoms of anxiety or insomnia in children. These are not isolated examples but pieces of a larger puzzle that forms the tapestry of natural remedies.

As parents, we are endowed with a powerful tool—our intuition. This innate sense often guides us in moments of uncertainty. When it comes to our children's health, this intuition becomes a beacon, guiding us towards the best course of action. Learning to trust this inner voice is an integral part of embracing natural remedies. It empowers us to become active participants in our children's health, rather than passive recipients of medical advice.

Natural remedies are not just about curing ailments; they are also about preventing them. The concept of "food as medicine" is deeply ingrained in the alkaline lifestyle. Foods like berries, leafy greens, and nuts are not just nutrient-dense; they are also medicinal. Incorporating these foods into your child's diet can act as a preventive measure, reducing the likelihood of common ailments.

As we delve deeper into the world of natural remedies for common childhood ailments, we'll explore a range of options—from herbal teas and tinctures to essential oils and alkaline foods. We'll learn how to prepare these remedies and how to administer them safely. But more importantly, we'll learn how to listen—to our children, to our intuition, and to the wisdom of nature.

In this chapter, we are not just sharing information; we are sharing a philosophy, a way of life that honors the innate wisdom of the body and the healing power of nature. It's a journey that promises not just better health for our children but a deeper, more meaningful connection with the natural world and with ourselves. So, let's take this first step together, hand in hand, as we embark on this transformative journey toward a healthier, happier future for our children.

The Art of Observation

As we delve deeper into the heart of holistic healing for children, it's essential to recognize that natural remedies are not just about the plants, herbs, or minerals we use. It's about the alchemy of nature and nurture, the magical blend of the right ingredients and the right care. This alchemy is what transforms a simple plant into a healing balm for your child's ailment. It's what turns a mother's touch into the ultimate comfort for a feverish child.

One of the most crucial skills in applying natural remedies is the art of observation. Children may not always be able to articulate what they're feeling, but their bodies often speak volumes. A flushed face, a restless night, or a sudden loss of appetite can all be signals that something is amiss. The alkaline lifestyle encourages us to be in tune with these subtle cues, to understand them not as isolated symptoms but as part of a larger pattern that points to an imbalance in the body.

The Healing Power of Plants

Let's consider the example of chamomile, a plant that has been cherished for centuries for its calming properties. A warm cup of chamomile tea can be a soothing ritual before bedtime, especially for a child who struggles with sleep. But the benefits of chamomile go beyond just inducing sleep; it can also alleviate digestive discomfort and reduce inflammation. It's a multi-faceted remedy that addresses the root cause of an issue rather than just masking the symptoms.

The alkaline approach to health is not just about what we put into our bodies; it's also about what we put into our minds. Stress and anxiety can manifest physically in children, often in the form of stomachaches or headaches. Techniques like deep breathing or grounding exercises can be incredibly effective in these situations. They serve as natural remedies that use the body's own resources to heal itself.

The Role of Diet in Natural Healing

The foods we eat play a significant role in our overall health, and this is especially true for children. An alkaline diet rich in fruits and vegetables can be a powerful tool in preventing common childhood ailments. For instance, berries are packed with antioxidants that boost the immune system, making them a natural defense against colds and flu. Similarly, leafy greens like spinach and kale are rich in iron and calcium, essential nutrients for a growing child.

Continuing our exploration of natural remedies, let's consider the incredible benefits of Eucalyptus oil. Just a few drops in a humidifier can clear up a stuffy nose and make breathing easier. Then there's the magic of honey, a natural sweetener that also acts as an antimicrobial agent. A spoonful of honey can soothe a sore throat and offer relief from coughing, making it a staple in many households.

While natural remedies offer a plethora of benefits, it's crucial to approach them with a sense of responsibility. Knowledge is your safety net here. Knowing the correct dosage, the right method of application, and when to seek professional medical advice can make all the difference. This is where the alkaline lifestyle shines, as it encourages continuous learning and empowers you to make informed decisions for your family's health.

The Community of Care

Natural remedies are not just individual choices; they are collective wisdom. They are the recipes passed down from grandmothers, the tips shared between friends, and the experiences discussed in community forums. This collective wisdom enriches our understanding and application of natural remedies, making each of us a link in a much larger chain of care.

As we use these natural remedies to care for our children, we're also passing down a legacy. It's a legacy of respect for nature, of trust in our own bodies, and of a holistic approach to health that goes beyond just treating symptoms. This legacy is what will empower the next generation to take control of their health, to live in harmony with nature, and to continue the cycle of healing and care.

In this central part of our exploration, we've journeyed through the multifaceted world of natural remedies for children, touching upon the importance of observation, the incredible healing power of plants, and the essential role of community and legacy. As we move forward, let's carry these insights with us, like precious gems, enriching not just our lives but also the lives of our children and the generations to come.

The Wisdom of Generations

As we draw this chapter to a close, it's essential to reflect on the wisdom that has been passed down through generations. The natural remedies we've discussed are not just a collection of herbs, oils, and practices; they are a legacy. They are the distilled wisdom of our ancestors, who understood the rhythms of nature and the human body long before modern medicine came into the picture. This wisdom is a gift, one that we have the privilege and responsibility to pass on to our children.

The concept of an alkaline family is not just about dietary choices or the pH level of the foods we consume. It's about creating a sanctuary—a safe space where holistic well-being is nurtured, where natural remedies are not just an alternative but a way of life. In this sanctuary, the child learns to trust the wisdom of their own body, to understand that they are not separate from nature but a part of it.

The Empowerment of Choice

One of the most empowering aspects of using natural remedies is the choice it offers. Unlike the often one-size-fits-all approach of conventional medicine, natural remedies offer a buffet of options. You can choose the remedy that resonates most with your child's needs, whether it's chamomile tea for a peaceful night's sleep or eucalyptus oil for a congested chest. This choice is empowering for parents and educational for children, who learn early on that they have agency over their own bodies.

The choices we make within our families have a ripple effect that extends far beyond the walls of our homes. When we choose natural remedies, we're also making an ecological choice. We're choosing sustainability over quick fixes, harmony over dissonance. This choice impacts not just our children but also the planet they will inherit. It's a step towards a more sustainable, equitable world, where the health of one is intrinsically linked to the health of all.

The Art of Being Present

In a world that's increasingly fast-paced and stressful, the act of administering a natural remedy is also an act of being present. It's a moment where you pause, connect, and focus entirely on your child's well-being. Whether it's the five minutes you spend massaging lavender oil into their temples or the half-hour bedtime routine that includes a warm mug of herbal tea, these are the moments that count. These are the moments that your children will remember and carry forward into their own families.

Natural remedies do more than just alleviate symptoms; they build resilience. They teach our children that their bodies are capable of healing, that they have an innate ability to restore balance. This resilience is not just physical but also emotional and psychological. It equips them to handle the challenges of life with a sense of capability and self-assurance.

The Tapestry of Community

As we've discussed, natural remedies are a collective wisdom, a tapestry woven from the threads of community knowledge. By embracing this wisdom, we're also embracing a community—a network of like-minded individuals who share our values and aspirations. This community is an invaluable resource, a wellspring of support and inspiration that can sustain us through the challenges of raising an alkaline family.

As we conclude this chapter, let's remember that this is not the end but a milestone on a lifelong journey. The natural remedies we've explored are stepping stones, guiding us towards a future where holistic health is not the exception but the norm. They are the seeds we plant today for a harvest of well-being that will nourish our children and generations to come.

The Legacy We Craft

In the end, the legacy we leave is not just in the remedies we use but, in the love, and wisdom with which we administer them. It's in the quiet moments of care, the whispered bedtime stories, the soft glow of a nightlight illuminating a room infused with the gentle aroma of calming herbs. This is the legacy we craft, one moment at a time, one choice at a time, one child at a time.

As you move forward, may you carry this legacy with you, nurturing it with the same love, wisdom, and care that you would a delicate seedling. May it grow into a towering tree, its roots deep in the earth, its branches reaching towards the sky, sheltering and nourishing all who seek its comfort.

Book 12: Social Challenges in Alkaline Living

Navigating Dining Out and Social Events

In a world where fast food joints are on every corner and social events often revolve around meals that are anything but alkaline-friendly, maintaining your commitment to an alkaline lifestyle can feel like an uphill battle. But let's get one thing straight: it's not just about the food on your plate; it's about the life you're choosing to live. And yes, you can absolutely live it fully without compromising your health goals.

The Social Quandary

Imagine this: you're at a friend's birthday party, and the table is laden with foods that are the antithesis of your alkaline diet. Fried chicken, cheesy pasta, and sugary desserts beckon. Your friends are diving in, and there's a palpable sense of enjoyment in the air. You feel the pressure, the temptation, but also a twinge of isolation. What do you do?

The key to navigating such scenarios lies in preparation. Before attending any social event, eat a small alkaline meal at home. This will not only curb your hunger but also give you the mental clarity to make better food choices. Carry alkaline-friendly snacks like raw almonds or a green smoothie as a backup. Trust me, your future self will thank you.

The Power of Choice

When you're at the event, scan the menu or buffet table for options that align with your alkaline lifestyle. Opt for salads, grilled vegetables, or lean proteins. If the choices are limited, don't hesitate to ask the chef to customize a dish for you.

Most restaurants are more than willing to accommodate dietary restrictions. Remember, you always have a choice, even when it seems like you don't.

Navigating social pressures is a dance, and like any dance, it requires finesse. Be honest but not preachy about your dietary choices. A simple "I feel better when I eat this way" is often enough to quell any questions. If someone insists on knowing why you're not partaking in the cheese platter, you can always say, "I'm focusing on foods that make me feel good right now." It's a statement that's hard to argue with.

But here's the thing: social events are not just about food; they're about connection, laughter, and shared experiences. Focus on the joy of being present in the moment, rather than what's missing on your plate. Engage in conversations, share stories, and create memories. After all, isn't that what life is truly about?

Living an alkaline lifestyle doesn't mean you have to live in a bubble. It's about balance, not perfection. It's about making conscious choices that honor both your body and your social well-being. And sometimes, it's about knowing when to bend the rules without breaking your commitment to yourself.

So the next time you find yourself in a social setting that challenges your alkaline lifestyle, remember: you're not just navigating a menu; you're navigating your life. And you have all the tools you need to do it successfully.

The Ripple Effect of Your Choices

As you continue to navigate the social landscape while maintaining an alkaline lifestyle, you'll notice something remarkable: the ripple effect of your choices. Your commitment to healthful living will not only benefit you but also subtly influence those around you. You'll become a beacon of wellness, a living testament to the vitality that comes from honoring your body with alkaline foods and practices.

The Emotional Aspect

Let's not overlook the emotional aspect of dining out and attending social events. Food is deeply tied to our emotions, and it's not uncommon to feel a sense of nostalgia or comfort from certain dishes. However, the key is to separate emotional eating from emotional well-being. You can still experience the joy of social gatherings without compromising your alkaline lifestyle. The emotional satisfaction derived from making healthful choices often outweighs the fleeting pleasure of indulgence.

Your alkaline lifestyle can also serve as a conversation starter, opening doors to meaningful dialogues about health and wellness. While you shouldn't turn every dinner invitation into a lecture on alkalinity, don't shy away from sharing your journey when asked. You never know who might be inspired by your story. And let's face it, in a world where chronic illnesses are on the rise, conversations about proactive health measures are not just timely; they're essential.

The Art of Saying No

Saying no is an art form that many of us struggle with, especially when it comes to food. The fear of offending someone often trumps our commitment to our health. But here's a liberating truth: saying no to something is actually saying yes to something else. When you decline that slice of cake, you're saying yes to better health, more energy, and a longer, more fulfilling life. And those are things worth saying yes to. As you navigate the complexities of social dining and events, always keep the bigger picture in mind. Your alkaline lifestyle is a long-term commitment, a marathon, not a sprint. There will be hurdles, but each one offers a lesson, an opportunity for growth. The challenges you face socially are but small bumps on the road to a life of optimal health and well-being.

The Final Takeaway

In the grand scheme of things, the food you choose to consume at a social event is just a small chapter in your larger life story. What truly matters is how you show up in the world, how you treat yourself and others, and how you contribute to the collective well-being of your community. Your alkaline lifestyle is not a limitation; it's an empowerment. It equips you with the energy, clarity, and vitality to live your best life, socially and otherwise.

So, the next time you find yourself at a crossroads, faced with a menu that challenges your alkaline commitments, remember this: you're not just making a choice for that moment; you're making a choice for your life. And when you choose wisely, you're not just nourishing your body; you're nourishing your soul.

In closing, navigating dining out and social events while living an alkaline lifestyle is not just doable; it's an enriching experience that adds layers of depth to your social interactions and personal growth. It's about striking a balance between social enjoyment and personal well-being, and in that balance, you'll find the true essence of a life well-lived.

Handling Criticism and Skepticism

The Inevitability of Criticism: A Universal Experience

If you've ever taken the road less traveled, you know it's not just a physical journey but an emotional one. The same holds true for adopting an alkaline lifestyle. While the physical benefits are transformative, the emotional landscape can be fraught with challenges, particularly when it comes to handling criticism and skepticism from others. It's a universal experience, one that transcends cultures, backgrounds, and lifestyles. Whether you're a seasoned advocate or a newcomer to alkaline living, criticism is an inevitable part of the journey.

Criticism carries an emotional weight that can be both disheartening and isolating. It's not just a matter of differing opinions; it's a clash of worldviews, a challenge to your deeply held beliefs and practices. And when that criticism comes from loved ones, friends, or even healthcare professionals, the emotional toll can be even greater. It's not just about defending your choices; it's about defending your identity, your commitment to a healthier, more balanced life.

The Psychology of Skepticism: Why People Resist Change

Skepticism, like criticism, is rooted in psychology. It's a defense mechanism, a way to resist change and maintain the status quo. When people encounter something that challenges their established beliefs or routines, skepticism is often the first line of defense. It's a protective barrier, a way to preserve one's sense of stability and control. And while skepticism is a natural human response, it can also be a significant obstacle in your journey toward alkaline living.

As counterintuitive as it may sound, criticism can serve as both an adversary and an ally. On one hand, it can be a source of emotional distress, a constant reminder of the societal norms and expectations you're challenging. On the other hand, it can be a catalyst for growth, a motivator that pushes you to refine your understanding, to deepen your commitment, and to become a more effective advocate for alkaline living.

The Art of Diplomacy: Navigating Difficult Conversations

Handling criticism and skepticism requires emotional resilience, a form of inner strength that allows you to navigate the emotional terrain with grace and poise. It's about developing a thick skin without becoming hard-hearted, about standing your ground without becoming confrontational. It's a delicate balance, one that requires both self-awareness and emotional intelligence.

One of the most effective ways to handle criticism and skepticism is to shift the narrative, to change the lens through which you view these challenges. Instead of seeing them as obstacles, see them as opportunities—opportunities to educate, to enlighten, and to empower. When you shift the narrative, you shift the emotional dynamics, transforming criticism and skepticism from emotional burdens into catalysts for change.

Handling criticism and skepticism often involves navigating difficult conversations, and that requires a certain level of diplomacy. It's about knowing when to speak and when to listen, when to assert your beliefs and when to seek common ground. It's an art form, one that requires practice, patience, and a deep understanding of human psychology.

The Emotional Toolkit: Strategies for Success

As we delve deeper into the intricacies of handling criticism and skepticism, we'll explore a range of strategies designed to equip you with the emotional toolkit you need for success. From effective communication techniques to psychological hacks, these strategies will empower you to handle criticism and skepticism with confidence, grace, and emotional resilience.

As we embark on this emotional journey, it's important to remember that criticism and skepticism are not just challenges to be overcome but integral parts of the human experience. They are the emotional hurdles that test our resolve, the societal norms that challenge our convictions, and the psychological barriers that shape our journey. And in overcoming these challenges, we don't just become better advocates for alkaline living; we become better, more resilient versions of ourselves.

The Emotional Intelligence Quotient: A Key Asset

One of the most potent tools in your arsenal for handling criticism and skepticism is emotional intelligence. This is the ability to recognize, understand, and manage our own emotions while also being sensitive to the emotions of others. When you're emotionally intelligent, you can defuse tension, navigate complex social situations, and turn potentially confrontational interactions into constructive dialogues. It's not about avoiding criticism but understanding its roots and addressing it in a way that fosters understanding and growth.

When faced with criticism or skepticism, our instinctual response may be to become defensive or to counter-attack. However, a more effective approach is to engage the critic in a dialogue. Utilize the Socratic method by asking questions that encourage them to elaborate on their views. This achieves two things: first, it forces them to think deeply about their criticisms, and second, it gives you valuable insights into the underlying issues that fuel their skepticism. Often, you'll find that their criticisms are based on misconceptions that can be easily clarified.

The Art of Storytelling: Humanizing Your Journey

Empathy is the ability to understand and share the feelings of another. When dealing with critics or skeptics, try to see the world from their perspective. What fears or concerns might be driving their skepticism? What experiences have shaped their views? By understanding where they're coming from, you can address their criticisms more effectively and perhaps even turn skeptics into allies.

People relate to stories far more than they do to abstract concepts or raw data. If you want to counter skepticism and criticism effectively, humanize your journey toward alkaline living. Share personal anecdotes that illustrate the challenges you've faced and the benefits you've gained. Make it relatable. When people can see themselves in your story, they're more likely to open their minds to new ideas.

The Importance of Credibility: Building Trust Through Transparency

Credibility is crucial when you're advocating for something as transformative as alkaline living. Be transparent about your sources of information, the experts you consult, and the scientific basis for your beliefs. The more credible you are, the less room there is for skepticism and criticism to take root.

There's strength in numbers, and this is particularly true when you're navigating the social challenges of alkaline living. Surround yourself with a supportive community of like-minded individuals. Not only can they provide emotional support, but they can also offer practical advice on how to handle criticism and skepticism. Sometimes, the collective wisdom of a community can be far more powerful than the insights of any single individual.

The Fine Line: Knowing When to Engage and When to Walk Away

It's essential to recognize that not all critics can be won over, and not all battles are worth fighting. Know when to engage and when to walk away. Some people are so entrenched in their views that no amount of evidence or reasoning will sway them. In such cases, it's more productive to disengage and focus your energies where they can make a real impact.

The Long Game: Persistence and Consistency

Handling criticism and skepticism is not a one-off event but an ongoing process. It requires persistence and consistency. Keep educating yourself, refining your arguments, and engaging with critics in a constructive manner. Over time, even the most ardent skeptics may start to see the value in what you're advocating, or at least respect the sincerity and depth of your convictions.

In the grand tapestry of life, criticism and skepticism are but threads that add complexity and depth to the overall design. They challenge us, shape us, and ultimately make us better advocates for the causes we hold dear. As you continue your journey in alkaline living, remember that every critic is a potential ally, every skeptic a possible convert. It's not about winning arguments, but about transforming lives—one conversation at a time.

The Alchemy of Criticism: Turning Lead into Gold

As we draw this chapter to a close, let's reflect on the transformative power of criticism and skepticism. These are not roadblocks on your journey toward alkaline living; they are stepping stones. Each critique, each skeptical question, is an opportunity for you to refine your understanding, deepen your commitment, and broaden your perspective. It's akin to the alchemical process of turning lead into gold. You take something that is seemingly negative and transform it into a valuable asset that enriches your life and the lives of those around you.

Resilience is not about avoiding criticism or skepticism; it's about learning how to deal with them effectively. It's about building an emotional armor that protects you but doesn't isolate you. This armor is made up of layers of understanding, empathy, and self-awareness. It allows you to engage with critics without losing your sense of self or your commitment to your alkaline lifestyle. And the more you engage, the stronger this armor becomes, reinforcing your resilience and equipping you to handle future challenges with grace and poise.

Your response to criticism and skepticism doesn't just affect you; it also shapes public perception of alkaline living as a whole. When you handle criticism poorly, it casts a shadow over the entire movement. But when you handle it well, you shine a light that can illuminate the path for others. You become a beacon of reason, integrity, and wisdom in a world that is often clouded by misinformation and prejudice. And in doing so, you elevate not just yourself but also the entire community of alkaline living advocates.

The Wisdom of Humility: Knowing You Don't Know It All

Humility is a virtue that is often overlooked in our quest for self-improvement and personal growth. But it's a crucial component of effectively handling criticism and skepticism. Acknowledging that you don't have all the answers, that you're still learning and growing, makes you more approachable and relatable. It opens the door for constructive dialogue and mutual growth. It also keeps you grounded, reminding you that the journey toward alkaline living is a lifelong pursuit, not a destination you reach and then abandon.

The Gift of Time: Patience as a Virtue

Time is a powerful ally in your quest to handle criticism and skepticism effectively. The initial sting of a critical comment may be painful, but with time, that pain subsides, giving way to understanding and insight. Time also allows you to see the long-term impact of your actions and choices. You'll find that the criticisms that once seemed so daunting are now mere footnotes in your larger journey, valuable lessons that have shaped you but no longer define you.

As you navigate the social challenges of alkaline living, remember that you're not just doing it for yourself; you're also doing it for future generations. The way you handle criticism and skepticism today will shape the way these issues are handled tomorrow. You're setting precedents, establishing norms, and, most importantly, serving as a role model for those who will follow in your footsteps. Your legacy is not just the health and wellness you achieve but also the wisdom and resilience you display in the face of social challenges.

The Final Takeaway: Your Journey, Your Rules

At the end of the day, your journey toward alkaline living is uniquely yours. You get to set the rules, define the milestones, and choose the paths you want to explore. Criticism and skepticism will be a part of this journey, but they don't have to dictate its course. You have the power to turn these challenges into opportunities for growth, learning, and transformation. And in doing so, you enrich not just your own life but also the lives of everyone you touch.

In closing, handling criticism and skepticism is not a detour on your journey toward alkaline living; it's an integral part of the road itself. It's a stretch of the path that tests your mettle, sharpens your skills, and ultimately makes you a stronger, wiser, and more resilient traveler. So the next time you encounter criticism or skepticism, don't sidestep it or shy away from it. Embrace it, engage with it, and transform it into another stepping stone on your lifelong journey toward health, wellness, and holistic living.

Building a Supportive Alkaline Community

The Power of Community: More Than Just a Buzzword

When we talk about a "community," it's not just a trendy term we throw around. It's the backbone of any significant change, especially when it comes to something as deeply personal and yet profoundly universal as our health. The journey towards alkaline living is not a solitary one, nor should it be. It's a collective endeavor, a shared mission that gains its strength from the community that supports it. The essence of building a supportive alkaline community is not just about gathering like-minded individuals; it's about creating a nurturing environment where each person's unique path to alkaline living is acknowledged, respected, and celebrated.

The Symbiosis of Shared Goals: A Collective Vision

Let's face it; we're emotional beings. We thrive on connection, understanding, and mutual respect. When we decide to make a significant lifestyle change, like adopting an alkaline diet, the emotional support we receive (or don't receive) can make or break our resolve. It's not just about having someone to share recipes with or go grocery shopping with; it's about having a safe space where you can express your doubts, share your triumphs, and navigate your failures without judgment. It's about knowing that you're not alone, that there are others who are walking the same path, facing the same challenges, and celebrating the same victories.

A supportive alkaline community is not just a group of individuals with similar interests; it's a collective with a shared vision. This vision is not imposed from the top down; it's organically developed from the ground up. It's a vision that respects individual autonomy while recognizing the power of collective action. It's a vision that understands that the whole is greater than the sum of its parts, that each member brings something unique to the table, and that these unique contributions enrich the community as a whole.

The Role of Leadership: Guiding Without Dictating

Support comes in many shapes and sizes, and in a community, it's often the small gestures that make the most significant impact. It could be as simple as sharing a tried-and-tested alkaline recipe, offering words of encouragement to someone who's struggling, or organizing a local meet-up to discuss challenges and solutions. These acts of support create a ripple effect, inspiring others to offer their support in return, thereby strengthening the community's fabric.

Every community needs leaders, but in a supportive alkaline community, leadership is not about dictating terms or imposing rules. It's about guiding, facilitating, and, most importantly, listening. It's about creating an environment where each member feels heard, valued, and empowered to contribute. It's about recognizing that leadership is not a position but a behavior, one that each member can embody in their unique way.

The Interplay of Individual and Community Growth

In today's digital age, the concept of community has expanded beyond geographical boundaries. Online platforms offer a unique opportunity to connect with like-minded individuals worldwide, providing a broader perspective and a more diverse range of experiences and insights. However, the principles of building a supportive community remain the same, whether online or offline. It's about creating a space that values authenticity, encourages openness, and fosters mutual respect.

One of the most beautiful aspects of a supportive community is the symbiotic relationship between individual and community growth. As individuals, we bring our unique skills, insights, and experiences to the community. In return, the community offers us a platform to grow, learn, and evolve, not just in our understanding of alkaline living but also in our interpersonal skills, emotional intelligence, and sense of social responsibility.

As we embark on this journey of building a supportive alkaline community, it's essential to remember that a community is not a static entity; it's a living, breathing organism that evolves over time. It's shaped by the people who are part of it, by the challenges it faces, and by the victories it achieves. It's an ever-changing landscape that requires constant nurturing, regular reassessment, and, above all, an unwavering commitment to the collective well-being.

In conclusion, building a supportive alkaline community is not a side project; it's a vital component of the alkaline living journey. It's the soil in which the seeds of individual efforts can take root, grow, and flourish. It's the sanctuary where we can find respite, inspiration, and the strength to continue on our path. And most importantly, it's the mirror that reflects the collective soul of all those who are part of it, reminding us that in this journey of alkaline living, we are never alone.

The Art of Listening: A Cornerstone of Community

In a world that's increasingly noisy, the art of listening has become a rare gem. A supportive alkaline community thrives on the ability of its members to listen—to listen to the struggles, the triumphs, and the nuanced experiences of each individual. Listening is not a passive act; it's an active engagement that fosters empathy, understanding, and, ultimately, support. When we listen, we're not just hearing words; we're creating a space for stories to unfold, for experiences to be shared, and for solutions to be discovered.

The collective wisdom of a community often surpasses that of any single individual. In a supportive alkaline community, shared knowledge becomes a powerful tool for personal and collective growth. Whether it's a new scientific study that sheds light on the benefits of alkaline living, a creative recipe that turns a bland meal into a culinary delight, or a personal anecdote that offers a fresh perspective, the value of shared knowledge cannot be overstated. It's the glue that binds the community, enriching the collective understanding and empowering each member to make informed choices.

Life is a roller coaster of ups and downs, and the journey towards alkaline living is no exception. Emotional resilience becomes crucial when facing the inevitable challenges and setbacks. A supportive community acts as a safety net, catching you when you fall and helping you bounce back with renewed vigor. It's the place where you can be vulnerable without the fear of judgment, where you can share your failures as openly as your successes, and where you can find the emotional strength to continue your journey, no matter the obstacles.

The Power of Storytelling: Humanizing the Experience

In any community, the role of mentors is pivotal. These are the individuals who have walked the path, faced the challenges, and reaped the rewards. They offer a wealth of experience and wisdom that can guide newcomers in their journey. But mentorship in a supportive alkaline community is not a one-way street; it's a dynamic relationship that benefits both the mentor and the mentee. The mentor gains a sense of purpose and the joy of seeing others grow, while the mentee receives invaluable guidance that can help navigate the complexities of alkaline living.

Stories have the power to humanize abstract concepts, making them relatable and accessible. In a supportive alkaline community, storytelling becomes a powerful medium for sharing experiences, imparting wisdom, and fostering a sense of belonging. Whether it's a story of overcoming health challenges through alkaline living, a narrative that demystifies complex scientific concepts, or a simple tale that brings a smile to someone's face, stories add a human dimension to the community, making it more than just a collection of individuals but a tapestry of interconnected lives.

The Importance of Celebrating Milestones: Small Wins, Big Impact

In the pursuit of long-term goals, it's easy to overlook the small victories that mark our progress. A supportive community recognizes the importance of celebrating these milestones, no matter how insignificant they may seem. Whether it's the first week of successfully sticking to an alkaline diet, the discovery of a new alkaline food that you enjoy, or the first time you feel the tangible benefits of your lifestyle changes, these small wins deserve celebration. They serve as reminders of the progress made and fuel the motivation to continue the journey.

The Dynamics of Inclusion: A Community for All

A supportive community is an inclusive community—one that welcomes individuals from all walks of life, regardless of their age, gender, ethnicity, or level of experience. Inclusion is not just a moral imperative; it's a practical necessity. A diverse community offers a richer tapestry of experiences, perspectives, and skills, making it more resilient, more adaptable, and more capable of facing the challenges that lie ahead.

A supportive alkaline community is not just inward-looking; it recognizes its responsibility towards the broader society and the planet. Whether it's advocating for sustainable farming practices, promoting ethical consumer choices, or engaging in community outreach programs, the ethical dimension adds a layer of depth and purpose to the community's mission.

In sum, building a supportive alkaline community is a multifaceted endeavor that goes beyond mere social interaction. It's about creating a nurturing ecosystem that fosters personal growth, emotional resilience, and collective wisdom. It's about recognizing the unique value that goes beyond mere social interaction. It's about creating a nurturing ecosystem that fosters personal growth, emotional resilience, and collective wisdom. It's about recognizing the unique value that each individual brings and leveraging this diversity for the greater good. And most importantly, it's about creating a space where the journey towards alkaline living becomes a shared experience, enriched by the stories, the wisdom, and the support of a community that cares.

The Lasting Impact: Sustaining and Nurturing a Supportive Alkaline Community

It's the kind word that lifts someone's spirits, the shared recipe that becomes a family favorite, or the personal story that inspires someone else to take the first step on their alkaline journey. Never underestimate the transformative power you hold as a member of this community. Your impact is not just a drop in the ocean; it's the ripple that can turn into a wave of change.

The Lifelong Commitment: Nurturing the Community's Growth

Building a community is not a one-time event but a lifelong commitment. It requires consistent nurturing, much like tending to a garden. The seeds have been sown, the plants are growing, but they need water, sunlight, and care to flourish. In the same vein, a supportive alkaline community needs ongoing engagement, open dialogue, and a continual influx of fresh ideas and perspectives. It's not just about reaching a destination; it's about enjoying and enriching the journey for everyone involved.

As the world changes, so do the needs and challenges of a community. What worked yesterday may not be effective tomorrow. A truly supportive alkaline community is adaptive in nature, willing to evolve and adjust its strategies to meet the changing landscape. Whether it's incorporating new scientific findings, adapting to technological advancements, or simply changing the way community meetings are held, flexibility is key. An adaptive community is a resilient community, one that can withstand the tests of time and circumstance.

The Power of Unity: Stronger Together

There's an old saying that goes, "United we stand, divided we fall." This couldn't be truer for a supportive alkaline community. The strength of the community lies in its unity, in the collective will of its members to support each other in the pursuit of a common goal. It's not about conforming to a single viewpoint or suppressing individuality. On the contrary, it's about harnessing the diverse talents, experiences, and perspectives of its members to create a unified force that can tackle any challenge.

Every community has a life cycle, and members will come and go. But what remains constant is the legacy that the community leaves behind. It's the wisdom passed down from mentors, the friendships that stand the test of time, and the positive changes that members have made in their lives and the lives of others. As you navigate your own alkaline journey, consider the legacy you want to leave. How will you pass the torch to the next generation? What values and lessons do you want to impart? Your legacy is your lasting imprint on the community, a testament to your contributions and impact.

The Ethical Footprint: A Broader Social Responsibility

While the primary focus of a supportive alkaline community is the well-being of its members, it also has a broader social responsibility. This extends to ethical consumer choices, advocating for sustainable practices, and contributing to social causes that align with the community's values. It's about recognizing that the community is part of a larger ecosystem and that its actions have repercussions that go beyond its boundaries.

One of the most rewarding aspects of being part of a supportive community is the joy of giving. Whether it's sharing knowledge, offering emotional support, or helping someone in need, the act of giving not only benefits the receiver but also enriches the giver. It creates a cycle of positivity and support that sustains the community's vitality.

As we conclude this exploration of building a supportive alkaline community, it's important to reflect on your personal role in this living tapestry. You are not just a passive observer; you are an active participant, a co-creator of this shared reality. Your actions, no matter how small, have the power to shape the community's future. So, take that step, however tentative. Share that story, however trivial it may seem. Offer that hand, however busy you are. Because in the end, it's the collective actions of individuals like you that make a community truly supportive, resilient, and enduring.

Book 13: Modern Medicine vs. Alkaline Practices

A Comparative Analysis of Treatment Modalities

The Crossroads of Tradition and Modernity

In the realm of healthcare, the debate between modern medicine and traditional, alkaline practices is as old as time. Yet, it's a conversation that has never been more relevant. As we navigate the complexities of the 21st century—a time of unprecedented technological advancements but also rising chronic illnesses—the question looms large: Which path offers not just a cure but true healing?

Modern medicine, often termed as 'Western medicine,' is rooted in scientific research and technological advancements. It's a system that has given us life-saving drugs, intricate surgeries, and the ability to combat diseases that were once considered fatal. The approach is predominantly reactive; you get sick, you get treated. The arsenal includes antibiotics, surgical procedures, and a plethora of pharmaceuticals designed to alleviate symptoms. It's a system built on the premise of quick fixes, often without delving into the root cause of the ailment.

The Essence of Alkaline Practices

On the flip side, alkaline practices, inspired by the teachings of visionaries like Dr. Sebi, take a more holistic approach. The focus is not just on treating the symptoms but on understanding the body as a complex, interconnected system. Alkalinity believes in the power of natural herbs, a balanced diet, and the importance of mental and spiritual well-being. It's proactive rather than reactive, emphasizing prevention over cure.

The Question of Efficacy

The most glaring difference between the two is their approach to the human body. Modern medicine often compartmentalizes the body, treating each organ or symptom in isolation. Alkaline practices, however, view the body as a whole. For instance, if you're experiencing chronic fatigue, a traditional doctor might prescribe you stimulants like caffeine pills. In contrast, an alkaline practitioner would look into your diet, your mental health, and even your daily routine to identify the root cause and treat it naturally.

One of the most contentious points in this debate is the question of efficacy. Critics of alkaline practices often argue that it lacks the empirical evidence that modern medicine boasts. However, this argument falls flat when you consider the countless testimonials and real-life stories of people who have found healing through alkaline methods. Moreover, the rise in chronic illnesses despite medical advancements raises questions about the long-term efficacy of modern treatments.

The Role of Lifestyle

Modern life is hectic. The stress, the lack of time for proper meals, and the sedentary lifestyle have led to an increase in lifestyle-related diseases. Here, the preventive and holistic nature of alkaline practices shines. It's not just about treating diseases; it's about creating a lifestyle that makes it hard for diseases to take root in the first place. Let's talk numbers. Healthcare is expensive, and not everyone has access to insurance or high-quality medical services. Alkaline practices offer a more accessible and often less expensive alternative. The focus on natural herbs and foods also makes it more sustainable in the long run.

In summary, both modern medicine and alkaline practices have their merits and demerits. The former excels in acute care and life-saving interventions, while the latter offers a more holistic and preventive approach. As we move forward, the ideal healthcare system would be one that integrates the strengths of both these worlds, offering a more rounded approach to health and well-being.

This comparative analysis serves as a starting point for anyone caught at the crossroads, offering insights into what each path has to offer. The choice, ultimately, is personal and should be made considering one's own body, beliefs, and lifestyle.

The Harmonization of Two Worlds: A Vision for the Future

As we delve deeper into the comparative analysis of modern medicine and alkaline practices, we cannot overlook the ethical dimension. Modern medicine often finds itself entangled in ethical dilemmas, from the overuse of antibiotics to the opioid crisis. Alkaline practices, grounded in natural healing, offer an ethical alternative that aligns with the principles of 'do no harm.' It's a path that respects not just the individual but also the environment, emphasizing sustainability and ethical sourcing of natural herbs and foods.

Health is not just a physical state but an emotional and psychological one. Modern medicine, with its clinical approach, often neglects this aspect. Patients are treated as cases, not as individuals with unique emotional landscapes. Alkaline practices, with their holistic approach, fill this gap. They consider the emotional and psychological well-being of the individual, offering a more compassionate form of care that resonates with many.

The Cultural Relevance

Culture plays a significant role in how we approach healthcare. Alkaline practices often resonate more with indigenous cultures and communities that have been marginalized by the mainstream healthcare system. It's a form of healthcare that respects cultural wisdom and traditional knowledge, offering a more inclusive approach.

The future of healthcare lies in a paradigm shift—a move away from the 'one-size-fits-all' approach to a more personalized form of medicine. Here, both modern medicine and alkaline practices have roles to play. Imagine a healthcare system where your treatment plan is tailored to your unique genetic makeup, lifestyle, and even your emotional state. A system that combines the diagnostic precision of modern medicine with the holistic wisdom of alkaline practices. That's not just healthcare; that's healing in its truest sense.

At the end of the day, the most empowering aspect of this comparative analysis is the power of choice it offers. You are not bound by a single path but have the freedom to choose a healthcare approach that aligns with your beliefs, lifestyle, and unique medical needs. Whether it's a life-saving surgery or a herbal remedy for stress relief, the choice is yours to make.

The Call to Action

As we conclude this comparative analysis, the call to action is clear: educate yourself. The more you know, the better choices you'll make. Whether you're a healthcare provider looking to offer more holistic options to your clients or an individual navigating the maze of modern healthcare, knowledge is your most potent weapon. Attend workshops, read research papers, join online forums—do whatever it takes to be informed.

In a world that's increasingly polarized, the integration of modern medicine and alkaline practices offers a beacon of hope. It shows us that it's not always about choosing sides but about finding a middle ground that offers the best of both worlds. As we stand at this intersection, the path forward is not one of division but of unity, collaboration, and a shared vision for a healthier, more holistic future.

So, as you ponder over this comparative analysis, remember that the ultimate goal is not to pit one against the other but to create a healthcare system that is as diverse, complex, and beautifully human as the individuals it serves.nal and should be made considering one's own body, beliefs, and lifestyle.

How to Integrate Alkaline Practices with Modern Medicine

The new frontier of health care

In a world where health care is often seen as a battleground of opposing ideologies, the idea of integration represents a beacon of hope. It is no longer a matter of choosing between modern medicine and alkaline practices, but of finding a harmonious blend that offers the best of both worlds. This is the new frontier of health care: a realm where science meets wisdom, where technology complements tradition, and where the focus shifts from simple treatment to holistic wellness.

The concept of integration is not to dilute one approach to fit the other, but to enhance the effectiveness of both. Modern medicine excels in diagnostics, emergency care and surgery. Alkaline practices shine in prevention, lifestyle management and chronic disease control. When these two come together, they create a model of health care that is not just reactive but proactive, not just curative but preventive.

The art of balance.

The first step in this integration is understanding the art of balance. Too often we swing like a pendulum: either we fully embrace drugs while neglecting natural remedies or we immerse ourselves in herbal treatments while ignoring medical advances. The art of balance teaches us to use modern medicine for acute conditions requiring immediate attention and to employ alkaline practices for long-term health and prevention. It is not an "either/or" scenario, but a judicious use of both.

The role of the physician

Health professionals play a key role in this integration. The modern physician must be open to the benefits of alkaline practices, just as practitioners of natural cures must appreciate advances in medical science. This mutual respect and understanding paves the way for collaborative care, in which the patient may be recommended for surgery but also guided to make lifestyle changes to prevent future complications.

The patient's journey

For the patient, this integration offers a more comprehensive and powerful health care experience. Imagine walking into a clinic where your doctor not only prescribes medication for high blood pressure, but also offers advice on alkaline foods that can help you control it. Or think of a scenario where your natural health practitioner works in tandem with your oncologist to create a cancer treatment plan that combines chemotherapy with herbal remedies to mitigate side effects.

One of the most interesting aspects of integrating alkaline practices with modern medicine is the ethical and sustainable dimension it adds to health care. Alkaline practices often involve the use of natural and environmentally friendly products and promote a lifestyle in harmony with nature. When combined with the ethical guidelines and rigorous testing that modern medicine adheres to, they result in a model of health care that is not only effective but also responsible.

The future is integrated

As we stand on the threshold of a health care revolution, the future undoubtedly belongs to an integrated approach. Research is already underway to understand how natural herbs can improve the effectiveness of chemotherapy drugs, how meditation can help recover faster after surgery, and how an alkaline diet can help in the management of autoimmune diseases.

The integration of alkaline practices with modern medicine is not a trend, but an evolution-an evolution toward a more inclusive, more holistic, and more humane health care system. It is a journey that each of us is a part of, whether we are health care providers, patients or simply individuals committed to living our best lives. So, as we navigate this exciting landscape, let us do so with an open mind, a collaborative spirit and a heart full of hope for a healthier tomorrow.

Final Thoughts on Integrating Alkaline Practices with Modern Medicine

The beauty of this integrated approach lies in the power of choice it offers. No longer are you confined to a single path; you have a myriad of options that can be tailored to your unique health needs. This is healthcare at its most democratic, a system that respects individuality while offering a collective wisdom that spans centuries and disciplines.

Integration also brings with it an ethos of personal responsibility. It's not just about following a doctor's orders or a natural healer's advice; it's about actively participating in your healthcare journey. You become a co-creator of your health, choosing alkaline foods to complement medication, or opting for meditation alongside a surgical procedure. This active role not only empowers you but also makes the healing process more effective and fulfilling.

The Healing Dialogue

One of the most transformative aspects of this integration is the dialogue it fosters—between healthcare providers, between different medical philosophies, and most importantly, between you and your own body. This dialogue is not just spoken but felt, as you start to listen to your body's signals, understanding when it needs medical intervention and when it can heal through natural remedies. This is the healing dialogue, a conversation that can change the course of your health and life.

The impact of this integrated approach goes beyond individual health; it has a ripple effect on the healthcare system and society at large. Imagine a world where hospitals have alkaline food cafeterias, where doctors prescribe mindfulness techniques as readily as they do antibiotics, where health insurance covers not just surgical procedures but also holistic therapies. This is not a utopian dream but a reachable reality, made possible through integration.

The term "synergy" is often thrown around, but in the context of integrating alkaline practices with modern medicine, it takes on a profound meaning. Synergy is not just about adding one approach to another; it's about the exponential power created when two different systems work in harmony. It's the magic that happens when a cancer patient finds their chemotherapy more effective because they've also been following an alkaline diet. It's the relief experienced by a chronic pain sufferer who discovers that their medication works better when complemented by herbal teas and mindfulness practices.

The Legacy of Integration

As we look toward the future, the legacy of this integrated approach will be measured not just in years added to life, but in the life added to those years. It will be seen in the smiles of individuals who found hope and healing through a balanced approach, in the stories of families who broke the cycle of chronic illness, and in the communities that embraced a more holistic, sustainable, and compassionate form of healthcare.

In conclusion, the integration of alkaline practices and modern medicine is not just a healthcare strategy; it's a philosophy, a lifestyle, and ultimately, a choice—a choice to live better, to heal better, and to be better. It's a choice that respects the past, leverages the present, and looks optimistically toward the future. It's a choice that recognizes that in the diversity of healing, there is unity, and in that unity, there is strength. So, as you turn the pages of this book and the chapters of your life, may you make the choice to integrate, to harmonize, and to heal. Because in that choice lies the promise of a healthier, happier you, and a better world for us all.

Real-Life Case Studies and Outcomes

The Tale of Two Paths

As we delve into the real-life case studies and outcomes, it's crucial to remember that behind every statistic, every percentage, and every medical term, there's a human story. These are not just numbers or isolated incidents; they are transformative journeys that individuals have undertaken, often in the face of overwhelming odds. The stories we're about to explore serve as living proof of the efficacy and potential of integrating alkaline practices with modern medicine.

Imagine two individuals, both diagnosed with the same chronic condition. One chooses the path of modern medicine alone, relying solely on pharmaceuticals and medical procedures. The other opts for an integrated approach, combining modern treatments with alkaline practices like dietary changes, herbal supplements, and mindfulness techniques. Over time, the latter not only experiences a significant improvement in symptoms but also enjoys enhanced overall well-being, from better mental health to increased physical stamina. This isn't a hypothetical scenario; it's a recurring narrative in the annals of holistic health.

The Resilience of Emily

Take Emily, a 42-year-old woman diagnosed with Type 2 diabetes. She was initially on a regimen of medication that included insulin injections and oral antidiabetic drugs. Despite this, her condition didn't improve significantly. Then she decided to integrate alkaline practices into her treatment plan. She switched to an alkaline diet rich in leafy greens and low-glycemic fruits, started practicing daily mindfulness, and incorporated herbal teas into her routine. Within months, her blood sugar levels stabilized, and her medication dosage was reduced. Today, Emily is a beacon of resilience and an advocate for the integrated approach.

The Transformation of Mark

Or consider Mark, a 35-year-old man grappling with chronic anxiety. Traditional medication provided him temporary relief but also brought along a host of side effects. Mark then chose to integrate alkaline practices into his life. He began with alkaline water and foods, moved on to herbal supplements, and started practicing yoga and meditation. The transformation was astounding. Not only did his anxiety levels plummet, but he also reported feeling more energized and focused than ever before.

These individual transformations often have a ripple effect, extending to families and communities. When one person adopts an integrated approach and witnesses remarkable improvements, it serves as a catalyst for others to explore this path. Families start making collective dietary changes, communities begin to discuss holistic health, and slowly but surely, a shift occurs. A shift towards a more balanced, more humane, and more effective approach to healthcare.

The Medical Community Takes Notice

It's not just patients and families who are taking note of these outcomes. The medical community is also beginning to recognize the value of an integrated approach. Doctors are now more open to discussing alkaline diets and herbal supplements as complementary treatments. Hospitals are even starting to incorporate mindfulness programs and alkaline food options. This change in attitude is a monumental step towards a healthcare system that values holistic well-being as much as it does medical intervention.

The Weight of Real-Life Evidence

While clinical trials and scientific studies provide the backbone of medical knowledge, real-life case studies offer something equally valuable—tangible evidence of how these practices impact everyday lives. These stories are the flesh and blood that wrap around the skeletal structure of scientific data, making it relatable, understandable, and ultimately, more compelling.

As we move forward, these real-life case studies serve as both inspiration and affirmation. They remind us that the path to optimal health doesn't have to be a one-way street paved solely with pharmaceuticals and surgical procedures. There's another path, one that's winding, scenic, and rich with possibilities. It's a path that recognizes the wisdom in both modern medicine and ancient alkaline practices, and it's a path that countless individuals are walking, with remarkable outcomes lighting their way.

In the pages that follow, we will delve deeper into these transformative journeys, exploring the nuances, the challenges, and the triumphs that come with choosing an integrated approach to health and well-being. The Lasting Impact: Real-Life Case Studies and Outcomes

As we draw this chapter to a close, it's essential to recognize the transformative power of personal narratives. These real-life case studies are not merely anecdotal evidence; they are the heartbeat of a movement that is redefining the landscape of healthcare. They offer a nuanced understanding that numbers and data often fail to capture—the emotional, psychological, and spiritual dimensions of healing and well-being. While the physical improvements in conditions like diabetes or anxiety are measurable and evident, the emotional and psychological benefits are often less visible but equally significant. For instance, the newfound sense of agency and empowerment that comes from taking an active role in one's health journey is immeasurable. It's not just about symptom relief; it's about reclaiming one's life, one's choices, and one's future.

The Domino Effect: From Individual to Collective Transformation

The impact of these case studies extends far beyond the individuals involved. When Emily or Mark share their stories, they're not just advocating for a particular diet or lifestyle; they're challenging the status quo. They're inviting us to question long-held beliefs about healthcare and to consider alternative paths that may be more harmonious, more holistic, and ultimately, more human. This ripple effect can lead to collective transformation, influencing healthcare policies, medical practices, and societal attitudes toward well-being.

Let's consider the journey of a skeptic, someone initially resistant to the idea of integrating alkaline practices with modern medicine. After witnessing the compelling outcomes in real-life case studies, éven the most hardened skeptic would find it difficult to dismiss the value of an integrated approach. These stories serve as a bridge, connecting the world of empirical evidence with the realm of lived experience, making the abstract tangible and the theoretical practical.

The Ethical Imperative: A Call to the Medical Community

The compelling outcomes we've discussed also present an ethical imperative for the medical community. When evidence—both scientific and anecdotal—points toward the benefits of an integrated approach, it becomes a moral obligation to consider these practices as viable treatment options. Ignoring them would be a disservice to patients who could benefit from a more holistic approach to health.

These real-life case studies and outcomes are not just isolated incidents; they're harbingers of a cultural shift. We're moving from a paradigm that views medicine and holistic practices as mutually exclusive to one that sees them as complementary. This shift is not just a trend; it's a revolution in how we understand and approach health and well-being. As we wrap up this chapter, let's reflect on the legacy that these real-life case studies leave behind. They serve as a testament to human resilience, the power of informed choices, and the profound impact of integrating mind, body, and spirit in the healing journey. These stories will continue to inspire, challenge, and guide us as we navigate the complex terrain of modern healthcare.

The Road Ahead: Your Story Awaits

Finally, as you turn the page, remember that your story is yet to be written. The real-life case studies and outcomes we've explored are not just tales of other people's journeys; they're signposts on your path. They offer hope, insight, and a roadmap for your own journey toward holistic well-being.

In the chapters that follow, we will continue to explore the multifaceted world of alkaline practices and modern medicine. But for now, let these real-life stories resonate with you, reminding you of the transformative power of an integrated approach to health. Your story could be the next one that inspires someone to take the first step on their journey to optimal health. And that, dear reader, is the ultimate outcome we all strive for.

Book 14: Debunking Myths and Misconceptions

Common Criticisms of the Alkaline Diet

The Inevitability of Doubt

In a world where information is abundant but often contradictory, skepticism is not only natural but also necessary. It's the tool we use to sift through the noise, to question what we're told, and to arrive at our own informed conclusions. The alkaline diet, despite its growing popularity and numerous success stories, is not immune to this scrutiny. In fact, it has become a subject of heated debate, drawing criticisms that range from mild skepticism to outright dismissal.

One of the most common criticisms of the alkaline diet is that it sounds "too good to be true." A diet that promises not just weight loss but also a cure for chronic conditions? It's easy to see why some people would raise an eyebrow. However, this criticism often stems from a misunderstanding of what the alkaline diet truly aims to achieve. It's not a magic bullet but a lifestyle change, one that encourages a holistic approach to health.

Another point of contention is the lack of extensive scientific research to back the claims made by proponents of the alkaline diet. Critics argue that while the idea of balancing your body's pH levels sounds plausible, there isn't enough empirical evidence to support it. This is a valid concern, but it's also worth noting that the absence of evidence is not evidence of absence. The field of nutritional science is ever-evolving, and what we don't know today might become the groundbreaking discovery of tomorrow.

The Complexity of Human Biology

Some critics point out that human biology is complex and that it's overly simplistic to attribute health or illness to the acidity or alkalinity of one's diet. They argue that the body has its own mechanisms for regulating pH levels and that dietary changes can have only a limited impact. While it's true that the body has its own regulatory systems, the alkaline diet doesn't claim to override them. Instead, it aims to support these natural processes, making it easier for the body to maintain its optimal state.

Another criticism often heard is that the alkaline diet, with its focus on fruits and vegetables, may lead to nutritional imbalances. Critics worry that followers might miss out on essential nutrients found in foods that are considered acidic. This concern, although understandable, often overlooks the diet's emphasis on balance and variety. The alkaline diet is not about eliminating food groups but about making more informed choices.

The Social Quandary: Is It Practical?

The economic aspect of the alkaline diet is also a point of criticism. Detractors argue that sourcing high-quality, organic, alkaline foods can be expensive and, therefore, unsustainable in the long run. While cost can be a concern, it's also an investment in long-term health, and there are ways to make it more affordable, such as community-supported agriculture or seasonal shopping.

Lastly, critics question the practicality of the alkaline diet in today's fast-paced world. They argue that it's too demanding, too restrictive, and incompatible with social events and dining out. However, any significant lifestyle change comes with its challenges, and the alkaline diet is no exception. The key is adaptability and finding a balance that works for you.

As we delve deeper into this chapter, we'll address these criticisms not as obstacles but as opportunities for clarification and growth. Skepticism can be a catalyst for deeper understanding, pushing us to question, research, and refine our beliefs. So let's embrace these criticisms, not as roadblocks, but as signposts guiding us toward a more nuanced and comprehensive understanding of the alkaline diet and its role in holistic health. After all, the journey to optimal health is not a straight path but a winding road, filled with questions that lead us to invaluable insights.

Navigating the Terrain of Skepticism Surrounding the Alkaline Diet

As we reach the conclusion of this chapter, it's essential to recognize that skepticism isn't inherently negative. In fact, it's a crucial part of any intellectual endeavor. The criticisms of the alkaline diet, as varied as they are, offer us a chance to deepen our understanding and refine our approach. They challenge us to look beyond the surface, to question the status quo, and to engage in a more nuanced dialogue about what it means to live an alkaline lifestyle.

While scientific evidence is a cornerstone of any health-related discussion, the power of personal experience cannot be discounted. For every critic who questions the efficacy of the alkaline diet, there are countless individuals who have experienced transformative changes in their health and well-being. These real-life stories serve as compelling counterpoints to the criticisms, offering a more holistic view that goes beyond the limitations of empirical data alone.

One of the most enriching aspects of adopting an alkaline lifestyle is the journey of self-discovery it entails. It's not just about changing what you eat; it's about changing how you think, how you feel, and how you interact with the world around you. This journey is deeply personal and varies from individual to individual, making it difficult to generalize or criticize. The criticisms often fail to capture this dynamic, evolving nature of the alkaline lifestyle, reducing it to a set of rigid rules or simplistic claims.

The Wisdom of Balance

Another aspect often overlooked by critics is the ethical dimension of the alkaline diet. It's not just about personal health; it's about making choices that are sustainable, ethical, and aligned with a broader vision of well-being. This includes everything from ethical sourcing of food to the environmental impact of our dietary choices. The alkaline diet encourages us to be mindful consumers, aware of the ripple effects our choices can have on the world around us.

Critics often portray the alkaline diet as extreme or imbalanced, but the essence of the diet is, in fact, balance. It's about creating an internal environment where your body can function at its best. This doesn't mean eliminating entire food groups or adhering to a rigid set of rules. It means making informed choices that bring you closer to your health goals while respecting your body's natural wisdom.

The Invitation to Explore

As we wrap up this chapter, let's acknowledge that the conversation around the alkaline diet is far from over. New research will emerge, opinions will evolve, and the dialogue will continue. And that's a good thing. It's through this ongoing conversation that we deepen our understanding, challenge our preconceptions, and arrive at a more nuanced, holistic view of health and well-being.

So, to the skeptics and critics, we extend an invitation: come explore this world with us. Bring your questions, your doubts, and your criticisms. They are the fuel that drives us to learn, to grow, and to strive for a deeper understanding of what it means to live a truly alkaline life.

In the end, the alkaline diet is not a dogma to be blindly followed but a pathway to explore. It's a journey filled with questions and discoveries, challenges and triumphs. And like any journey, it's best undertaken with an open mind, a curious spirit, and a willingness to embrace the complexity and beauty of the human experience.

Scientific Evidence Supporting Alkaline Living

The Confluence of Science and Alkaline Living: A New Paradigm

In a world where scientific evidence is often considered the gold standard for truth, the alkaline diet has found itself under the microscope. Critics and skeptics have questioned its efficacy, often demanding rigorous scientific proof. As we delve into this chapter, let's explore the scientific evidence that not only supports alkaline living but also elevates it from a mere dietary fad to a lifestyle backed by empirical data.

The Biochemical Basis: Understanding pH Levels

At the core of the alkaline diet is the concept of pH levels—potential of hydrogen—a measure of the acidity or alkalinity of a solution. Our body operates optimally at a slightly alkaline pH level of around 7.4. Deviations from this can lead to a host of health issues, from inflammation to chronic diseases. Scientific studies have shown that an alkaline diet can help maintain this delicate balance, thereby supporting overall health.

One of the most compelling pieces of scientific evidence supporting alkaline living comes from the study of metabolic processes. Research has shown that an alkaline diet can positively impact cellular respiration and energy production. This is crucial because efficient cellular function is the cornerstone of good health. When cells function optimally, they can better combat disease, repair damage, and contribute to a state of well-being.

Minerals like calcium, potassium, and magnesium play a pivotal role in maintaining an alkaline environment in the body. These minerals act as "buffers," neutralizing excess acidity. Numerous studies have demonstrated that an alkaline diet rich in these minerals can improve bone density, reduce muscle wasting, and even enhance the body's ability to absorb essential nutrients.

The Cardiovascular Connection

Cardiovascular health is another area where the alkaline diet shines. Scientific research has shown that an alkaline diet can help lower blood pressure and reduce cholesterol levels. These are significant markers for cardiovascular health, and their improvement through an alkaline diet provides strong evidence for its benefits.

The Gut-Brain Axis: Mental Health Implications

Emerging research in the field of neuroscience has begun to explore the gut-brain axis, the biochemical signaling that occurs between the gastrointestinal tract and the central nervous system. Preliminary studies suggest that an alkaline diet can positively influence this axis, potentially improving mental health conditions such as depression and anxiety.

The Cancer Conundrum: A Ray of Hope

While it's crucial to note that no diet can "cure" cancer, some scientific studies suggest that an alkaline environment may inhibit the growth of cancer cells. This is a burgeoning area of research, and while definitive conclusions are yet to be drawn, the initial findings are promising.

The Immunity Boost: Beyond Anecdotal Evidence

The alkaline diet's impact on the immune system has also been the subject of scientific scrutiny. Research indicates that an alkaline diet can enhance the body's natural defense mechanisms, making it more resilient to infections.

Bridging the Gap: Science Meets Lifestyle

As we navigate the labyrinth of health and wellness, it's easy to get lost in the cacophony of diets, trends, and fads. But when a lifestyle like alkaline living finds support in scientific evidence, it offers us a unique opportunity to bridge the gap between traditional wisdom and modern science. It allows us to approach health holistically, armed with the best of both worlds.

In conclusion, the scientific evidence supporting alkaline living is not just a collection of isolated facts but a harmonious symphony of interconnected truths. It invites us to look beyond the skepticism and embrace a lifestyle that is not only intuitively appealing but also empirically validated. As we continue to explore the nuances of alkaline living, let this chapter serve as a cornerstone, grounding our journey in the bedrock of scientific understanding.

Scientific Evidence Supporting Alkaline Living

Part II: The Conclusive Insights

In recent years, the alkaline diet has gained significant attention, with proponents touting its myriad health benefits. But what does science say about alkaline living? Let's delve deeper into the evidence that supports the benefits of maintaining an alkaline balance in the body.

Our body operates optimally within a narrow pH range, with blood pH hovering around 7.4. Any significant deviation from this can lead to metabolic acidosis or alkalosis, both of which can have detrimental effects on health. The body has intricate mechanisms to maintain this balance, including the respiratory and renal systems. However, the foods we consume can influence this balance, either by producing acid or alkaline residues after metabolism.

Bone Health and Alkalinity

One of the most debated topics in the realm of alkaline living is its impact on bone health. Some studies suggest that consuming an acid-forming diet can lead to calcium loss from bones, increasing the risk of osteoporosis. The rationale is that the body may use bone minerals to neutralize excess acid. A review published in the Journal of Environmental and Public Health found that alkaline diets might improve bone health by reducing bone resorption, a process where bones break down and release minerals into the bloodstream.

Muscle Mass Preservation

As we age, the loss of muscle mass becomes a concern. A study in the American Journal of Clinical Nutrition found that alkaline diets might benefit muscle mass in older adults. The research suggests that when the body is in a chronic acidic state, it may lead to muscle wasting. An alkaline diet, rich in fruits and vegetables, can help counteract this effect.

Improved Cardiovascular Health

Cardiovascular diseases remain a leading cause of death worldwide. Research indicates that an alkaline diet, rich in potassium, magnesium, and calcium, can lead to improved heart health. These minerals are vital for heart function and can help reduce blood pressure and the risk of stroke.

Chronic Disease and Inflammation

Chronic inflammation is a root cause of many diseases, including cancer, diabetes, and heart disease. Alkaline foods, especially green leafy vegetables and fruits, are rich in antioxidants that combat oxidative stress and reduce inflammation. A study in the Journal of Inflammation found that an alkaline diet might reduce inflammation and the risk of chronic diseases.

Cognitive Function and Alkalinity

Emerging research suggests that an alkaline diet might benefit brain health. Acidic diets, high in processed foods and sugars, have been linked to reduced cognitive function and an increased risk of neurodegenerative diseases. Alkaline foods, on the other hand, are rich in nutrients that support brain health, such as omega-3 fatty acids, antioxidants, and vitamins.

The Final Verdict

While the alkaline diet has its critics, a growing body of scientific evidence supports its benefits. It's essential to approach the topic with an open mind and a critical eye, understanding that while the diet may offer several health advantages, it's not a panacea. As with any dietary approach, individual responses can vary.

In conclusion, the alkaline diet, grounded in scientific evidence, offers a holistic approach to health. By focusing on whole foods and reducing processed, acid-forming foods, individuals can harness the benefits of alkaline living. As always, it's crucial to consult with healthcare professionals before making significant changes to one's diet.

Remember, the journey to optimal health is a continuous one, and while the alkaline diet provides a roadmap, it's the daily choices we make that determine our health trajectory. Embrace the science, listen to your body, and embark on a path of holistic well-being.

Addressing Doubts and Concerns

The Fear of the Unknown

Let's face it, skepticism is a natural part of the human experience. When we're presented with a new idea, especially one that challenges our long-held beliefs, it's normal to have doubts and concerns. The alkaline lifestyle, despite its growing popularity and scientific backing, is no exception.

One of the most significant barriers people face when considering the alkaline lifestyle is the fear of the unknown. "What will happen to my body? Will I be able to sustain this lifestyle? What if it doesn't work for me?" These are valid questions, and it's okay to ask them. The fear of the unknown can be paralyzing, but it's also an opportunity for growth and enlightenment.

The Skepticism of Science

Another common concern is the skepticism surrounding the scientific evidence that supports alkaline living. While it's true that more research is needed to fully understand the long-term effects and benefits, numerous studies have shown promising results. For instance, research has indicated that an alkaline diet can help improve bone health, reduce muscle wasting, and even mitigate chronic diseases like hypertension and diabetes.

Let's not forget the social aspect. Adopting an alkaline lifestyle often means going against the grain, and that can be socially isolating. The fear of judgment from friends and family can be a significant hurdle. It's crucial to remember that your health journey is personal. While social acceptance is essential, it should not come at the expense of your well-being.

The perceived financial burden is another concern that many people have. Organic fruits, vegetables, and alkaline water can be more expensive than their non-organic counterparts. However, it's essential to view this as an investment in your health. The long-term benefits, both physically and mentally, can far outweigh the initial costs.

Change is hard; there's no sugar-coating it. Transitioning to an alkaline lifestyle is not just a dietary change; it's a lifestyle overhaul. It requires commitment, discipline, and a willingness to step out of your comfort zone. But remember, every significant change starts with the decision to try.

The Power of Personal Experience

While scientific evidence provides a strong foundation, personal experience is just as valuable. Countless testimonials speak to the transformative power of alkaline living. These are real people who have experienced real changes. Their stories serve as both inspiration and validation for those looking to embark on this journey.

It's easier to address doubts and concerns when your part of a community. Whether it's online forums, social media groups, or local meetups, find your tribe. Share your fears, ask your questions, and celebrate your victories, no matter how small.

Conclusion: Embrace the Journey, Doubts and All

Doubts and concerns are not roadblocks; they're signposts. They guide us, challenge us, and ultimately help us grow. So, as you consider stepping into the world of alkaline living, don't let your doubts hold you back. Instead, let them propel you forward, armed with questions, open to discoveries, and ready for a transformative experience.

In the end, addressing these doubts and concerns is not just about providing answers; it's about encouraging a mindset shift. It's about moving from a place of hesitation to a space of confident, informed action. And that, dear reader, is where the real magic happens.

Winston Churchill once said, "Success is not final, failure is not fatal: It is the courage to continue that counts." Your doubts and concerns are not a sign of failure; they are a natural part of the human experience. What matters is your courage to continue, to explore, and to grow.

Book 15: Grow Your Own – The Alkaline Garden

Basics of Alkaline Farming and Gardening

The symphony of soil and soul

Imagine entering a garden where every plant, every flower and even the soil beneath your feet resonates with the natural rhythm of your body. This is not the scene of a utopian novel: it is the essence of alkaline farming and gardening. It is a practice that not only nourishes the body but also the soul, creating a harmonious relationship between you and the Earth.

The cornerstone of alkaline farming is soil. Soil is not just soil; it is a living, breathing entity. It is the womb in which seeds are nurtured to life. Alkaline soil, rich in minerals such as calcium and magnesium, provides an optimal environment for plant growth. But how do you turn your garden soil into this alkaline paradise? The answer lies in understanding the current pH level and taking steps to adjust it. Lime, wood ash and bone meal are some of the natural substances that can help raise the pH of the soil, making it more alkaline.

The rhythm of the seasons and choosing plants

Once the soil has been prepared, the next step is to choose the right plants. Not all plants are suitable for alkaline conditions. Some plants, such as lavender, thyme and oregano, not only thrive in alkaline soils but also offer medicinal benefits. These plants become the brushstrokes of color on the canvas of your alkaline garden, each contributing to a masterpiece of health and wellness.

Nature has its own rhythm, a cycle of seasons that influences the growth and decay of all living things. Alkaline farming and gardening are no different.

Understanding the rhythm of the seasons allows you to plant at the right time, harvest at maximum nutritional value, and prepare the soil for the next cycle. This cyclical approach ensures a sustainable and fruitful relationship with your garden.

The dance of water and light

Water and sunlight are to plants what love and care are to humans. The quality of water used for irrigation can affect the alkalinity of the soil. Rainwater, being naturally slightly acidic, can balance a highly alkaline soil. Sunlight, on the other hand, plays a key role in photosynthesis, the process by which plants convert light into energy. The right balance of water and light can make your alkaline garden a sanctuary of health.

Sustainability is not just a buzzword, but a commitment to future generations. In alkaline farming, sustainability means practices such as composting, crop rotation, and natural pest control. These practices not only maintain the alkaline balance, but also enrich the soil, making it a legacy to be passed on to future generations.

The harvest of an alkaline garden is not just a harvest of fruits and vegetables, it is a harvest of well-being. The foods grown will be rich in essential nutrients, sure, but the very act of gardening is therapeutic. It is a form of meditation, a break from the hectic pace of modern life. It is a space in which one can breathe, reflect and reconnect with one's self.

The journey ahead: Your garden, your sanctuary

As we delve into the complexities of alkaline farming and gardening in the coming chapters, remember that it is not just about growing food. It is about cultivating a life in harmony with nature. It is about creating a sanctuary where every plant, every flower and every crop is a celebration of the natural balance of life.

So, as you stand on the threshold of this exciting journey, know that you are not just a gardener; you are an artist, a healer and a guardian of the Earth. And that, dear reader, is just the beginning. Welcome to the world of alkaline farming and gardening-a world where the earth is your canvas, the plants are your palette, and your hands are the tools of creation.

The Symbiotic Relationship: Soil, Plants, and You

As you stand in your alkaline garden, you're not merely an observer; you're a participant in a grander scheme. The soil nurtures the plants, the plants nourish you, and you, in turn, care for the soil. It's a symbiotic relationship, a closed loop of life that transcends the boundaries of traditional farming. This is not just agriculture; it's a form of alchemy where elements transform into something more valuable, both nutritionally and spiritually.

Your garden speaks to you, not in words but in signs. A drooping leaf, a yellowing bud, or even the vibrancy of a flower can tell you about the soil's health and the plant's needs. The art of observation is crucial in alkaline farming. It's akin to a doctor diagnosing a patient, where the smallest symptom can reveal a lot. By being attuned to these signs, you can address issues before they escalate, ensuring that the alkaline balance is maintained.

The fruits and vegetables you harvest are laden with nutrients, but let's not overlook the emotional harvest. The joy of seeing a seed sprout, the satisfaction of plucking a ripe fruit, and the peace that comes from digging your hands into the earth—these are emotional nutrients. They feed your soul and combat the stress and anxiety that often accompany a fast-paced lifestyle. Your alkaline garden becomes a sanctuary, a place where you can reclaim your emotional equilibrium.

In the enthusiasm of creating an alkaline garden, it's easy to get carried away. However, wisdom lies in understanding limitations. Not every plant will align with the alkaline philosophy. Some plants may even disrupt the soil's pH balance.

Knowing what not to grow is as important as knowing what to grow. This discernment ensures that your garden remains a true alkaline environment, without the risk of unintentional sabotage.

The Legacy of Seeds: The Future of Your Alkaline Garden

Every seed you plant is a promise to the future. By choosing organic, non-GMO seeds, you're making a commitment to sustainability. These seeds will one day grow into plants that will produce seeds of their own, continuing the cycle. Your alkaline garden, thus, becomes a legacy, a gift to future generations. It's a testament to a life lived in harmony with nature, a life that respects the delicate balance of the earth.

As the seasons change and years pass, your alkaline garden will evolve, and so will you. The person who first tilled the soil will not be the same person who enjoys the harvests year after year. You'll find that you've not only grown food but also grown in wisdom, patience, and gratitude. Your relationship with your garden will mirror your relationship with life—deep, meaningful, and richly rewarding.

The Closing Chapter: An Invitation to a Lifelong Journey

As we close this chapter on the basics of alkaline farming and gardening, remember that this is not an end but a beginning. Your garden is a living, evolving entity, and your journey with it is lifelong. With each seed you plant, you sow not just a crop but a new experience, a new lesson. Your alkaline garden is not just a plot of land; it's a classroom, a therapist's office, and a temple.

So, as you step back into your garden, trowel in hand and heart full of dreams, know that you're stepping into a world of endless possibilities. You're not just a gardener; you're a steward of the earth, a student of life, and a harvester of dreams. And in this role, you'll find that the most beautiful blooms are not always in your garden; sometimes, they're in you. Welcome to the lifelong journey of alkaline farming and gardening—a journey that promises not just abundant harvests but also abundant life.

Sourcing Seeds and Plants: Organic and Non-GMO

The Genesis of Every Garden: The Seed

Every garden, no matter how expansive or modest, begins with a simple seed. It's a tiny capsule of potential, holding within its shell the blueprint for vibrant blooms, lush foliage, and nutritious fruits and vegetables. But not all seeds are created equal. In the realm of alkaline gardening, the quality of your seeds and plants is not just a matter of good gardening practice; it's a cornerstone of holistic health.

When you opt for organic seeds, you're making a conscious choice to steer clear of synthetic pesticides, herbicides, and genetically modified organisms (GMOs). These chemicals not only disrupt the natural pH balance of the soil but also introduce toxins into your food supply. Organic seeds are harvested from plants that have been nurtured in balanced soil, free from harmful chemicals. They are the custodians of a nutrient-rich lineage, promising a harvest that is as pure as nature intended.

The Non-GMO Commitment: A Stand for Health and Integrity

GMOs are often touted as the future of agriculture, engineered for higher yields and resistance to pests. However, the long-term health implications of GMOs are still not fully understood. By choosing non-GMO seeds, you're not just planting a garden; you're taking a stand. You're saying yes to biodiversity, yes to ecological balance, and yes to health. It's a commitment to the integrity of your food and the sanctity of your body.

Finding a reputable source for organic, non-GMO seeds and plants is akin to finding a trusted family doctor. You're entrusting the vitality of your garden to this source. Local farmers' markets, specialized online stores, and community seed banks are excellent places to start your search. Always look for certifications and don't hesitate to ask questions. Your due diligence today will bear fruits—quite literally—in seasons to come.

Heirloom seeds are the jewels of the gardening world. These are varieties that have been passed down through generations, each seed carrying the wisdom and resilience of its ancestors. Unlike hybrid seeds, which are often sterile and short-lived, heirlooms can be saved and replanted year after year. They are a living legacy, a link to an age-old agricultural heritage that honored the earth and its cycles.

Seeds and plants are living entities, sensitive to the rhythms of nature. Buying your seeds too early or too late can compromise their vitality. Align your purchasing schedule with the natural cycles of the season. This alignment is not just practical; it's also symbolic. You're syncing your gardening activities with the cosmic dance of the earth and sun, a ritual as old as time.

The Community Connection: Seed Swaps and Sharing

Gardening is not a solitary endeavor; it's a community act. Participating in seed swaps or sharing surplus seeds and plants with neighbors not only enriches your garden but also strengthens community bonds. It's a form of social permaculture, where relationships are nurtured alongside plants.

Your choices as a consumer have a ripple effect, impacting lives and ecosystems far removed from your immediate environment. Opting for fair trade seeds and plants ensures that the farmers who have toiled to bring you these botanical wonders are compensated fairly. It's an ethical dimension to gardening that elevates it from a hobby to a humanitarian act.

The Sacred Act: Setting Intentions for Your Garden

As you hold a seed in your hand, ready to plant it in the soil, pause for a moment. This is a sacred act, a covenant between you and the earth. Set an intention for your garden. Whether it's health, peace, or abundance, let that intention infuse every seed, every plant, and every harvest. Your garden will not just be a plot of land; it will be a sanctuary of your highest aspirations.

In the end, sourcing organic and non-GMO seeds and plants is not just a chapter in a gardening manual; it's a manifesto for life. It's about making choices that honor the earth, nourish your body, and enrich your soul. As you embark on this journey, know that each seed you plant is a declaration of your values, a testament to your vision for a healthier, more harmonious world. Welcome to the transformative power of conscious gardening.

The Garden as a Reflection of Self

As you stand amidst the lush greenery of your alkaline garden, each leaf and bloom is a testament to the choices you've made. The organic, non-GMO seeds and plants you've carefully sourced have not only flourished but have also become an extension of your own commitment to holistic health. Your garden is not just a collection of plants; it's a living, breathing manifestation of your values.

The beauty of an organic, non-GMO garden extends far beyond its visual appeal. Each fruit, vegetable, and herb you harvest carries a nutritional profile that is markedly superior. Free from synthetic chemicals and genetic modifications, these plants offer a cornucopia of essential nutrients, antioxidants, and phytochemicals. It's not just food; it's medicine, nurtured by the earth and curated by you.

Your choice to go organic and non-GMO is also a choice to be an environmental steward. Organic farming practices enhance soil fertility, promote biodiversity, and reduce water pollution. By opting for non-GMO seeds, you're also helping to preserve the genetic diversity of plant species, a critical factor in the resilience of ecosystems. Your garden becomes a microcosm of a more sustainable and harmonious world, a legacy that you can pass on to future generations.

Gardening is often described as therapeutic, but when your garden is rooted in the principles of organic and non-GMO practices, this therapy takes on a deeper dimension. The act of planting, nurturing, and harvesting becomes a meditative practice, a dialogue between you and the natural world. The garden responds to your care, but it also cares for you, offering emotional and spiritual sustenance that is as vital as the nutritional benefits.

The Culinary Alchemy: Transforming Harvest into Health

The fruits of your labor are not just to be admired but to be consumed. As you bring your harvest into the kitchen, you have the opportunity to transform these raw ingredients into culinary masterpieces. Whether it's a simple salad or an elaborate meal, the flavors are more vibrant, the textures more robust, and the nutritional value uncompromised. Each bite is a celebration of your garden's integrity and your own commitment to holistic health.

Your garden can serve as an inspiration to others, a living example of what is possible when intention aligns with action. Friends, family, and even casual visitors will notice the difference, not just in the quality of your produce but in the quality of your life. You become a silent ambassador for organic and non-GMO living, sowing seeds of change in the minds and hearts of those you touch.

The Lifelong Commitment: Beyond the Current Season

As the seasons change, your garden will go through cycles of growth, harvest, and renewal. Yet, your commitment to sourcing organic and non-GMO seeds and plants remains constant. It's a lifelong journey, one that evolves with each passing year, offering new challenges and new rewards. But the core principles remain unchanging: a dedication to health, sustainability, and the sheer joy of nurturing life in its purest form.

As you stand in your garden, you realize that each plant is a note in a grand symphony, a symphony composed of choices and rewards. The organic, non-GMO seeds and plants you've sourced have not only enriched your garden but have also enriched your life in ways both tangible and intangible. It's a harmonious cycle of giving and receiving, a testament to the transformative power of conscious choices.

In closing, sourcing organic and non-GMO seeds and plants is not a mere gardening tip; it's a philosophy, a way of life that reverberates through every aspect of your being. It's a commitment to a higher standard of living, a pledge to honor the sanctity of life in all its forms. As you nurture your garden, you nurture yourself, and in doing so, you nurture the world. Welcome to the fulfilling journey of conscious, holistic living.

The Joy of Foraging and Wildcrafting

The Call of the Wild: Reconnecting with Our Roots

Imagine stepping into a verdant forest, the air tinged with the earthy scent of moss and damp soil. Sunlight filters through the canopy of leaves, casting dappled shadows on the forest floor. You're not just a visitor; you're a participant in an ancient ritual that dates back to the dawn of humanity: foraging and wildcrafting. This practice is not just about gathering food or medicinal herbs; it's a transformative experience that reconnects us with our ancestral roots and the natural world.

As you venture deeper into the woods, your senses come alive. Your eyes scan the foliage for the vibrant hues of edible berries, your nose picks up the subtle fragrance of medicinal herbs, and your ears tune into the rustle of leaves, signaling the presence of a nearby creature. Each step is a dance, a delicate balance between observation and intuition, as you learn to read the subtle cues of nature.

Foraging and wildcrafting are not just about what you take; they're about what you give back. As you carefully pick a berry or snip a medicinal herb, you're engaging in a form of alchemy, transforming the raw elements of nature into something more valuable. But this alchemy is reciprocal. By understanding the cycles of growth and decay, you learn to harvest sustainably, ensuring that the plants you gather today will be replaced by new growth tomorrow.

The Spiritual Harvest: Nourishing the Soul

The forest is not just a source of food; it's a pharmacy stocked with a myriad of medicinal plants and herbs. From the anti-inflammatory properties of willow bark to the immune-boosting benefits of elderberries, nature offers a treasure trove of remedies that have been used for centuries. As you gather these natural medicines, you're not just benefiting your health; you're tapping into the collective wisdom of generations who have walked this earth before you.

But the benefits of foraging and wildcrafting extend beyond the physical. There's a spiritual dimension to this practice, a sense of communion with the land that nourishes the soul as much as the body. Each plant you gather carries the energy of the place where it grew, a unique vibrational signature that resonates with your own. As you incorporate these plants into your alkaline diet, you're not just consuming nutrients; you're absorbing the very essence of the land.

The Community of Life: A Web of Interconnectedness

As you forage and wildcraft, you become acutely aware of your place in the larger community of life. You're not an isolated individual but a part of a complex web of interconnectedness that includes not just humans but animals, plants, and even the soil itself. This awareness fosters a sense of responsibility, a commitment to stewardship that goes beyond mere conservation. It's a call to action, a mandate to protect and preserve the delicate balance of life on this planet.

Part of the joy of foraging and wildcrafting is the element of surprise, the thrill of discovering something new. Whether it's a rare mushroom hidden beneath a fallen log or a patch of wild strawberries nestled in a sunny clearing, each find is a revelation, a moment of pure delight that rekindles the sense of wonder we often lose in adulthood.

The Art of Mindfulness: The Here and Now

In a world that constantly pulls us in different directions, foraging and wildcrafting offer a rare opportunity for mindfulness. As you focus on the task at hand, all other concerns fade away, leaving you fully present in the moment. It's a form of meditation, a practice that not only calms the mind but also sharpens the senses, making you more attuned to the subtle beauty of the world around you.

It's a journey into the heart of nature, a voyage of discovery that challenges us, nurtures us, and ultimately transforms us. As you step back into the world, basket in hand, you carry with you not just the fruits of your labor but the invaluable lessons of the land. Welcome to the enriching world of foraging and wildcrafting, where every step is a step closer to your true self.

The Joy of Foraging and Wildcrafting: Embracing Nature's Bounty

In the heart of nature, where the earth meets the sky and the wind whispers tales of yore, there lies a secret. A secret that our ancestors knew, that indigenous tribes honor, and that many of us, in our modern, fast-paced lives, have forgotten. This secret is the joy of foraging and wildcrafting.

Foraging is not just an act; it's a dance with nature. It's about understanding the rhythms of the seasons, knowing when the wild berries will ripen, when the mushrooms will sprout after a rain, and when the herbs are at their most potent. It's about walking through the woods, meadows, and along riverbanks with an open heart and a keen eye, ready to discover the treasures that Mother Nature has scattered in her wake.

Wildcrafting, on the other hand, is the art of harvesting these wild plants sustainably. It's about taking only what you need, leaving plenty behind for wildlife and for the plant to continue its life cycle. It's about understanding that we are a part of this intricate web of life, and our actions have consequences.

The Healing Power of Wild Plants

The plants that grow wild, untouched by pesticides, fertilizers, or human intervention, often have a potency that cultivated plants lack. They have battled the elements, fought for their place under the sun, and in doing so, have developed a resilience that they pass on to us when we consume them.

Take, for instance, the humble dandelion. Often dismissed as a pesky weed, this plant is a powerhouse of nutrition. Its leaves are rich in vitamins and minerals, its roots cleanse the liver, and its flowers are a favorite among bees. And yet, how often do we walk past a field of dandelions without giving them a second glance?

Reconnecting with Our Roots

Foraging and wildcrafting are not just about collecting food or medicine. They are about reconnecting with our roots, with a time when humans lived in harmony with nature. They remind us that we are not separate from the earth, but a part of it. That the health of the planet and our health are intertwined.

As we kneel to pick a berry or pluck a herb, we are participating in an age-old tradition. We are walking in the footsteps of our ancestors, experiencing the same wonder and gratitude that they must have felt as they gathered nature's bounty.

There's a meditative quality to foraging. As we walk silently, attuned to our surroundings, we enter a state of flow. The chatter of our minds quietens, and we are present in the moment. Each leaf, each bird song, each rustle in the underbrush becomes magnified. We realize the beauty and abundance that surrounds us, and how often we take it for granted.

Foraging also teaches us humility. Nature doesn't bend to our will. We can't force a plant to grow or a berry to ripen. We have to adapt to nature's timetable, to learn patience and respect.

In Conclusion

The joy of foraging and wildcrafting is multi-faceted. It's the thrill of discovery, the satisfaction of self-sufficiency, the deep connection with nature, and the myriad health benefits of consuming wild plants. But more than anything, it's a reminder. A reminder of our place in the world, of the wisdom of ancient traditions, and of the beauty that lies in the simple act of walking, observing, and being one with nature.

As we move forward in our fast-paced lives, let's take a moment to pause. To look around and truly see the wonders that nature offers. And maybe, just maybe, rediscover the joy of foraging and wildcrafting.

Book 16: Dr. Sebi's Global Footprint

How Different Cultures Embraced Dr. Sebi's Teachings

The teachings of Dr. Sebi have transcended borders, cultures, and languages, leaving an indelible mark on the global health landscape. His philosophy of alkaline living has resonated with people from all walks of life, and it's fascinating to see how different cultures have adopted, adapted, and integrated these teachings into their own unique ways of life.

Dr. Sebi's message is fundamentally a universal one: the body is a temple that thrives in an alkaline environment. This message has been embraced by cultures that already have a deep-rooted understanding of the body's connection to nature. For instance, in India, the ancient practice of Ayurveda shares similarities with Dr. Sebi's teachings. Both philosophies emphasize the importance of maintaining a balanced internal environment for optimal health.

The African Connection

In Africa, where Dr. Sebi's lineage traces back, the teachings have been welcomed as a return to ancestral wisdom. Traditional African medicine often incorporates herbs and natural remedies, aligning closely with Dr. Sebi's herbal treatments. Communities across the continent have started incorporating his recommended alkaline foods into their diets, seeing it as a way to reclaim their health sovereignty.

The Latin American Embrace

In Latin America, where natural healing practices like curanderismo have been passed down through generations, Dr. Sebi's approach has found a receptive audience. The use of herbs like Damiana and Sarsaparilla, which are native to Latin America and also feature in Dr. Sebi's herbal list, has strengthened the connection. People have started to merge these ancient practices with Dr. Sebi's guidelines, creating a holistic health model that honors both tradition and modern understanding.

The Western World's Awakening

In the Western world, where pharmaceuticals often overshadow natural remedies, Dr. Sebi's teachings have sparked a renaissance of interest in holistic health. Amidst the backdrop of rising chronic illnesses, many in Europe and North America have turned to Dr. Sebi's alkaline diet as an alternative to conventional treatment methods. The teachings have also found resonance within vegan and vegetarian communities, who see it as an extension of their own ethical and health-conscious choices.

The Asian Integration

In Asia, where traditional medicine like Traditional Chinese Medicine (TCM) and Ayurveda have been practiced for centuries, Dr. Sebi's teachings have been integrated rather seamlessly. The emphasis on herbal remedies and the balance of bodily energies aligns well with existing philosophies. In Japan, for example, the concept of "Hara," or the body's center, shares similarities with Dr. Sebi's focus on the gut as the core of overall health.

What's remarkable is the formation of a global community that transcends geographical and cultural boundaries. Social media platforms and online forums dedicated to Dr. Sebi's teachings have become melting pots of cultural exchange. People from around the world share their experiences, recipes, and success stories, enriching each other's journey toward alkaline living.

In conclusion, the global footprint of Dr. Sebi's teachings is a testament to their universal applicability and transformative power. Different cultures have not just embraced these teachings but have enriched them by integrating their own traditional wisdom. It's a beautiful tapestry of global unity, woven together by the common thread of a desire for holistic well-being. And in a world that often highlights differences, the universal acceptance of Dr. Sebi's teachings serves as a poignant reminder of the shared human quest for health, happiness, and a life in harmony with nature.

This is just the beginning of an exploration into how Dr. Sebi's teachings have been adopted worldwide. The stories are as diverse as the people who share them, and they all contribute to the ever-expanding legacy of a man whose life mission was to heal humanity, one person at a time.

The Resonance of Dr. Sebi's Teachings Across the Globe

As we delve deeper into the global impact of Dr. Sebi's teachings, it's essential to recognize that the embrace of his philosophy is not merely an act of adoption but a profound transformation. Different cultures have not just accepted his teachings; they've made them their own, tailoring the principles to fit into their existing health paradigms. This adaptability is perhaps the most compelling testament to the universal truth that Dr. Sebi sought to share: the power of alkalinity to heal and harmonize the human body.

The Cultural Tapestry of Alkaline Living

In the Middle East, where herbal medicine has been a cornerstone of health for centuries, Dr. Sebi's herbal recommendations have found a natural home. The region's rich biodiversity offers a plethora of herbs that align with Dr. Sebi's guidelines, and people have begun to incorporate these into their traditional remedies. It's a beautiful blend of ancient wisdom and modern understanding, creating a holistic health model that is both timeless and timely.

The Indigenous Embrace

Among Indigenous communities worldwide, Dr. Sebi's teachings have been seen as an affirmation of their ancestral knowledge. These communities have always lived in harmony with nature, and the alkaline diet resonates with their traditional foods and natural remedies. The teachings have empowered these communities to resist the encroachment of processed foods and pharmaceuticals, preserving their health and heritage.

Educational initiatives have also played a significant role in spreading Dr. Sebi's teachings. From workshops in Australia that focus on alkaline superfoods to seminars in Europe discussing the science of body pH, the educational landscape has become a fertile ground for sowing the seeds of alkaline living. These initiatives have helped demystify the science behind the diet, making it more accessible to people who are new to the concept.

The Digital Bridge

The digital age has been a boon for the global spread of Dr. Sebi's philosophy. Online platforms have become the new town squares where people from diverse backgrounds come together to share their alkaline journey. These digital communities offer support, advice, and most importantly, a sense of global camaraderie that transcends geographical and cultural barriers.

The global embrace of Dr. Sebi's teachings has had a ripple effect, influencing even the medical community to reevaluate its stance on natural healing. While the journey is far from over, the increasing number of healthcare professionals advocating for an alkaline lifestyle indicates a promising shift. It's a slow but steady movement toward a more holistic approach to health, one that considers the individual as an integral part of the natural world rather than a subject to be treated in isolation.

As we conclude this exploration, it's clear that Dr. Sebi's global footprint is not just a historical account but an ongoing narrative. The teachings continue to evolve as they spread, enriched by the cultural diversity and individual experiences of those who adopt them. It's a living legacy, one that honors the man who started it all and the global community that carries it forward.

In the end, the universal embrace of Dr. Sebi's teachings is not just about the adoption of an alkaline diet or the use of herbal remedies. It's about a collective awakening to the innate power we all possess to heal ourselves and live in harmony with nature. It's a journey of empowerment, a global movement that is redefining the way we think about health, community, and the very essence of human life. And in that sense, Dr. Sebi's teachings have not just crossed borders; they've dissolved them, uniting us all in a shared quest for holistic well-being.

The Spread and Influence of Alkaline Practices Worldwide

The Eastern Embrace: A Harmonious Fusion

As the sun rises over different parts of the world, it illuminates a global community united by a shared commitment to alkaline living. This is not a fleeting trend or a niche lifestyle; it's a worldwide awakening to the transformative power of alkalinity. Dr. Sebi's teachings have transcended borders, languages, and cultures, becoming a universal language of health and well-being. This chapter aims to explore the global spread and influence of alkaline practices, a phenomenon that has redefined the way we approach health on a planetary scale.

While Dr. Sebi's teachings originated in the West, their influence has permeated every corner of the globe. From the bustling streets of Tokyo to the serene landscapes of New Zealand, the alkaline lifestyle has found a home. It's essential to dispel the notion that this is a Western-centric movement. The universality of the alkaline approach to health speaks to its adaptability and relevance across diverse cultural contexts.

In Eastern cultures, where traditional medicine like Ayurveda and Traditional Chinese Medicine have reigned for centuries, the alkaline diet has been welcomed as a complementary practice. These ancient systems already emphasize balance and harmony, making the alkaline lifestyle a natural fit. In India, for example, alkaline foods are being incorporated into Ayurvedic diets, creating a holistic approach that honors both tradition and modernity.

Africa: Returning to Roots

In Africa, the cradle of humanity, the alkaline lifestyle is seen as a return to ancestral ways of living. Indigenous diets were naturally alkaline, rich in fruits, vegetables, and herbs. The introduction of processed foods disrupted these traditional diets, but the alkaline movement is helping to restore that balance. From community workshops in Nairobi to alkaline food markets in Accra, Africa is reclaiming its heritage through alkaline living.

Latin America: A Cultural Resonance

In Latin American countries, where herbal remedies and natural foods are deeply ingrained in the culture, Dr. Sebi's teachings have found fertile ground. The focus on natural healing and prevention resonates with the Latino ethos of 'buen vivir' or 'good living.' The alkaline lifestyle is not seen as an imposition but as an enhancement of existing cultural practices.

Europe: The Intersection of Tradition and Innovation

In Europe, a continent steeped in history yet driven by innovation, the alkaline lifestyle has been embraced as a progressive approach to health. Countries like Germany and Sweden, known for their advanced healthcare systems, are now integrating alkaline practices into their wellness programs. It's a marriage of cutting-edge science and age-old wisdom, creating a healthcare model for the future.

The Global Community: United in Diversity

What's truly remarkable about the global spread of alkaline practices is the sense of community it has fostered. People from different walks of life, disparate cultures, and opposite ends of the world are finding common ground in their pursuit of holistic health. Online forums, international workshops, and global health retreats are just some of the platforms where this global community converges, sharing experiences, knowledge, and support.

The Future is Alkaline

As we stand at this pivotal moment in history, it's clear that the alkaline movement is not just a passing fad but a lasting shift in global health consciousness. Its rapid spread and universal embrace are not merely indicators of its popularity but testaments to its efficacy. The world is waking up to the power of alkaline living, and this awakening is both a collective achievement and a promise of a healthier future for all.

In this ever-connected world, the spread and influence of alkaline practices serve as a beacon, guiding us towards a unified vision of health and well-being. It's a vision that honors our diversity, celebrates our unity, and holds the promise of a healthier, happier world for generations to come.

The Ripple Effect: The Lasting Impact of Alkaline Practices Across the Globe

As we've journeyed through the global landscape of alkaline living, it's evident that this is more than just a dietary shift; it's a catalyst for transformative change. The alkaline lifestyle has become a vehicle for social empowerment, environmental stewardship, and spiritual awakening. It's not just about what we consume; it's about how we live, how we connect with others, and how we contribute to the world.

One of the most compelling aspects of the alkaline lifestyle is its economic viability. Unlike fad diets or expensive wellness programs, alkaline living is accessible and sustainable. It encourages local farming, supports small businesses, and promotes ethical consumerism. From farmers' markets in Sydney to organic co-ops in Buenos Aires, the economic ripple effect is both local and global.

The Environmental Footprint: A Commitment to the Earth

The alkaline lifestyle is intrinsically linked to environmental consciousness. By advocating for organic farming, reducing waste, and promoting sustainable living, it contributes to a healthier planet. This is not just an individual choice but a collective commitment. As more communities worldwide adopt alkaline practices, we're seeing a reduction in soil degradation, water pollution, and carbon emissions.

In a world often divided by differences, the alkaline lifestyle serves as a unifying force. It transcends political boundaries, religious beliefs, and cultural norms, creating a global community bound by the shared goal of holistic well-being. This sense of unity is not just theoretical; it's palpable. From international alkaline cuisine festivals to global wellness retreats, the social fabric of alkaline living is rich, diverse, and inclusive.

The Spiritual Dimension: A Journey Within

While the physical benefits of alkaline living are well-documented, its spiritual implications are profound yet understated. It's not just about bodily health; it's about achieving a state of inner equilibrium. The principles of alkalinity align with spiritual tenets found in various philosophies and faiths, from the Buddhist concept of 'Middle Way' to the Sufi philosophy of balance. This spiritual dimension adds depth to the alkaline lifestyle, making it a holistic journey of body, mind, and soul.

The Legacy of Dr. Sebi: A Global Movement

As we reflect on the global footprint of Dr. Sebi's teachings, it's clear that his legacy is not confined to books, lectures, or products. His legacy is alive in the hearts and lives of millions around the world who have embraced the alkaline lifestyle. It's a legacy of empowerment, a legacy of community, and above all, a legacy of holistic health.

As we look to the future, the prospects for alkaline living are not just promising; they are transformative. With advancements in research, growing public awareness, and increasing global collaboration, the alkaline lifestyle is poised to become a cornerstone of global health initiatives. It's not a question of if but when.

In the grand tapestry of life, each thread—each choice, each action, each voice—contributes to the overall pattern. The global spread and influence of alkaline practices are akin to a symphony, where each note, no matter how subtle, adds to the collective melody. It's a symphony of well-being, a harmonious blend of individual choices and collective actions that resonate across the globe.

Continuing the Legacy: Alkaline Advocates Around the Globe

A Global Community United by Purpose

In the realm of health and wellness, the alkaline lifestyle has transcended its origins to become a global phenomenon. It's not just a diet or a regimen; it's a movement. And like any movement, its strength lies in its advocates—those individuals who not only embrace these principles but actively spread them. These are the torchbearers of Dr. Sebi's legacy, a diverse group of men and women who are united by a common purpose: to live better and to help others do the same.

The journey often starts with a personal transformation. Imagine a 45-year-old corporate executive from New York, burdened by chronic stress and poor health, who discovers the alkaline lifestyle. Within months, the transformation is so profound that it becomes a personal mission to share this newfound knowledge.

He starts by influencing his immediate circle, then his community, and eventually finds himself advocating for alkaline living at international health forums. His story, like many others, adds a new chapter to Dr. Sebi's global footprint.

The Role of Digital Advocacy

In today's interconnected world, the power of digital advocacy cannot be overstated. Social media platforms have become fertile ground for sharing success stories, recipes, and tips related to alkaline living. A mom from London sharing her journey of overcoming postpartum depression through an alkaline diet can inspire a young woman in Mumbai dealing with similar challenges. The ripple effect of such digital connections creates a global network of alkaline advocates, each contributing to the larger narrative.

While digital platforms offer a broad reach, grassroots movements remain the heartbeat of alkaline advocacy. These are community-led initiatives that organize workshops, seminars, and farmer's markets to promote alkaline living. For instance, a group of college students in Nairobi might start an alkaline food co-op, sourcing directly from local organic farmers. Their efforts not only promote health but also contribute to sustainable agriculture, thereby hitting two birds with one stone.

The Professional Advocates: Integrating Alkalinity into Healthcare

One of the most fascinating aspects of this global advocacy is the intersection of culture and alkalinity. In Japan, for example, the principles of alkaline living are finding resonance with the traditional philosophy of "Hara Hachi Bu," or eating until you are 80% full. Similarly, in Mediterranean regions, the emphasis on fresh fruits, vegetables, and olive oil aligns seamlessly with alkaline principles. This cultural integration makes the advocacy not just a health movement but a cultural exchange, enriching it in ways previously unimagined.

Beyond individual advocates, there's a growing number of healthcare professionals who are integrating alkaline principles into their practice.

Nutritionists, naturopaths, and even some forward-thinking physicians are recognizing the value of an alkaline approach to health. They serve as critical validators of the lifestyle, giving it the scientific backing and credibility that attract even the skeptics.

As the movement grows, so does the responsibility that comes with advocacy. It's crucial to approach it with a sense of ethics and integrity. Misinformation can be as viral as information, and therefore, the onus is on each advocate to be well-informed, transparent, and honest. This ethical dimension adds a layer of gravitas to the advocacy, making each proponent not just a follower but a custodian of Dr. Sebi's legacy.

The Road Ahead: A Collective Journey

As we stand at this juncture, what's clear is that the journey ahead is not a solitary one. It's a collective endeavor, fueled by the passion and commitment of alkaline advocates around the globe. Each story, each initiative, and each advocate add a unique flavor to this global tapestry. And as this tapestry expands, so does the legacy of Dr. Sebi, alive and thriving in the hearts and lives of millions worldwide.

In this ever-expanding global community, each one of us has a role to play. Whether you're a beginner just starting your alkaline journey or a seasoned advocate, your voice matters. Your experiences, your challenges, and your triumphs contribute to this global narrative. And it's this collective narrative that will define the future of alkaline living—a future that promises not just better health but a better world for us all.

The Unifying Thread: A Legacy in Motion

The alkaline lifestyle has become more than a health regimen; it's a catalyst for change, a transformative force that transcends geographical boundaries. It's a lifestyle that has been embraced by people from all walks of life, from the bustling streets of New York to the tranquil villages of Bali. The universal appeal of alkalinity lies in its simplicity, its rootedness in nature, and its profound impact on well-being. It's a lifestyle that doesn't just add years to your life, but life to your years.

The alkaline community is a resilient one, often rising above the challenges posed by a world that is increasingly commercialized and industrialized. Advocates are not just passive consumers of information; they are active participants, contributors, and even creators of knowledge. They share their personal stories, their struggles, and their triumphs, adding a layer of authenticity that no marketing campaign can replicate. This resilience is what keeps the community vibrant, engaged, and ever-expanding.

The Emotional Quotient: Compassion and Empathy

Mentorship plays a crucial role in the alkaline community. Seasoned advocates often take it upon themselves to guide newcomers, offering them not just tips and recipes, but also emotional support and encouragement. This mentor-mentee relationship is a two-way street, enriching both parties involved. The mentors gain a sense of fulfillment and purpose, while the mentees receive invaluable guidance that helps them navigate the complexities of alkaline living.

What sets the alkaline advocacy apart is its emotional quotient. It's not just about disseminating information; it's about doing so with compassion and empathy. Advocates understand that each individual's journey is unique, fraught with its own set of challenges and triumphs. They approach advocacy with an open heart, offering not just solutions but also a listening ear. This emotional connection is what turns casual followers into lifelong advocates.

The Future: A Legacy Unfolding

Every advocate adds a ripple to the ever-expanding ocean of alkaline living. Each story, each testimonial, each act of advocacy has a multiplier effect, inspiring others to take the plunge. Imagine a woman in her 40s who overcame chronic fatigue through alkaline living. Her story could inspire her neighbor, her colleague, or even a stranger halfway across the globe. This ripple effect is the essence of grassroots advocacy, and it's what keeps the movement dynamic, relevant, and impactful.

As we look to the future, the legacy of Dr. Sebi and the alkaline lifestyle is not set in stone; it's a tapestry that's still being woven, one thread at a time. It's a legacy that's not confined to the pages of a book or the walls of a seminar room; it's a living, breathing entity that exists in the hearts and minds of its advocates. And as this community of advocates continues to grow, so does the scope and impact of alkaline living.

The future is not just about expanding the community but enriching it, adding more colors to the tapestry, more voices to the chorus. It's about creating a legacy that's as diverse as it is unified, as global as it is personal. And in this endeavor, each one of us has a role to play. Whether you're a seasoned advocate or a newcomer, your voice, your story, and your advocacy matter. You are a part of this unfolding legacy, a legacy that promises a future of health, wellness, and holistic living for generations to come.

So, as we stand on the shoulders of giants like Dr. Sebi, let's not just be content with where we are. Let's strive for more. Let's dream bigger, aim higher, and work harder. Because the legacy of alkaline living is not just Dr. Sebi's legacy; it's ours to shape, ours to nurture, and ours to pass on. And in this collective endeavor, each one of us is both a student and a teacher, both a follower and a leader, both a beneficiary and a benefactor. It's a collective journey, and it's a journey that's just getting started.

Book 17: Tools, Resources, and Continued Learning

Dr. Sebi's Product Recommendations and Reviews

The Curated Path

In a world inundated with health products, supplements, and quick-fix solutions, making an informed choice is not just a luxury; it's a necessity. The alkaline lifestyle, as championed by Dr. Sebi, is not merely a diet but a holistic approach to well-being. It's a journey that requires not just the right mindset but also the right tools. And that's where Dr. Sebi's product recommendations come into play. These are not just products; they are lifelines that can either make or break your journey toward optimal health.

When it comes to health and wellness, trust is not given; it's earned. Dr. Sebi earned this trust over decades of research, practice, and most importantly, results. His recommendations are not based on fads or trends but on a deep understanding of human biology, herbal medicine, and the science of alkalinity. When Dr. Sebi recommends a product, it comes with a seal of approval that is backed by years of efficacy and countless testimonials.

The Personal Touch: Tailored Recommendations

In today's market, terms like 'organic,' 'natural,' and 'holistic' are often thrown around loosely, creating a fog of confusion for consumers. Dr. Sebi's product recommendations cut through this fog, offering clarity and assurance. These products are rigorously tested for quality, efficacy, and most importantly, alignment with the principles of alkaline living. They are free from harmful additives, preservatives, and artificial ingredients that can counteract the benefits of an alkaline lifestyle.

One size doesn't fit all, especially when it comes to health and wellness. Dr. Sebi understood this, and his product recommendations reflect this understanding. Whether you're dealing with specific health issues like diabetes or hypertension, or you're simply looking to enhance your overall well-being, there's a product tailored to meet your needs. These recommendations take into account not just your health status but also your lifestyle, your dietary preferences, and even your emotional well-being.

The Power of Synergy: Complementary Products

Dr. Sebi's approach to health was always holistic, and this is evident in his product recommendations. You'll find that these products often work best when used in synergy, complementing each other to provide a comprehensive solution for your health needs. For instance, a detoxifying tea may be recommended alongside a nutrient-rich supplement to enhance your body's natural cleansing processes. This synergistic approach ensures that you're not just addressing symptoms but tackling the root causes of your health issues.

Dr. Sebi's product recommendations don't exist in a vacuum; they are part of a vibrant community of alkaline advocates who share their experiences, reviews, and insights. This community-driven approach adds an extra layer of credibility and relatability to the products. It allows you to hear real stories from real people who have walked the path you're embarking on. These shared experiences serve as both a guide and a source of inspiration, making your alkaline journey less daunting and more achievable.

The Long Game: Sustainability and Ethical Practices

In a world grappling with environmental degradation and ethical dilemmas, Dr. Sebi's product recommendations offer a breath of fresh air. These products are not just good for you; they're good for the planet. Sourced sustainably and produced ethically, they align with the broader goals of environmental conservation and social responsibility. This makes your journey towards alkaline living not just a personal quest for health but a contribution to the greater good.

As you delve deeper into the world of alkaline living, these product recommendations serve as your compass, guiding you through the maze of choices and helping you make decisions that align with your health goals. They are more than just products; they are partners in your journey towards optimal health, holistic well-being, and a life of vitality and vigor. So, as you take this crucial step in your alkaline journey, know that you're not alone; you're backed by the wisdom, experience, and trust that Dr. Sebi's recommendations bring. And in this journey, that makes all the difference.

The Lasting Impact: Dr. Sebi's Product Recommendations and Reviews

As you navigate the labyrinth of health and wellness, Dr. Sebi's product recommendations serve as your North Star. They are not just items on a shelf but signposts on a journey of self-discovery. This journey is not a sprint but a marathon, requiring sustained effort, commitment, and the right resources. Dr. Sebi's recommendations are not just about what to consume but also about what to embody—values of authenticity, integrity, and holistic well-being.

In a world awash with information, discernment becomes a prized skill. Dr. Sebi's product recommendations are not just about telling you what to buy; they're about teaching you how to make choices. Choices that resonate not just with your body but also with your soul. It's about understanding the 'why' behind the 'what.' Why this herb over that one? Why this supplement and not that vitamin? The answers lie not just in the products themselves but in the philosophy that underpins them—a philosophy rooted in nature, science, and ancestral wisdom.

The Lifelong Commitment: It's Not a Phase, It's a Lifestyle

Your choices don't just affect you; they create ripples that extend to your family, your community, and even the planet. When you choose a product recommended by Dr. Sebi, you're not just investing in your health; you're investing in a vision of wellness that transcends individual boundaries. You become part of a collective endeavor to redefine health, challenge the status quo, and create a paradigm shift that could benefit generations to come.

Dr. Sebi's product recommendations are not a one-time affair. They are part of a lifelong commitment to excellence, purity, and vitality. This is not about quick fixes or temporary solutions. It's about building a lifestyle that stands the test of time, stress, and societal pressures. It's about creating a sanctuary of wellness in a chaotic world, a sanctuary built on the solid foundation of quality products, informed choices, and unwavering commitment.

The Legacy: Carrying the Torch Forward

Dr. Sebi left us with more than just a list of recommended products; he left us with a legacy—a legacy of empowerment, enlightenment, and eternal wellness. When you use a product that carries Dr. Sebi's endorsement, you're not just a consumer; you're a torchbearer. You're carrying forward a legacy that could illuminate lives and heal our planet. It's a responsibility, yes, but also a privilege—one that comes with the joy of knowing that your part of something much larger than yourself.

As we conclude this exploration of Dr. Sebi's product recommendations and reviews, let's remember that every choice we make is a vote for the kind of world we want to live in. A world of health, happiness, and holistic well-being. Dr. Sebi's recommendations are not just products; they are a philosophy, a lifestyle, and ultimately, a legacy. They are a testament to a life well-lived and a journey well-traveled. So, as you make these choices, know that you're not alone. Your part of a global community of enlightened individuals who have chosen to walk the path of wellness, wisdom, and wonder. And on this path, every step you take is not just for you; it's for all of us. The Unquenchable Thirst for Knowledge

The journey towards holistic health and well-being is akin to a river that never ceases to flow. It's a lifelong quest for wisdom, a thirst for understanding that can't be quenched by merely following a set of dietary guidelines or adopting a new lifestyle. This is where the importance of further reading—books, journals, and research papers—comes into play. These resources are the tributaries that feed into the river of your understanding, enriching it with diverse perspectives, scientific rigor, and a depth of knowledge that can't be found elsewhere.

Further Reading: Books, Journals, and Research Papers

The Power of Books: Your Personal Mentors

Books are more than just a collection of printed pages; they are your personal mentors guiding you through the complexities of holistic health. They offer you the wisdom of experts who have dedicated their lives to understanding the intricacies of the human body, the healing power of nature, and the profound impact of lifestyle choices on our well-being. When you delve into a well-researched book, you're not just reading; you're engaging in a dialogue with the author, questioning your preconceptions, and emerging with a more nuanced understanding of what it means to live a truly healthy life.

Journals: The Cutting Edge of Science

While books provide a broad overview, scientific journals are where you'll find the cutting edge of research. These are the platforms where scientists and researchers share their latest findings, often after years of meticulous study. Journals offer you a glimpse into the future, showing you what's on the horizon in the field of holistic health. They challenge you to keep up-to-date, to understand the evolving nature of scientific knowledge, and to apply this understanding in a practical, day-to-day context.

If journals are the cutting edge, then research papers are the finely honed blade. These are highly specialized publications that delve into the minutiae of specific topics. Whether it's the impact of a particular herb on cellular health, the physiological effects of an alkaline diet, or the psychological benefits of mindfulness, research papers offer you the most detailed, up-to-date information available. They are not for the faint-hearted but for those who wish to delve deep, to understand not just the 'what' but also the 'how' and the 'why.'

The Responsibility of Knowledge

The beauty of further reading lies in the synergy that arises from multiple sources. Books give you the broad strokes, journals fill in the details, and research papers offer you the microscopic view. Together, they form a comprehensive, multi-dimensional picture of holistic health that is far greater than the sum of its parts. This is not just about gathering information; it's about synthesizing knowledge, about understanding the interconnectedness of all things, and about applying this understanding in a way that is both practical and profoundly transformative.

With great knowledge comes great responsibility. The more you read, the more you realize that holistic health is not just a personal endeavor but a collective one. It's about making choices that not only benefit you but also have a positive impact on your community and the world at large. It's about becoming an advocate for a healthier, more sustainable way of living and inspiring others to join you on this journey.

As we embark on this section of our book, consider it an invitation to dive deeper into the ocean of knowledge that awaits you. The resources we'll explore are not just optional extras but essential tools for anyone serious about mastering the art of holistic health. They are your companions on a journey that has no final destination but offers endless opportunities for growth, discovery, and transformation. So, let's turn the page and begin this exciting new point in your lifelong journey towards holistic health and well-being.

The Evergreen Nature of Knowledge

As we approach the end of this chapter, it's crucial to understand that the last page is not the end but a new beginning. The world of holistic health is ever-evolving, and the knowledge we have today may be refined, expanded, or even contradicted by the discoveries of tomorrow. This is why the role of further reading—be it books, journals, or research papers—cannot be overstated. These resources are your gateway to the evergreen nature of knowledge, a way to keep your understanding fresh, relevant, and deeply rooted in scientific credibility.

In the age of information overload, the challenge is not just to read but to read wisely. Not all books are created equal, and the same goes for journals and research papers. The art of selective reading involves discerning the quality of the source, the credibility of the author, and the relevance of the content to your personal journey towards holistic health. It's about asking the right questions before you turn the page: "Is this source reliable? Does it add value to my understanding? Does it resonate with my personal experiences and observations?"

The Dynamic Interplay of Theory and Practice

Reading is not a passive act but a dynamic interplay between theory and practice. It's about taking the abstract concepts, scientific data, and expert opinions you encounter and translating them into actionable steps in your daily life. This is where the real magic happens. It's one thing to read about the benefits of an alkaline diet, the healing properties of herbs, or the psychological impact of mindfulness. It's another thing entirely to apply this knowledge in a way that transforms your health, enriches your life, and empowers you to make informed choices.

One of the most rewarding aspects of further reading is the opportunity it provides to share wisdom. Knowledge, when shared, has a ripple effect that extends far beyond the individual. Whether it's recommending a groundbreaking book to a friend, discussing the latest research findings in a community forum, or even writing a review to guide others, the act of sharing amplifies the impact of what you've learned. It's a way to contribute to the collective understanding of holistic health and to inspire a culture of continuous learning.

The Ethical Dimension of Informed Choices

As you deepen your understanding through further reading, you'll find that your choices take on an ethical dimension. You become more aware of the impact of your lifestyle not just on your health but on society and the planet. Whether it's choosing organic, locally-sourced produce, advocating for ethical practices in the pharmaceutical industry, or raising awareness about the importance of mental health, informed choices are ethical choices. They reflect a commitment to a greater good, a sense of responsibility that transcends the individual and touches the lives of others.

As we close this chapter, let's embrace the unfinished symphony that is lifelong learning. The notes may change, the tempo may vary, but the music plays on. Your journey towards holistic health is a composition in progress, a melody that evolves with each new piece of information, each fresh perspective, each moment of insight. Further reading is not an optional extra but an essential instrument in your orchestra of well-being.

Let the reading continue, let the learning flourish, and let the journey unfold.

Online Platforms, Forums, and Communities for Support

The New Age of Connection

In a world that's increasingly digital, the essence of community has evolved but not diminished. The hearth around which we gather has transformed from a physical space to a digital platform, yet the warmth of shared experience and collective wisdom remains. This chapter aims to explore the significance of online platforms, forums, and communities in your journey toward holistic health and alkaline living. These digital spaces are not just repositories of information; they are vibrant ecosystems where learning is reciprocal, and support is mutual.

Imagine having a question about the alkaline diet or a specific herb in Dr. Sebi's catalog. You could spend hours sifting through articles and research papers, or you could post your question in a dedicated forum and receive answers from those who have walked the path before you. The collective wisdom found in these online communities often transcends what you can find in formal publications. It's real, it's lived, and it's generously shared.

Holistic health is not just about physical well-being; it's a blend of emotional, mental, and spiritual equilibrium. Online communities often serve as emotional anchors. Whether you're celebrating a milestone in your alkaline journey or seeking comfort during a challenging phase, the emotional support you find in these spaces is invaluable. It's a reminder that you're not alone, that others share your struggles and triumphs, and that your journey is a shared human experience.

In a world awash with information, the challenge often lies in discerning the authentic from the misleading. Online platforms dedicated to alkaline living and Dr. Sebi's teachings often have stringent moderation policies to ensure that the information shared is accurate and reliable. These platforms become trusted spaces where you can safely seek advice, share experiences, and expand your understanding without the fear of misinformation.

The Ethical Responsibility of Digital Citizenship

There's a unique synergy that emerges when individuals with shared goals come together. Online communities focused on alkaline living become think tanks where new ideas are born, refined, and disseminated. Whether it's a novel way to incorporate alkaline foods into your diet or a groundbreaking interpretation of Dr. Sebi's teachings, the innovation that stems from these communities is a testament to the power of collective thinking.

One of the most fascinating aspects of online platforms is their ability to transcend geographical boundaries. You could be in New York seeking advice from someone in Tokyo about sourcing specific alkaline ingredients. The global reach of these platforms enriches your perspective, exposing you to different cultural nuances and broadening your understanding of holistic health as a universal pursuit.

Participation in online communities comes with an ethical responsibility. The anonymity of the internet should not be an excuse for harmful behavior. As digital citizens in the realm of holistic health, it's our collective responsibility to maintain the integrity of these spaces. This means respecting differing opinions, providing constructive feedback, and reporting any form of misinformation or abuse.

Weaving Your Own Narrative in Online Communities

As you navigate the labyrinth of online platforms, forums, and communities, it's essential to approach them with a sense of mindfulness. These spaces are not just bulletin boards where you pin questions and wait for answers. They are dynamic ecosystems where your active participation can either enrich or deplete the collective experience. Mindfulness in this context means being aware of the energy you bring into these spaces. Are you contributing positively, or are you merely a spectator? The quality of your engagement will often mirror the value you derive from these communities.

In a digital world where anonymity is often the norm, trust becomes a valuable currency. How do you establish trust in a community where faces are replaced by usernames, and tone is often lost in text? The answer lies in consistency and authenticity. When you consistently contribute valuable insights, ask thoughtful questions, and respect the guidelines of the community, you build a reputation that turns your username into a trusted brand within that space.

Your queries may echo the silent questions of others, and your answers may illuminate someone else's path. The beauty of online communities is that they serve as living archives. Long after you've moved on, your contributions continue to educate and inspire. It's a form of digital legacy that underscores the importance of thoughtful participation.

The Unspoken Etiquette of Digital Spaces

While it's natural to seek answers to your specific questions, it's equally important to contribute to the collective good of the community. This doesn't mean you need to have all the answers. Sometimes, sharing your personal experiences, successes, and even failures can offer invaluable insights to others. The balance between seeking and giving is what sustains the vitality of these communities.

Every community, digital or otherwise, operates on a set of unspoken rules. While guidelines and policies are explicitly stated, the etiquette often remains implied. It's crucial to observe and understand the dynamics of the community before diving into discussions. Knowing when to speak, when to listen, and how to disagree respectfully are skills that elevate the quality of discourse and foster a nurturing environment for all members.

The Exit Strategy: Knowing When to Step Back

Digital communities are not static; they evolve, and so do you. There may come a time when you feel the need to step back or move on. Whether it's because you've outgrown the space or because you find that it no longer aligns with your journey, the grace with which you exit speaks volumes about your digital citizenship. A simple thank-you post acknowledging the value the community has added to your life can serve as a beautiful full-circle moment.

In the grand tapestry of your holistic health journey, online platforms serve as intricate patterns that add depth and color. They are not the entire picture but rather a vital part of it. As you weave in and out of these digital spaces, remember that each thread you add enriches not just your own narrative but also those of others in this shared journey toward optimal health and well-being.

As we close this chapter, let's acknowledge that the digital hearth remains ever-lit, ever-welcoming, and ever-evolving. It's a space where you can always return for wisdom, solace, and the comforting sense of community. Your seat by this modern hearth is always reserved, inviting you to partake in the eternal dance of give-and-take that is the essence of human connection.

Book 18: Personal Transformation Chronicles

Real-Life Journeys of Health and Healing

The Mosaic of Transformation

Welcome to a chapter that serves as the beating heart of this book—where the abstract becomes tangible, where theories manifest into lived experiences. Here, we delve into the real-life journeys of individuals who have walked the path of alkaline living and emerged transformed. These stories are not just testimonials; they are intimate portraits of resilience, courage, and the indomitable human spirit.

Change is an alchemical process, a transformation that begins at the cellular level and radiates outward, touching every aspect of our lives. It's not just about altering what's on your plate; it's about reshaping your relationship with your body, your mind, and the world around you. The individuals whose stories we share have undergone this alchemy. They've turned the leaden aspects of their lives—be it illness, stress, or dissatisfaction—into golden opportunities for growth and healing.

In a world obsessed with instant gratification, we often see the 'before' and 'after' but overlook the 'during.' The 'during' is where the magic happens. It's where we grapple with challenges, confront our limitations, and unearth our potential. It's messy, it's uncomfortable, but it's also incredibly enriching. The stories in this chapter honor the 'during,' giving you a glimpse into the struggles that often remain unseen but are integral to the journey.

The Power of Vulnerability

Sharing one's journey, especially the bumps and bruises along the way, requires a certain level of vulnerability. It's an act of courage to say, "This is where I was, this is where I am, and this is how I got here." Vulnerability is not a sign of weakness; it's a testament to strength. It's an invitation for others to say, "Me too," and find solace in shared experiences.

Each story is a pebble thrown into the lake of collective consciousness, creating ripples that extend far beyond the individual. You may find pieces of yourself in these stories. You may find the inspiration to embark on your own journey or the courage to continue one you've already begun. The ripple effect of these personal chronicles can be profoundly impactful, not just for you, but for those in your life who also seek a path to better health and well-being.

The Intersection of Science and Spirituality

What makes these journeys compelling is the seamless blend of science and spirituality. It's not just about pH levels, herbal supplements, or dietary changes. It's also about a deeper connection to oneself and the universe. It's about finding a harmonious balance that honors both the tangible and the intangible aspects of well-being.

The stories you'll encounter are as diverse as the individuals who lived them. They come from different backgrounds, cultures, and walks of life. Yet, they all share a common thread—a quest for a life of vitality, clarity, and holistic health. This diversity serves as a powerful reminder that the path to alkaline living is not a one-size-fits-all journey; it's a tapestry woven from a myriad of individual experiences.

The Invitation to Your Own Odyssey

As we delve into these transformative stories, consider this chapter an invitation. An invitation to reflect on your own journey, to find resonance in the experiences of others, and perhaps, to share your own story someday. After all, every transformation begins with a single step, and your odyssey towards health and healing could very well be the next story that inspires others to embark on their own.

In this chapter, we're not just sharing stories; we're building a community of kindred spirits, united in their quest for a life less ordinary. So, let's turn the page and step into the world of real-life journeys, where each story serves as both a mirror and a window—reflecting your own potential and offering a glimpse into what's possible when you commit to the path of alkaline living.

The Last Mile: The Transformative Power of Resilience and Community

As we near the end of this chapter, it's crucial to acknowledge the resilience that each individual demonstrated in their journey towards health and healing. Resilience isn't just about bouncing back; it's about growing through what you go through. It's about-facing setbacks with grace, embracing challenges as opportunities, and emerging stronger than before. The stories we've shared are testaments to the transformative power of resilience, a quality that turns obstacles into stepping stones on the path to holistic well-being.

The Healing Power of Community

No one walks this journey alone. Behind each story of transformation is a community that provided support, encouragement, and sometimes, a loving nudge in the right direction. Whether it's a spouse who joins you in adopting an alkaline diet, a friend who becomes your yoga buddy, or an online group that offers valuable tips and resources, the role of community in these journeys cannot be overstated. It's a reminder that while the journey is personal, the road is often shared.

There's a unique wisdom that comes from lived experience, a wisdom that transcends textbooks and scientific studies. It's the wisdom of the body listening to its innate needs, the wisdom of the mind finding peace amid chaos, and the wisdom of the soul connecting with something greater than itself. This wisdom is the golden thread that weaves through each story, offering insights that are both deeply personal and universally relevant.

The Gift of Perspective

One of the most profound gifts these stories offer is perspective. They allow us to step out of our own experiences and see the world through another's eyes. This shift in perspective can be a catalyst for change, inspiring us to reevaluate our priorities, reassess our beliefs, and perhaps, rewrite our own stories. It's an invitation to look beyond the surface, to dig deeper, and to discover the transformative potential that lies within each of us.

Each story is not just an endpoint but a beginning, a legacy of change that inspires others to embark on their own journeys. These are not just individual triumphs; they are collective victories that elevate the discourse on health, wellness, and the human potential for transformation. They serve as beacons, lighting the way for others and proving that change is not just possible; it's achievable.

The Unfolding Journey: Your Chapter Awaits

As we close this chapter, remember that your journey is continually unfolding. Each day presents a new opportunity to make choices that align with your highest good, to learn from your experiences, and to grow in ways you never thought possible. Your story is still being written, and it's yours to shape in any way you choose.

In sharing these real-life journeys of health and healing, we hope to have ignited a spark within you—a spark that fuels your quest for a life of vitality, purpose, and holistic well-being. May these stories serve as both a mirror reflecting your own potential and a compass guiding you towards your true north.

ChalleOvercoming nges: Personal Stories of Resilience

The Resilient Spirit: Unveiling the Human Capacity for Overcoming Challenges

Resilience is not just a buzzword; it's a deeply ingrained human quality that has been the cornerstone of our survival and evolution. It's the invisible force that propels us forward, especially when the odds are stacked against us. In the context of personal transformation, resilience takes on a nuanced meaning. It becomes the bedrock upon which the edifice of change is built, the catalyst that turns setbacks into comebacks.

The Stories We Tell Ourselves

The narratives we internalize play a significant role in shaping our resilience. These are not just stories we tell others; these are the stories we tell ourselves, about ourselves. They can either be limiting beliefs that hold us back or empowering narratives that propel us forward. The individuals whose stories we've chronicled in this book have rewritten their narratives, choosing to author a story of triumph over adversity.

Adversity, in many ways, is like the crucible in which the metal of our character is tested and purified. The people we've profiled have faced challenges that range from debilitating illnesses to life-altering events. Yet, they've emerged not just unscathed but transformed. They've turned their adversities into opportunities for growth, their challenges into stepping stones toward holistic well-being.

One of the most striking aspects of these stories is the profound mind-body connection that is evident in each journey. The resilience demonstrated is not just mental or emotional; it's physical. The body, too, has its own language of resilience. It's in the way it adapts to a new, alkaline-rich diet, the way it responds to herbal treatments, and the way it thrives when aligned with the mind and spirit.

The Role of Choice

At the heart of each story is a pivotal moment of choice. It's the moment when the individual decides to take control of their destiny, to be an active participant in their journey toward health and healing. This choice is often made in the face of overwhelming odds, and it's this act of choosing that sets the stage for resilience to unfold. While the journey is deeply personal, it's rarely undertaken alone.

The role of a supportive community—be it family, friends, or even online forums—is invaluable. It serves as both a safety net and a sounding board, providing the emotional sustenance that is often needed when the road gets tough.

The Transformative Power of Small Steps

Resilience is not a giant leap but a series of small, intentional steps. It's in the daily choices we make, the habits we form, and the rituals we adopt. Each step, no matter how small, is a testament to the human spirit's indomitable will to not just survive but thrive.

In sum, resilience is not an abstract concept but a lived reality. It's the thread that weaves through the tapestry of human experience, giving it texture, depth, and strength. As we delve into these personal stories of resilience, let's remember that they are not just tales of individual heroism but collective testaments to the transformative power of the human spirit. They serve as both inspiration and affirmation, reminding us that no matter the challenge, we have within us the resilience to overcome.

The Resilient Journey: The Road to Transformation

As we delve deeper into these personal stories of resilience, it's crucial to recognize that each journey is unique, yet there are common threads that bind them. These threads form a sort of "resilience blueprint," a guide that can be adapted to fit individual circumstances. This blueprint is not a one-size-fits-all solution but a flexible framework that allows for personalization. It's a tool that empowers you to take charge of your life, to navigate the complexities of health and well-being with confidence and grace.

One of the most transformative aspects of these stories is the role of reflection. It's through introspection that these individuals were able to identify the limiting beliefs holding them back, the toxic patterns affecting their health, and the untapped potential within them. Reflection is not a passive act; it's an active engagement with oneself, a deep dive into the soul that brings clarity and purpose. It's the mirror that reveals not just who we are but who we could become.

Time is often viewed as an enemy, especially when dealing with health challenges. Yet, in these stories, time emerges as an ally. It's the space that allows for growth, the canvas upon which the masterpiece of resilience is painted. Time is not to be rushed; it's to be respected. It's the medium through which transformation occurs, the vessel that carries us from the realm of possibility to the domain of reality.

The Courage to Change

Change is never easy; it's fraught with uncertainty and risk. Yet, it's also the only constant, the inevitable outcome of a life well-lived. The courage to change is a recurring theme in these stories, a testament to the indomitable human spirit. It's the courage to question conventional wisdom, to challenge the status quo, and to venture into the unknown. It's the audacity to dream big, to aim high, and to reach for the stars, even when the world tells you to stay grounded.

The impact of these stories extends far beyond the individuals involved. It creates a ripple effect that touches lives, transforms communities, and shifts paradigms. It's a reminder that resilience is not a solitary endeavor but a collective journey. Your story of overcoming challenges can inspire others to do the same, creating a virtuous cycle of growth and transformation. It's the legacy you leave, the footprint you make, and the difference you create.

The Resilient Future

As we conclude this chapter, let's not view it as an end but as a beginning, a launching pad for your own journey of resilience. The stories shared here are not just narratives of overcoming challenges; they're blueprints for a resilient future. They're the stepping stones that pave the way for a new era of holistic health and well-being, an era where resilience is not just a trait but a way of life.

In the grand tapestry of human experience, your story is a vital thread, woven with the fibers of resilience, courage, and transformation. As you turn the pages of your life, may you write a story that not only stands the test of time but also serves as a beacon of resilience for generations to come.

The Alkaline Renaissance

In a world where quick fixes and fad diets often take center stage, a quiet revolution is taking place. It's a revolution not led by celebrities or high-profile influencers but by everyday people—men and women who have discovered the transformative power of alkaline living. This growing community of alkaline advocates is not just a trend; it's a movement. A movement that is reshaping our understanding of health, wellness, and the very fabric of our lives.

What starts as a personal quest for better health often turns into a universal journey, impacting families, communities, and eventually society at large. The beauty of this alkaline movement is its grassroots nature. It's not dictated from the top down but rather grows organically from the ground up. People share their stories, their struggles, and their triumphs, and in doing so, they create a ripple effect that extends far beyond their immediate circle.

In this community, the language is not one of deprivation or restriction but of abundance and empowerment. It's a language that speaks to the soul, resonating with our deepest desires for health, happiness, and fulfillment. It's a language that transcends age, gender, and cultural boundaries, uniting us in a common quest for a better, healthier life. And it's a language that is increasingly being heard, not just in health forums and social media groups but in mainstream conversations around the world.

The Power of Shared Wisdom

One of the most remarkable aspects of this growing community is the collective wisdom that emerges from individual experiences. Each person's journey adds a unique piece to the puzzle, contributing to a larger, more comprehensive picture of what alkaline living truly means. This shared wisdom is not just theoretical; it's practical, actionable, and incredibly potent. Its wisdom born out of trial and error, out of personal challenges and victories, and out of a deep-seated commitment to holistic well-being.

Another fascinating dimension of this movement is the way it bridges the gap between science and spirituality. It's not just about pH levels and nutrient profiles; it's about the mind-body-spirit connection. It's about understanding how our thoughts, emotions, and beliefs impact our physical health and vice versa. This holistic approach is what sets the alkaline community apart, elevating it from a dietary fad to a comprehensive lifestyle.

The Growing Community of Alkaline Advocates

The Alkaline Renaissance

In a world where quick fixes and fad diets often take center stage, a quiet revolution is taking place. It's a revolution not led by celebrities or high-profile influencers but by everyday people—men and women who have discovered the transformative power of alkaline living. This growing community of alkaline advocates is not just a trend; it's a movement. A movement that is reshaping our understanding of health, wellness, and the very fabric of our lives.

What starts as a personal quest for better health often turns into a universal journey, impacting families, communities, and eventually society at large. The beauty of this alkaline movement is its grassroots nature. It's not dictated from the top down but rather grows organically from the ground up. People share their stories, their struggles, and their triumphs, and in doing so, they create a ripple effect that extends far beyond their immediate circle.

In this community, the language is not one of deprivation or restriction but of abundance and empowerment. It's a language that speaks to the soul, resonating with our deepest desires for health, happiness, and fulfillment. It's a language that transcends age, gender, and cultural boundaries, uniting us in a common quest for a better, healthier life. And it's a language that is increasingly being heard, not just in health forums and social media groups but in mainstream conversations around the world.

The Power of Shared Wisdom

One of the most remarkable aspects of this growing community is the collective wisdom that emerges from individual experiences. Each person's journey adds a unique piece to the puzzle, contributing to a larger, more comprehensive picture of what alkaline living truly means. This shared wisdom is not just theoretical; it's practical, actionable, and incredibly potent. Its wisdom born out of trial and error, out of personal challenges and victories, and out of a deep-seated commitment to holistic well-being.

Another fascinating dimension of this movement is the way it bridges the gap between science and spirituality. It's not just about pH levels and nutrient profiles; it's about the mind-body-spirit connection. It's about understanding how our thoughts, emotions, and beliefs impact our physical health and vice versa. This holistic approach is what sets the alkaline community apart, elevating it from a dietary fad to a comprehensive lifestyle.

The Catalyst for Change

As this community continues to grow, it serves as a catalyst for broader societal change. It challenges the status quo, questions conventional wisdom, and pushes the boundaries of what's possible. It's a community that doesn't just accept things as they are but strives to make them better. And in doing so, it paves the way for a new era of health and wellness—an era where the focus shifts from merely treating symptoms to addressing the root causes, from temporary fixes to sustainable solutions, and from isolated efforts to collective action.

As we delve deeper into the stories and insights that make up this vibrant community, let's remember that this is just the beginning. The alkaline movement is still in its infancy, and its full potential is yet to be realized. But one thing is clear: it's a movement that is here to stay. It's a movement that is changing lives, transforming communities, and shaping the future of health and wellness.

The Resonance of Real Stories

The most compelling aspect of the alkaline community is its authenticity. These are not tales scripted for dramatic effect but real-life narratives of transformation. The community thrives on the genuine experiences of its members, each one contributing a thread to the ever-expanding tapestry of alkaline living. This tapestry is rich in its diversity, vibrant in its colors, and intricate in its patterns. It reflects the complexity and beauty of human life, capturing the essence of what it means to embark on a journey toward holistic well-being.

The Ripple Effect of Advocacy

The power of advocacy within this community cannot be overstated. When one person shares their story of overcoming chronic illness or achieving mental clarity through alkaline living, it resonates. It resonates not just because it's a success story, but because it's relatable. It's a story that could belong to any one of us, and that's what makes it so impactful. Each story serves as a catalyst, inspiring others to take action, to explore the possibilities, and to dare to dream of a healthier, happier life.

There's a certain alchemy that occurs when people come together with a shared purpose. In the case of the alkaline community, this alchemy is transformative. It turns skepticism into belief, challenges into opportunities, and individuals into a collective force for change. The community serves as both a sanctuary and a laboratory—a place where people can seek refuge and support, as well as experiment and innovate. It's a dynamic, evolving space that welcomes everyone, regardless of where they are on their alkaline journey.

In this community, wisdom is not a static entity but a dynamic interplay between knowledge and action. People learn from each other, adapt this knowledge to their unique circumstances, and then share their new insights with the community. This creates a symbiotic relationship where wisdom and action feed off each other, leading to more effective and sustainable outcomes. It's a model that challenges the traditional hierarchy of expertise, placing equal value on lived experience and academic knowledge.

The Horizon of Possibilities

As we look toward the future, it's clear that the growing community of alkaline advocates is leaving an indelible mark on the world. They are the pioneers of a new health paradigm, the torchbearers of a legacy that will benefit generations to come. But this legacy is not just about the dissemination of information; it's about the transformation of lives. It's about empowering people to take control of their health, to break free from the limitations of conventional wisdom, and to explore the boundless potential of human vitality.

So, as we stand on the cusp of this new era, let's take a moment to honor the incredible journey that has brought us here. Let's honor the courage, the resilience, and the unwavering commitment of this growing community of alkaline advocates. And let's look forward to the horizon of possibilities that lies ahead—a horizon that is not defined by the limitations of the past but by the potential of the future.

In the end, the true power of this community lies not in its numbers but in its spirit. It's a spirit of curiosity, of compassion, and of relentless pursuit of a better way. It's a spirit that challenges us to question, to explore, and to grow. And it's a spirit that invites us all to be part of something greater than ourselves—a movement that is not just changing diets but changing lives.

Book 19: The Intersection of Technology and Alkalinity

Digital Tools for Tracking and Promoting Alkaline Living

The Confluence of Tradition and Technology

In a world where technology often seems to be at odds with tradition, the intersection of digital tools and alkaline living presents a harmonious confluence. It's like a symphony where each instrument plays its part, contributing to a magnificent whole. The digital age, often criticized for distancing us from nature, can actually bring us closer to our roots—our roots of holistic well-being, that is.

Imagine having a compass in your pocket, not one that points north, but one that directs you toward better health. That's what digital tools for alkaline living can be—a guide that helps you navigate the complexities of modern life while staying true to your alkaline goals. Whether it's an app that tracks your pH levels or a platform that offers personalized alkaline meal plans, these tools are designed to make your journey easier and more effective.

One of the most transformative aspects of integrating technology into alkaline living is the ability to receive real-time feedback. Gone are the days when you had to wait for your annual check-up to know if your lifestyle changes were making a difference. Now, with wearable devices and mobile apps, you can monitor your progress in real-time. This immediate feedback loop not only keeps you motivated but also allows you to make timely adjustments, fine-tuning your approach for optimal results.

Digital platforms have democratized access to expertise. You no longer need to travel miles to consult with a nutritionist or spend hours in a library to access valuable information. Online courses, webinars, and even social media groups have brought the experts to your fingertips. This democratization has made alkaline living more accessible, breaking down barriers of geography, time, and even socio-economic status.

The Virtual Alkaline Community

While nothing can replace the warmth of human interaction, virtual communities offer a different kind of value. They provide a space for people from diverse backgrounds and geographies to come together, united by their commitment to alkaline living. These platforms offer more than just information; they offer emotional support, accountability, and a sense of belonging. It's a global village where everyone speaks the language of health and wellness.

As we embrace these digital tools, it's crucial to consider the ethical implications. Data privacy, for instance, is a significant concern. When we use apps to track our health metrics, where does this data go? Who has access to it? These are questions we must ask as responsible consumers. The goal is to use technology as an enabler, not as a tool for exploitation.

The Future is Now

We stand at a pivotal moment in history, a moment where technology and tradition have the potential to come together in a dance of possibilities. The digital tools available to us today are not just gadgets; they are instruments of change. They have the power to amplify our efforts, to accelerate our progress, and to deepen our understanding of what it means to live an alkaline life.

In this digital symphony, each one of us is both a musician and a conductor. We choose the instruments, we set the tempo, and we create the music. It's a collaborative composition, one that evolves with each note, each chord, and each crescendo. And as we look to the future, one thing is clear: this is just the prelude. The most beautiful parts of the symphony are yet to come.

So, let's embrace these digital tools with open arms but also with discerning minds. Let's use them to enhance, not replace, the wisdom of alkaline living. And as we do, let's remember that the ultimate goal is not just to live but to thrive—in harmony with ourselves, with each other, and with the world around us.

The Digital Frontier: A New Dawn for Alkaline Living

In the realm of alkaline living, the digital age has ushered in an era of unprecedented personalization. Imagine a world where your smartphone knows your pH levels better than you do, where it nudges you to hydrate just when your body needs it, and even suggests a recipe for an alkaline smoothie tailored to your current health metrics. This is not science fiction; it's the reality we're stepping into. Digital tools are not just tracking devices; they're becoming our personalized health consultants.

As we integrate these digital tools into our lives, we must also become stewards of our own digital footprints. The data we generate has immense value, not just for us but for the broader healthcare ecosystem. It's crucial to be vigilant about how this data is used and shared. The digital age offers us tools of empowerment, but with great power comes great responsibility. We must be the guardians of our own digital sanctuaries, ensuring that our data serves us and not the other way around.

While digital tools offer convenience and efficiency, they also come with the risk of becoming yet another source of stress. The constant pings and notifications can easily turn from helpful reminders into nagging digital voices. The key is mindful usage. Setting boundaries with our devices allows us to use them as tools for betterment rather than as instruments of distraction. Remember, the goal is to enhance our alkaline lifestyle, not to create a digital dependency.

The Digital-Physical Loop

One of the most exciting developments in this space is the creation of a digital-physical loop. Wearable devices can now sync with smart home systems to create an environment that actively supports your alkaline lifestyle. Picture this: your wearable detects a drop in your hydration levels and signals your smart home system to start the water purifier, ensuring that a glass of alkaline water is ready for you as soon as you walk into the kitchen. This seamless integration of the digital and physical worlds is not just convenient; it's revolutionary.

In this digital journey, let's not forget the human element. Technology can guide, assist, and even prod us in the right direction, but the choices ultimately lie in our hands. The apps and devices are facilitators; we are the executors. It's our commitment, our discipline, and our desire for a healthier life that turns these digital tools into catalysts for real-world change.

The Horizon Ahead

As we stand on the cusp of this digital frontier, it's exhilarating to think about the possibilities that lie ahead. Artificial Intelligence and Machine Learning are set to take these tools to the next level, offering predictive analytics and even more personalized recommendations. But as we look forward to these advancements, let's also take a moment to look inward, to ensure that our digital evolution aligns with our core values and goals.

In the grand composition of life, digital tools for alkaline living are like the latest instruments added to an ancient orchestra. They bring a new texture, a new range, and a new depth to the music. But the essence of the melody—the core principles of alkaline living—remains unchanged. As we embrace these new tools, let's not lose sight of the age-old wisdom that forms the foundation of this lifestyle. Let's use technology to amplify our efforts, not to overshadow them. And as we do, let's create a symphony that's not just harmonious but also profoundly healing.

Online Courses, Webinars, and Workshops

The Virtual Classroom: A New Frontier in Alkaline Living

In a world where information is at our fingertips, the quest for optimal health has never been more accessible. The digital age has democratized education, breaking down barriers that once made the pursuit of wellness a privilege for the few. Nowhere is this more evident than in the realm of alkaline living, where online courses, webinars, and workshops are revolutionizing how we learn, connect, and evolve on our health journeys.

Gone are the days when wisdom was confined to the pages of a dusty book or the walls of a classroom. Today's virtual sages are dynamic, interactive, and available at the click of a button. These digital platforms offer a rich tapestry of knowledge, from beginner courses that demystify the basics of pH balance to advanced webinars that delve into the biochemistry of alkaline living. The virtual classroom is as diverse as it is expansive, catering to a wide range of learning styles and needs.

The Power of Community in Digital Spaces

One of the most transformative aspects of online education is the sense of community it fosters. Virtual workshops not only serve as educational platforms but also as social hubs where like-minded individuals can connect, share experiences, and offer support. This sense of community is invaluable, especially when navigating the complexities of an alkaline lifestyle. It provides a safety net of collective wisdom, where the challenges of one become the lessons for many.

In a digital landscape teeming with information, not all courses are created equal. Authenticity becomes a crucial factor in choosing the right educational platform. Look for courses led by certified professionals, backed by scientific research, and enriched by real-life testimonials. The credibility of the instructor and the quality of the content can make or break your learning experience.

One of the most compelling advantages of online courses is the flexibility they offer. In a world where time is a luxury, the ability to learn at your own pace is a game-changer. Whether you're a busy professional juggling work commitments or a parent navigating the demands of family life, digital platforms offer the freedom to tailor your learning journey to fit your schedule.

The Synergy of Theory and Practice

What sets digital education apart is its ability to seamlessly integrate theory with practice. Interactive webinars often include live demonstrations, Q&A sessions, and even virtual lab exercises that allow you to apply what you've learned in real-time. This dynamic approach ensures that the knowledge you gain is not just theoretical but immediately applicable to your daily life.

Let's talk about the elephant in the room: cost. Traditional educational platforms can be prohibitively expensive, making them inaccessible to many. Online courses, on the other hand, often offer a more cost-effective alternative without compromising on quality. Many platforms even offer free introductory courses, making it easier for you to dip your toes into the world of alkaline living without breaking the bank.

As we stand on the threshold of this digital renaissance in health education, the possibilities are limitless. Virtual reality workshops, AI-driven personalized courses, and blockchain-secured certificates are not far-off dreams but imminent realities. As technology continues to evolve, so will the ways we engage with it to enhance our health and well-being.

The digital age has redefined the boundaries of what's possible in health education, offering us a plethora of tools to enrich our understanding of alkaline living. As we navigate this brave new world, let's do so with discernment, flexibility, and an open heart, knowing that each click, each course, and each connection brings us one step closer to our most vibrant selves.

The Lasting Impact: How Digital Learning Shapes Our Alkaline Journey

As we've navigated the labyrinth of online courses, webinars, and workshops, it's essential to pause and reflect on the transformative power of digital learning. The knowledge we acquire doesn't merely reside in the recesses of our minds; it manifests in the choices we make, the foods we consume, and the lifestyles we adopt. The ripple effect of a single webinar can extend far beyond the confines of a computer screen, influencing not just the individual but also their families, communities, and ultimately, the world at large.

Completing an online course or workshop is not the end but rather a milestone on a lifelong journey toward alkaline mastery. The 'End Course' button is not a full stop but an ellipsis, a pause before the next chapter. The real work begins when the screen goes dark, and you're left with the newfound wisdom to integrate into your daily life. It's a commitment that requires diligence, consistency, and an unwavering dedication to your well-being.

With knowledge comes responsibility—the ethical obligation to share what you've learned. Whether it's recommending a course to a friend struggling with health issues or hosting a community webinar to discuss the benefits of alkaline living, your actions can serve as a beacon for others. You become not just a student but a teacher, an advocate, and a catalyst for change. In this way, the cycle of learning and teaching becomes a virtuous circle, enriching lives and elevating consciousness.

The Personal Touch: Customizing Your Digital Experience

One of the most exciting aspects of digital learning is the ability to customize your educational journey. Many platforms offer advanced features that allow you to bookmark sections, make notes, and even interact with instructors in real-time. These personalized touches make the learning experience not just educational but deeply engaging, ensuring that the lessons resonate on a personal level.

While technology can sometimes feel impersonal, the best online platforms strive to create an emotionally enriching experience. From instructors who share personal anecdotes to forums where students can share their struggles and triumphs, digital empathy is a cornerstone of effective online education. It's this emotional connection that transforms a mere course into a life-changing experience.

In an era where sustainability is more than a buzzword, digital learning offers an eco-friendly alternative to traditional education. The carbon footprint of a webinar is significantly lower than a physical seminar, making it a choice that aligns not just with your health goals but also with the well-being of the planet.

The Future Beckons: The Uncharted Territories of Digital Alkaline Education

As we look to the horizon, the future of digital alkaline education is shimmering with possibilities. Imagine virtual reality cooking classes where you can virtually step into a chef's kitchen or AI-powered apps that tailor a learning curriculum based on your health metrics. The confluence of technology and alkalinity is not a fleeting trend but a paradigm shift, one that promises to redefine how we approach health and wellness in the years to come.

The digital realm of online courses, webinars, and workshops is more than a convenient alternative to traditional learning; it's a transformative force that empowers, enlightens, and elevates. As we close this chapter, let's carry forth the wisdom we've gained, sharing it generously and applying it conscientiously, ever mindful of the profound impact our choices have on our health and the world around us.

The Future of Alkaline Advocacy in the Digital Age

The Digital Frontier: A Canvas for Change

As we stand on the precipice of a new decade, the digital landscape has never been more fertile for the seeds of change. The intersection of technology and alkalinity is not just a convergence of two worlds; it's the birth of a new frontier—a frontier where advocacy takes on a form as dynamic and fluid as the digital bytes that carry its message.

The Human Element: Advocacy in the Age of Algorithms

In a world increasingly governed by algorithms and data analytics, the human element remains the cornerstone of effective advocacy. The digital age offers a plethora of tools to amplify our voices, but it's the authenticity, the raw human emotion, that turns a post into a movement, a tweet into a revolution. Alkaline advocacy in the digital realm is not about leveraging technology to replace the human touch; it's about using it to amplify our innate desire for health and well-being.

One of the most compelling aspects of digital advocacy is the power of storytelling. The stories we share—of transformation, of overcoming adversity, of the sheer joy that comes from living an alkaline lifestyle—these are the narratives that resonate. They transcend the limitations of traditional media, reaching people in the most intimate spaces of their lives—their homes, their phones, their moments of solitude. It's in these quiet moments that change happens, that people are moved to act, to explore, and to transform.

The Social Media Paradox: Navigating the Double-Edged Sword

Social media is a double-edged sword. On one hand, it offers unprecedented reach, connecting us to like-minded individuals across the globe. On the other, it's a landscape fraught with misinformation, where myths can spread as quickly as truths. The challenge for alkaline advocates is to navigate this complex terrain with integrity, ensuring that the information we disseminate is not just compelling but also scientifically sound.

One of the most transformative aspects of digital advocacy is the democratization of knowledge. No longer confined to academic journals or elite conferences, the wisdom of alkaline living is now accessible to anyone with an internet connection. This level of accessibility is not just a technological achievement; it's a societal shift, one that empowers individuals to take control of their health and well-being.

With great power comes great responsibility. The digital realm offers a megaphone to anyone willing to use it, but it's crucial to wield this power with ethical consideration. Advocacy is not about pushing an agenda; it's about educating, enlightening, and empowering. It's about providing people with the tools they need to make informed decisions, free from coercion or manipulation.

The Future Unveiled: A Glimpse into Tomorrow

As we look toward the future, the possibilities for alkaline advocacy in the digital age are boundless. Imagine a world where AI-powered apps provide personalized alkaline meal plans, where virtual reality seminars offer immersive educational experiences, where blockchain technology ensures the ethical sourcing of alkaline products. This is not the realm of science fiction; it's the next chapter in our collective journey toward holistic health and well-being.

The future of alkaline advocacy in the digital age is a tapestry yet to be woven, but the threads are already in our hands. It's a future that beckons us to be not just consumers of technology but also creators, not just followers but leaders, not just advocates but pioneers. As we step into this brave new world, let us carry forth the wisdom of alkalinity with the innovation of technology, ever mindful of the profound impact we can have on the world and on ourselves.

The Ethos of Digital Responsibility

As we navigate the digital seas of the 21st century, we must not lose sight of our ethical compass. The digital realm is a powerful tool, but it's also a reflection of our collective consciousness. The content we create, the messages we amplify, and the communities we build are all imbued with our values, our beliefs, and our aspirations. In the realm of alkaline advocacy, this means adhering to principles of integrity, transparency, and inclusivity. It means ensuring that the digital platforms we use are not just conduits for information but also catalysts for positive change.

In the digital age, the impact of our actions can ripple out far beyond our immediate sphere of influence. A single tweet can spark a global conversation; a well-crafted blog post can inspire a movement. But it's not just about the grand gestures; it's also about the small, everyday actions that contribute to a larger narrative. Responding to a comment, sharing a personal story, or even just liking a post—all of these actions have the potential to make a difference. They are the building blocks of a digital advocacy ecosystem that is both robust and resilient.

The Art of Digital Listening

Advocacy is not a one-way street; it's a dialogue, a conversation that requires both speaking and listening. In the digital realm, listening takes on a new dimension. It's not just about monitoring mentions or tracking hashtags; it's about tuning into the subtle frequencies of human emotion and experience. It's about understanding the needs, the fears, and the aspirations of those we seek to serve. Digital listening is an art form, one that requires empathy, intuition, and a deep understanding of the human condition.

In a world of viral trends and fleeting moments, how do we ensure the longevity of our advocacy efforts? The answer lies in building sustainable digital ecosystems—platforms and communities that are designed to evolve, adapt, and grow. This means investing in quality content, fostering meaningful relationships, and staying committed to the principles that guide us. It's not about chasing likes or views; it's about creating a lasting impact that stands the test of time.

The Final Frontier: The Uncharted Territories of Digital Advocacy

As we look to the future, we find ourselves standing on the edge of uncharted territories. Advances in artificial intelligence, augmented reality, and blockchain technology offer unprecedented opportunities for innovation and impact. But they also raise important ethical questions that we must grapple with. How do we ensure that these technologies are used for the greater good? How do we navigate the ethical dilemmas that arise from the convergence of technology and health? These are the questions that will shape the future of alkaline advocacy in the digital age.

As we close this chapter, let us not forget that the journey is far from over. The future of alkaline advocacy in the digital age is a story still being written, a path still being paved. It's a journey that invites us all to be pioneers, explorers, and visionaries. It's a journey that challenges us to be better, to do better, and to create a world that reflects our highest ideals. So let us step boldly into the future, armed with the wisdom of alkalinity and the power of technology, ever mindful of the profound impact we can have on the world and on ourselves. The digital age is not just a chapter in the story of alkaline advocacy; it's a whole new book waiting to be written. And in that book, each and every one of us has a role to play.

Book 20: Advocacy, Legacy, and Making a Difference

How to Become an Advocate for Alkaline Living

Call to Advocacy

You've felt it, haven't you? That subtle pull toward something greater, a cause that resonates with your very core. It's not just about you anymore; it's about the collective well-being of humanity. You've experienced the transformative power of alkaline living, and now you're ready to share it with the world. But where do you begin? Advocacy is a journey, one that requires courage, commitment, and a deep sense of purpose. It's a path that beckons you to step out of your comfort zone and into the realm of possibility.

Advocacy isn't just about talking; it's about doing. It's about embodying the principles you stand for and letting your life be a testament to the transformative power of alkaline living. It's about walking the talk, day in and day out, in ways both big and small. Whether it's making conscious choices about the food you eat, the products you use, or the messages you share, every action counts. And it's these actions, collectively, that create a ripple effect, inspiring others to embark on their own journey toward alkaline living.

Every advocate has a story to tell, a narrative that serves as the foundation for their advocacy efforts. Your story is your most potent weapon, a tool that can inspire, educate, and mobilize. It's not just about recounting your personal experiences; it's about framing them in a way that resonates with others. It's about finding the universal truths in your unique journey and using them to connect with people on a deeper level. Storytelling is an art, one that requires authenticity, vulnerability, and a keen understanding of human psychology.

Building Bridges: The Role of Empathy in Advocacy

Empathy is the cornerstone of effective advocacy. It's the ability to step into someone else's shoes, to see the world from their perspective, and to understand their needs, fears, and aspirations. Empathy is what allows you to connect with people on a human level, transcending the barriers of language, culture, and ideology. It's what enables you to find common ground, even in the face of seemingly insurmountable differences. And it's this common ground that serves as the foundation for meaningful change.

Advocacy is not a solo endeavor; it's a collective effort that requires collaboration, support, and a shared vision for the future. Finding your tribe—those who share your passion for alkaline living—is crucial to the success of your advocacy efforts. Whether it's joining online forums, attending workshops, or simply connecting with like-minded individuals in your community, building a strong support network is essential. Your tribe will not only provide you with the emotional support you need but also amplify your efforts, helping you reach a wider audience and make a more significant impact.

The Long Game: Commitment and Resilience

Advocacy is a long game, one that requires unwavering commitment and resilience. It's about staying the course, even when the odds are stacked against you. It's about-facing setbacks with grace and turning challenges into opportunities for growth. And most importantly, it's about never losing sight of why you started this journey in the first place. Your commitment to alkaline living is not just a personal choice; it's a declaration of your values, your beliefs, and your vision for a healthier, happier world.

As you stand on the precipice of this exciting new chapter, take a moment to reflect on the journey that brought you here. You are not the same person you were when you started; you are an advocate in the making, armed with the knowledge, the passion, and the purpose to make a difference. So take that first step with confidence, knowing that you are part of a growing movement that is changing the world, one choice, one action, one story at a time. Welcome to the tribe. Welcome to the world of alkaline living advocacy.

The Culmination: Your Lasting Impact as an Advocate for Alkaline Living

You've walked the path, you've told your story, and you've connected with your tribe. Now, it's time to amplify your voice and make it resonate in the hearts and minds of others. Influence isn't about imposing your beliefs; it's about inspiring change through authentic engagement. It's about creating compelling narratives that not only inform but also empower. Your voice is your most potent tool in this advocacy journey. Use it wisely, use it consistently, and most importantly, use it authentically.

Never underestimate the power of small actions. Whether it's a blog post, a community workshop, or even a simple conversation with a friend, each interaction is an opportunity to plant a seed. And each seed has the potential to grow into something extraordinary—a movement, a community, a global shift towards alkaline living. The ripple effect starts with you. Your actions, no matter how small, can set off a chain reaction that extends far beyond your immediate circle.

Effective advocacy requires more than just passion; it requires skill. Mastering the art of communication is crucial in conveying your message in a way that's not only compelling but also relatable. Whether it's public speaking, social media engagement, or one-on-one conversations, each platform offers a unique opportunity to connect and influence. Invest in honing these skills, perhaps through courses or mentorship, as they will serve you well in your advocacy journey.

In a world rife with misinformation, maintaining ethical integrity is non-negotiable. Your credibility is your currency in the realm of advocacy. Always strive for accuracy in the information you share and be transparent about your sources. Acknowledge the limitations of your knowledge and be open to learning and evolving. Integrity is not just about being honest; it's about being accountable—to yourself, to your community, and to the cause you represent.

As you navigate the complexities and joys of advocacy, take a moment to ponder the legacy you wish to leave behind. Legacy is not about fame or recognition; it's about impact. It's about the lives you touch, the minds you open, and the communities you empower. Your legacy is the sum total of the ripples you create, extending far beyond your lifetime. So, what will your legacy be? How will you be remembered in the annals of alkaline living advocacy?

The Final Mile: A Call to Perseverance

Advocacy is a marathon, not a sprint. There will be hurdles, setbacks, and moments of doubt. But remember, the final mile is often the hardest, and it's also the most rewarding. Perseverance is your steadfast ally in this journey. When the going gets tough, dig deep into your reservoir of passion and purpose, and you'll find the strength to carry on.

The Horizon Awaits: Your Next Steps in Alkaline Living Advocacy. You stand now at a pivotal juncture, armed with the tools, the tribe, and the tenacity to make a lasting impact. The horizon is wide open, teeming with possibilities and opportunities for growth. As you take your next steps, carry with you the wisdom of your journey and the fervor of your convictions. The world is ready for your message, and the time for action is now. Go forth and be the advocate for alkaline living that you were destined to be. Your journey has only just begun. Welcome to your future in making a difference.

Organizing Community Events, Workshops, and Seminars

The Heartbeat of Advocacy: Organizing Community Events, Workshops, and Seminars

Imagine a room filled with like-minded individuals, all gathered for a singular purpose—to learn, to grow, and to embrace the transformative power of alkaline living. This is the magic of community events. They serve as a crucible for change, a space where ideas can be exchanged, questions can be answered, and lives can be changed. But organizing such events isn't just about booking a venue or creating a Facebook event page; it's about crafting an experience that leaves a lasting impact.

Before you dive into the logistics, take a step back and ask yourself some fundamental questions. What is the core message you want to convey? Who is your target audience? What format—be it a workshop, seminar, or community gathering—would best serve your objectives? Your answers to these questions will serve as the blueprint for your event, guiding every decision you make, from the speakers you invite to the topics you cover.

The logistics: Navigating the Nitty-Gritty

The success of any event hinges on the quality of the experience you provide. This goes beyond the content; it's about creating an atmosphere that fosters engagement and encourages interaction. Utilize different formats like panel discussions, interactive workshops, and Q&A sessions to keep the energy high and the audience engaged. Remember, the goal is not just to inform but to inspire action.

While the vision and strategy are crucial, the devil is in the details. This is where your organizational skills come into play. From securing a venue to coordinating with speakers, from promoting the event to managing registrations, each aspect requires meticulous planning. Don't shy away from seeking help; a well-coordinated team can be your greatest asset in pulling off a successful event.

The Human Touch: Building Authentic Connections

In our digitally connected world, the value of face-to-face interaction cannot be overstated. Use your event as an opportunity to build authentic connections. Whether it's through networking sessions or informal conversations during coffee breaks, encourage attendees to share their stories, challenges, and aspirations. These connections often serve as the catalyst for lasting change, both at an individual and community level.

Success isn't just measured by the number of attendees or the amount of positive feedback you receive. The true impact of your event lies in the ripple effect it creates. Did attendees leave with actionable insights they can apply in their lives? Have you equipped them with the tools to become advocates themselves? The answers to these questions will determine the long-term success of your advocacy efforts.

The Legacy: Planting Seeds for Future Gatherings

As the event comes to a close, take a moment to reflect on the seeds you've planted. Each attendee leaves as a potential ambassador for alkaline living, armed with knowledge, inspired by experiences, and connected to a community. Your event may be over, but its legacy is just beginning to unfold.

You've now taken a significant step in your advocacy journey. The event you've organized is not an end but a beginning—a launching pad for broader conversations, deeper engagements, and more impactful community actions. As you move forward, carry with you the lessons learned, the connections made, and the lives touched. Your role in shaping the narrative around alkaline living is far from over; in fact, it's just getting started. Welcome to the next chapter of your advocacy story.

The Lasting Echo: Sustaining the Impact of Your Community Events, Workshops, and Seminars

As the applause fades and the last attendee walks out the door, you might feel a mix of relief and accomplishment. But remember, the end of your event is just the beginning of its impact. The real work starts now—how do you capture that essence, that afterglow, and turn it into a sustainable movement?

The Feedback Loop: Listening to Your Audience

One of the most valuable resources you'll have post-event is the feedback from your attendees. This isn't just about what went well; it's also about what could be improved. Create a simple, yet comprehensive, feedback form and encourage everyone to fill it out. This will not only help you gauge the success of the event but also provide insights for future endeavors.

The Digital Footprint: Extending the Conversation Online

In today's interconnected world, the conversation doesn't have to end when the event does. Utilize social media platforms to keep the dialogue going. Share highlights, key takeaways, and even recordings of the event for those who couldn't attend. This extends the life of your event and broadens its reach, turning a one-time gathering into an ongoing conversation.

The Community Hub: Creating a Space for Continued Engagement

Consider creating a digital community hub—a website or a dedicated social media group—where attendees can continue to engage, ask questions, and share their own experiences and insights. This becomes a self-sustaining ecosystem that not only keeps the community engaged but also serves as a valuable resource for newcomers.

The true measure of your event's success is how well it empowers others to take action. Encourage attendees to host their own mini-events, workshops, or discussion groups, guided by the principles and insights gained from your event. Offer to provide resources or even act as a mentor. This creates a ripple effect, turning each attendee into an advocate and multiplying the impact of your efforts.

The Legacy Project: Documenting and Sharing the Journey

Consider creating a "Legacy Project" that documents the entire journey of your event, from inception to impact. This could be a video documentary, a series of blog posts, or even a digital magazine. Not only does this serve as a testament to what you've achieved, but it also becomes a blueprint that others can follow.

As you reflect on the success and learnings of your event, start thinking about the next chapter. What topics or issues were left unexplored? What new challenges has your community identified? Use these as starting points for planning your next event, thus ensuring that your advocacy is not a one-off but a sustained campaign.

The Infinite Loop: Advocacy as a Way of Life

In the end, advocacy isn't just something you do; it's a way of life. It's a commitment to continuous learning, to growing as a community, and to making a tangible difference in the world. Your event is a milestone on this journey, a marker of what you've achieved and a signpost pointing the way to what still needs to be done.

As you close this chapter, remember that your part of a larger narrative—a tapestry of efforts aimed at promoting alkaline living and holistic health. Each thread, each color, each knot in this tapestry adds depth and richness to the larger picture. Your event, your advocacy, is one such vibrant thread. So take a bow, but don't exit the stage. The curtain hasn't fallen; in fact, it's just rising on a world of possibilities.

The Path Forward: Spreading Awareness and Education

The Lasting Echo: Sustaining the Impact of Your Community Events, Workshops, and Seminars

As the applause fades and the last attendee walks out the door, you might feel a mix of relief and accomplishment. But remember, the end of your event is just the beginning of its impact. The real work starts now—how do you capture that essence, that afterglow, and turn it into a sustainable movement?

The Feedback Loop: Listening to Your Audience

One of the most valuable resources you'll have post-event is the feedback from your attendees. This isn't just about what went well; it's also about what could be improved. Create a simple, yet comprehensive, feedback form and encourage everyone to fill it out. This will not only help you gauge the success of the event but also provide insights for future endeavors.

The Digital Footprint: Extending the Conversation Online

In today's interconnected world, the conversation doesn't have to end when the event does. Utilize social media platforms to keep the dialogue going. Share highlights, key takeaways, and even recordings of the event for those who couldn't attend. This extends the life of your event and broadens its reach, turning a one-time gathering into an ongoing conversation.

The Community Hub: Creating a Space for Continued Engagement

Consider creating a digital community hub—a website or a dedicated social media group—where attendees can continue to engage, ask questions, and share their own experiences and insights. This becomes a self-sustaining ecosystem that not only keeps the community engaged but also serves as a valuable resource for newcomers.

The true measure of your event's success is how well it empowers others to take action. Encourage attendees to host their own mini-events, workshops, or discussion groups, guided by the principles and insights gained from your event. Offer to provide resources or even act as a mentor. This creates a ripple effect, turning each attendee into an advocate and multiplying the impact of your efforts.

The Legacy Project: Documenting and Sharing the Journey

Consider creating a "Legacy Project" that documents the entire journey of your event, from inception to impact. This could be a video documentary, a series of blog posts, or even a digital magazine. Not only does this serve as a testament to what you've achieved, but it also becomes a blueprint that others can follow.

As you reflect on the success and learnings of your event, start thinking about the next chapter. What topics or issues were left unexplored? What new challenges has your community identified? Use these as starting points for planning your next event, thus ensuring that your advocacy is not a one-off but a sustained campaign.

The Global Stage

In the end, advocacy isn't just something you do; it's a way of life. It's a commitment to continuous learning, to growing as a community, and to making a tangible difference in the world. Your event is a milestone on this journey, a marker of what you've achieved and a signpost pointing the way to what still needs to be done.

As you close this chapter, remember that your part of a larger narrative—a tapestry of efforts aimed at promoting alkaline living and holistic health. Each thread, each color, each knot in this tapestry adds depth and richness to the larger picture. Your event, your advocacy, is one such vibrant thread. So take a bow, but don't exit the stage. The curtain hasn't fallen; in fact, it's just rising on a world of possibilities.

The Path Forward: Spreading Awareness and Education

As we've navigated the labyrinth of advocacy, one thing becomes clear: the impact of a single voice can be exponential. Your voice, imbued with the wisdom and experience of alkaline living, can be the catalyst that sparks a chain reaction. But it's not enough to merely speak; we must also listen. Listen to the questions, the concerns, and even the skepticism of those around us. It's in this dialogue that we find the fertile ground for change.

Persuasion isn't about manipulation; it's about connection. It's about finding the common ground that allows us to communicate the profound benefits of alkaline living in a language that resonates with others. This could mean tailoring your message to address the specific health concerns of your audience or sharing personal anecdotes that humanize the often-abstract concepts of holistic health. The key is to be relatable, to be human, and to speak from a place of genuine concern and understanding.

Advocacy is not a sprint; it's a marathon. It's about the long-term vision, the legacy we leave behind. This means thinking beyond immediate impact to sustainable change. How can we ensure that the awareness we've raised transforms into lasting habits and lifestyle changes? One approach is mentorship. By taking someone under your wing and guiding them through the initial stages of their alkaline journey, you're not just creating a convert; you're nurturing a future advocate.

The Power of Collaboration: Unity in Diversity

No man is an island, and no movement can thrive in isolation. Collaboration is the lifeblood of any successful advocacy effort. This could mean partnering with healthcare professionals to lend credibility to the alkaline message or teaming up with local businesses to sponsor community health events. The diversity of voices and perspectives can only enrich the message and broaden its appeal.

As advocates, we bear a significant ethical responsibility. The advice we give and the information we share can have real-world consequences. This makes it imperative to stay updated with the latest research, to be transparent about the limitations of alkaline living, and most importantly, to admit when we don't have all the answers. Integrity is not just a virtue; it's a non-negotiable component of effective advocacy.

The Final Mile: A Personal Commitment

As we reach the end of this chapter, let's make a personal commitment. A commitment to be the change we wish to see, to be the voice that breaks the silence, to be the hand that lifts others up. Let's commit to stepping out of our comfort zones, to challenging the status quo, and to questioning the accepted narratives.

Imagine a world where alkaline living is not an alternative but the norm, where holistic health is not a luxury but a fundamental right. This is the world we're striving to create. And while the path may be fraught with challenges, the rewards are immeasurable. We're not just improving lives; we're transforming futures. We're not just spreading awareness; we're educating generations.

In this grand symphony of life, each of us plays a unique role. Your role, should you choose to accept it, is that of a maestro, orchestrating a movement that harmonizes the melodies of awareness and education into a rhapsody of change. So pick up your baton, step onto the podium, and let the music begin. For the path forward is not a solitary journey but a collective endeavor. And it starts with you.

Book 21: The Future Landscape of Alkaline Living

Predicting Trends in Alkaline Health and Wellness

The Winds of Change: A New Era in Health and Wellness

As we stand on the precipice of a new decade, the landscape of health and wellness is undergoing a seismic shift. No longer confined to the fringes, alkaline living is poised to enter the mainstream consciousness. But what does the future hold? How will this ancient wisdom, reinvigorated by modern science, shape our lives in the years to come? Let's embark on a journey to explore the emerging trends that promise to redefine the contours of alkaline health and wellness.

The Confluence of Tradition and Technology

One of the most exciting developments is the marriage of traditional alkaline practices with cutting-edge technology. Imagine a world where your smartwatch not only tracks your steps but also monitors your body's pH levels in real-time. Or consider the rise of AI-powered nutrition apps that curate personalized alkaline meal plans based on your unique health profile. Technology is not just amplifying the message; it's revolutionizing the way we engage with it.

The Democratization of Alkaline Living

For too long, holistic health has been the preserve of the privileged few. But the winds of change are blowing. The democratization of alkaline living is on the horizon. Community gardens are sprouting up in urban landscapes, offering access to organic, alkaline-rich produce. Telehealth platforms are making it easier for people in remote areas to consult with alkaline nutrition experts. The future is inclusive, and it's a trend that's here to stay.

The Rise of Alkaline Gastronomy

The culinary world is also catching on to the alkaline wave. We're witnessing the emergence of alkaline gastronomy, where Michelin-starred chefs are crafting gourmet meals that are as nourishing as they are delicious. This is not just food; it's medicine for the soul. And as this trend gains momentum, we can expect to see a proliferation of alkaline restaurants, cookbooks, and even cooking shows that bring this culinary art form into our homes.

Mindfulness: The Missing Link

The holistic nature of alkaline living extends beyond diet. The future will see a greater emphasis on the role of mindfulness in maintaining an alkaline state. Stress, after all, is acidic to the body. Mindfulness techniques, integrated into our daily routines, will become the norm rather than the exception. From corporate boardrooms to elementary school classrooms, the practice of mindfulness will be as ubiquitous as taking a daily vitamin.

The Green Revolution: Sustainability and Alkaline Living

As we grapple with the existential threat of climate change, sustainability is no longer an option; it's a necessity. And here, alkaline living offers a blueprint for a sustainable future. From eco-friendly farming practices to zero-waste lifestyles, the principles of alkaline living are intrinsically aligned with environmental stewardship. This convergence of personal health and planetary well-being is a trend that promises to gain significant traction.

The Medical Establishment: A Paradigm Shift

Perhaps the most transformative trend is the gradual thawing of the medical establishment's stance towards alkaline living. While skepticism still exists, a growing body of research is hard to ignore. We're already seeing the integration of alkaline therapies in the treatment of chronic conditions, and this trend is likely to accelerate. The day is not far off when your physician prescribes an alkaline diet as readily as they do medication.

As we navigate the labyrinth of the future, one thing is clear: the tapestry of alkaline health and wellness is rich and varied, woven with threads of innovation, inclusivity, and integrity. It's a future that beckons with promise and potential, inviting each of us to play our part in this unfolding narrative. So as we stand at this crossroads, let's choose the path that leads to a healthier, happier, and more harmonious world. For in that choice lies not just our well-being, but the well-being of generations yet unborn.

The Path Forward: Spreading Awareness and Education

As we've explored the emerging trends in alkaline health and wellness, it's crucial to remember that the future is not a distant realm; it's a tapestry woven from the threads of individual choices. Each decision to opt for alkaline water over soda, each moment spent in mindful meditation, and every plate filled with alkaline-rich foods is a step toward a future where alkaline living is the norm, not the exception. Your choices matter, and they're part of a collective momentum that's pushing society toward a healthier, more balanced existence.

The Role of Education and Advocacy

While individual choices are the building blocks, education and advocacy serve as the scaffolding for this emerging structure. The power of knowledge can't be overstated. As more people become educated about the benefits of alkaline living, the ripple effect will be profound. Schools will start incorporating nutrition education that goes beyond the food pyramid, focusing on pH balance and alkaline diets. Wellness coaches and healthcare providers will become invaluable assets, guiding people through the maze of misinformation to credible, science-backed alkaline practices.

The Media's Influence: A Double-Edged Sword

The media, with its far-reaching influence, plays a pivotal role in shaping public perception. While it can be a double-edged sword, the increasing coverage of alkaline living in reputable outlets will lend credibility and spur interest among the masses. Documentaries, podcasts, and feature articles will delve into real-life success stories, demystifying the alkaline lifestyle and making it more accessible. The narrative will shift from a niche health trend to a mainstream wellness philosophy.

The Corporate Conundrum: Ethical Responsibility vs. Profit

As alkaline living gains traction, corporations will inevitably jump on the bandwagon. While this could lead to greater accessibility of alkaline products, it also poses the risk of commercialization and dilution of core principles. The challenge will be to hold these entities accountable, ensuring that they adhere to ethical practices. Consumer demand for transparency will drive companies to source sustainably, label accurately, and invest in quality.

The Global Perspective: A Universal Human Right

Health is not a luxury; it's a universal human right. As the alkaline movement gains global momentum, it's imperative to ensure that it doesn't become a privilege reserved for the affluent. International collaborations can play a role here, sharing resources and knowledge to make alkaline living attainable for all, regardless of socio-economic status. Imagine a world where alkaline filtration systems are as common as wells in developing countries, where the right to health transcends borders.

The Final Mile: Your Role in this Journey

As we look toward the horizon, your role in this transformative journey becomes clear. You are not just a passive observer; you're an active participant. Whether you're sharing an alkaline recipe on social media, participating in community wellness programs, or simply making mindful choices in your daily life, you're contributing to a larger narrative. It's a narrative of empowerment, of taking control of your health and inspiring others to do the same.

As we close this point on predicting trends in alkaline health and wellness, let's remember that every ending is a new beginning. The future is not set in stone; it's a living, breathing entity that we're shaping with our actions, right here, right now. So let's embrace the uncertainty, armed with the knowledge and conviction that alkaline living offers a path to a better tomorrow. It's a path that promises not just longevity but a quality of life that we all aspire to. And that, dear reader, is a future worth striving for.

The Role of Research and Science in Shaping the Future

The Nexus of Science and Alkaline Living

As we venture into the uncharted territories of the future landscape of alkaline living, it's imperative to recognize the role that research and science will play in shaping this evolving narrative. Science isn't just a collection of facts or theories; it's a dynamic process, a method of inquiry that allows us to test, validate, and refine our understanding of the world. In the context of alkaline living, science serves as both a compass and a catalyst, guiding us toward a deeper understanding while accelerating the pace of innovation and discovery.

For years, the alkaline lifestyle has been buoyed by anecdotal evidence—personal testimonials, word-of-mouth recommendations, and the lived experiences of its proponents. While these stories are compelling, they often lack the rigorous scrutiny that only scientific research can provide. As we move forward, it's crucial to transition from a narrative dominated by anecdotes to one fortified by empirical evidence. Clinical trials, peer-reviewed studies, and interdisciplinary research will serve as the bedrock upon which the credibility of alkaline living will be built.

The Interplay of Disciplines: A Holistic Approach

The beauty of science lies in its ability to draw from multiple disciplines to create a more comprehensive picture. Nutrition science can tell us about the biochemical effects of an alkaline diet, psychology can explore the mental health benefits, and environmental science can assess the sustainability of alkaline practices. By integrating insights from these diverse fields, we can develop a holistic understanding of alkaline living that transcends the limitations of any single discipline.

As the scientific community delves deeper into the intricacies of alkaline living, ethical considerations must take center stage. Research should be conducted with the utmost integrity, transparency, and respect for human and environmental well-being. This ethical imperative extends to the dissemination of findings. The public deserves access to clear, unbiased information that empowers them to make informed choices about their health and lifestyle.

One of the most exciting prospects of scientific research in this field is the potential for personalization. Advances in genomics and data analytics could enable us to tailor alkaline diets and lifestyle interventions to individual genetic profiles, optimizing outcomes and minimizing risks. Imagine a future where your healthcare provider can prescribe a personalized alkaline regimen based on your unique genetic makeup, lifestyle factors, and health history.

The Global Context: Science as a Unifying Force

In a world rife with division, the universal language of science has the power to unite us. Alkaline living is not confined to any one culture, geography, or demographic; it's a global movement with universal implications for human health and planetary sustainability. International collaborations in research can foster a sense of global community, transcending borders and breaking down barriers to access and information.

As we stand on the cusp of a new era in alkaline living, the role of research and science has never been more critical. It's not just about validating what we already believe; it's about pushing the boundaries of what we know, challenging our assumptions, and daring to imagine new possibilities. Each scientific inquiry is a step toward a future where alkaline living is not just a lifestyle choice but a well-researched, widely-accepted, and deeply-embedded part of our collective consciousness.

In closing, the future of alkaline living is not a foregone conclusion; it's a living tapestry that we are all weaving together. And science, with its rigorous methods and relentless quest for truth, will be one of our most valuable tools in crafting a future that is not only healthier but also more equitable, sustainable, and fulfilling for all.

The role of research and science in shaping the future

As we contemplate the future of alkaline life, it is essential to recognize that scientific research is not an isolated activity conducted in ivory towers. It is a collective activity that thrives on the democratization of knowledge. Open access journals, community-led research initiatives, and citizen science projects are breaking down barriers between experts and the public. This democratization ensures that the benefits of alkaline life science discoveries are accessible to all, not just a privileged few.

The future will be shaped by collaborative efforts that transcend academic disciplines, cultural boundaries, and socioeconomic statuses. Public-private partnerships could fund innovative research, while international coalitions of scientists could address global health challenges. The ethos of collaboration will serve as a cornerstone, ensuring that alkaline life science evolves in inclusive, equitable, and impactful ways.

The pulse of innovation and the human element

At a time when technology is advancing at an unprecedented pace, its role in shaping the future of the alkaline lifestyle cannot be overstated. From artificial intelligence-driven data analysis to virtual reality simulations, technology will revolutionize the way research is conducted and disseminated. These advances will not only make research more efficient but also more precise, enabling real-time adjustments and adaptations that could save lives and preserve health.

While the scientific method is rooted in objectivity, the application of research findings must be guided by emotional intelligence. Understanding the human element-our fears, hopes and motivations-is critical to translating scientific data into actionable insights. As we navigate the complexities of a rapidly changing world, the ability to connect with people emotionally will be just as important as the ability to innovate scientifically.

The final frontier: The unknown and the unknowable

As we move forward, the moral implications of our scientific endeavors must be at the forefront of our minds. Sustainability is not just an environmental buzzword, but an ethical imperative. Research on alkaline life must be conducted in a way that respects not only human life but also the planet that sustains it. This moral compass will guide us through ethical dilemmas and ensure that the pursuit of knowledge does not come at the expense of our ethical integrity.

Science is a journey into the unknown, a quest to push the boundaries of the possible. When we look to the future, we must embrace the mysteries that lie ahead. The unknown is not a void to be feared, but a canvas to be painted. And while science can illuminate the path forward, the brushstrokes of that future will be colored by our courage, imagination and humanity.

In the great tapestry of human history, the role of research and science in shaping the future of alkaline life is akin to a symphony: a harmonious blend of different instruments, each contributing to a larger whole. It is a symphony of progress, where each note resonates with the promise of better health, greater understanding, and a more equitable world.

Your Personal Role in the Global Alkaline Movement

The Power of One: A Ripple in the Ocean

You may wonder, "What can one person do?" The answer is, a lot more than you think. Each of us is a ripple in the ocean of change, and when those ripples converge, they form waves—waves that have the power to reshape landscapes. Your personal role in the global alkaline movement is not just a matter of choice; it's a calling, a responsibility that beckons you to be part of something greater than yourself.

It's one thing to know about the benefits of alkaline living; it's another to put that knowledge into action. The alchemy of transformation occurs when you take the first step, whether it's swapping out processed foods for natural alternatives or incorporating alkaline water into your daily routine. These seemingly small actions are the building blocks of a larger revolution, one that starts within the walls of your home and extends far beyond.

The Echo Chamber: Amplifying Your Voice

In this digital age, your voice has the potential to reach corners of the world you've never even heard of. Social media platforms, blogs, and community forums are not just spaces for idle chatter; they're powerful tools for advocacy. By sharing your journey, your challenges, and your triumphs, you amplify the message of alkaline living. You become a beacon of inspiration for others who are just starting their journey, and in doing so, you strengthen the collective voice advocating for a healthier, more holistic way of life.

Trust is the currency of influence, and authenticity is its cornerstone. People are more likely to listen to someone they can relate to, someone who has walked the path they're considering. Your personal story, replete with its ups and downs, serves as a testament to the transformative power of alkaline living. By being open, honest, and vulnerable, you build trust, and that trust translates into influence.

The Symbiosis of Community: We're All in This Together

Never underestimate the impact of small actions. The butterfly effect posits that a single flap of a butterfly's wings can set off a tornado miles away. Similarly, your choices, no matter how insignificant they may seem, have far-reaching consequences. By choosing to live an alkaline lifestyle, you're not just improving your health; you're setting an example for your family, your community, and yes, even the world.

The global alkaline movement is not a solo endeavor; it's a collective undertaking that thrives on community. Whether it's participating in local workshops, joining online forums, or simply engaging in meaningful conversations with friends and family, community involvement enriches your experience and adds a layer of accountability to your journey. It's a symbiotic relationship where your growth fuels the community's progress and vice versa.

The Vanguard of Change: You

As we stand on the cusp of a new era in health and wellness, you are the vanguard of change. Your actions, your voice, and your choices serve as the catalysts that will propel the global alkaline movement into the mainstream consciousness. You are not just a passive consumer of information; you are an active participant in a revolution that has the potential to redefine our understanding of health, wellness, and quality of life.

As we delve into the future landscape of alkaline living, remember that this is not just a theoretical discussion; it's a call to action. Your personal role in the global alkaline movement is not a footnote; it's the headline. So, as you turn the pages of this book and absorb its wisdom, know that the most important chapter is the one you're about to write—your own.

In this grand narrative of transformation, you are both the author and the protagonist. Your choices will pen the script, and your actions will breathe life into the characters. So, pick up that pen, step onto that stage, and let your life be the masterpiece that inspires a new chapter in the global alkaline movement.

Your Personal Role in the Global Alkaline Movement: The Final Act

As we draw the curtain on this chapter, let's consider your role as a unique instrument in the grand symphony of alkaline living. Just as a violin or a trumpet has its distinct sound, your journey has its unique timbre. Your experiences, your struggles, and your triumphs add a unique note to this collective melody. And when we all play in harmony, the music we create can stir souls and inspire change.

Alkaline living is not a sprint; it's a marathon. The initial enthusiasm is crucial, but what truly counts is your sustained commitment. It's easy to be a zealot for a week, but it takes dedication to make it a lifetime commitment. The beauty of this lifestyle is that the more you invest in it, the more it gives back to you—in terms of health, vitality, and well-being. Your continued commitment not only benefits you but also serves as a living testament to the efficacy and transformative power of alkaline living.

The Ripple Effect: Your Impact on the Micro and Macro

Your choices don't just affect you; they have a ripple effect that extends outward, influencing those around you and even impacting the larger ecosystem. When you choose organic, alkaline foods, you're supporting sustainable farming practices. When you share your alkaline recipes or wellness tips, you're contributing to a body of knowledge that can help others. Your actions, both big and small, contribute to a larger narrative, one that transcends individual benefit and contributes to collective well-being.

Every movement has its heroes, its advocates who take up the mantle and push the boundaries. In the realm of alkaline living, you have the opportunity to be one of those heroes. Your advocacy doesn't have to be grandiose; it can be as simple as sharing your story, mentoring someone new to the lifestyle, or even organizing a community clean-up. The legacy you leave behind will be composed of these small but significant acts of advocacy.

The alkaline movement, like any other, is not static; it's dynamic and ever-evolving. New research will emerge, new foods will be classified, and new techniques will be developed. Your role in this movement is not just to follow but to evolve with it. Stay updated, keep learning, and be willing to adapt. Your flexibility not only enriches your own journey but also makes you a valuable asset to the community.

The Final Note: Your Role in the Tapestry of Change

As we conclude this book, remember that you are an integral thread in the tapestry of this movement. Your color, texture, and pattern add richness to the overall design. Your role is not peripheral; it's central. You are not just a spectator; you are a participant, an actor on this grand stage.

So, as you step into the world armed with the knowledge and inspiration you've gained, remember that the spotlight is on you. You have the script, you know your lines, and the stage is set. It's time to give the performance of a lifetime, one that not only enriches your life but also elevates the global alkaline movement to unprecedented heights.

In this narrative of transformation and hope, you are not just a chapter; you are a volume. Your actions, your advocacy, and your commitment have the power to write a story that future generations will read with awe and gratitude. So, take that pen, embrace your role, and let's write a future that's not just alkaline but also genuinely divine.

Conclusion

The Lifelong Journey of Alkaline Mastery

The Road Less Traveled: Embracing the Alkaline Way

As we close the final chapter of this transformative journey, let's pause and reflect on the road less traveled—the alkaline way. This isn't just a diet or a fad; it's a lifelong commitment to holistic well-being. It's about understanding that the choices you make today will echo in the corridors of your future, shaping not just your health but your very essence.

The Alchemist Within: Turning Challenges into Gold

Life will throw curveballs at you. Stress, work pressures, and the chaos of a fast-paced life can make it tempting to veer off the alkaline path. But remember, mastery isn't about avoiding challenges; it's about turning them into opportunities. Like an alchemist, you have the power to turn the lead of adversity into the gold of wisdom and resilience. Each challenge you face and overcome fortifies your commitment to this lifestyle, making you an undeniable master of your own destiny.

The Living Library: Continuous Learning and Adaptation

Alkaline mastery is not a static achievement; it's a dynamic process. The world of holistic health is ever-evolving, with new research and discoveries continually enriching our understanding. Being a master means being a perpetual student. It means staying curious, staying hungry, and most importantly, staying humble in the face of the vast ocean of knowledge that lies ahead.

The Symphony of Balance: Harmonizing Mind, Body, and Spirit

True mastery in alkaline living transcends the physical realm; it permeates the mental and spiritual dimensions of your existence. It's about achieving a harmonious balance that resonates in every fiber of your being. This is not just about what you eat but also about how you think, how you feel, and how you connect with the world around you. It's about crafting a life symphony where each note, each chord, and each melody resonates with the frequency of alkaline balance.

The Legacy of Mastery: Inspiring the Next Wave

Your journey toward alkaline mastery is not just your own; it's a beacon for others who are seeking the light. The wisdom you gain, the challenges you overcome, and the balance you achieve serve as a living testament to the transformative power of this lifestyle. You become a lighthouse, guiding others through the fog of misinformation and doubt, toward the shores of alkaline enlightenment.

The Final Milestone: A Life Well Lived

As we wrap up this odyssey, let's not forget that the ultimate milestone of alkaline mastery is a life well lived. It's a life rich in vitality, brimming with purpose, and radiant with the glow of holistic well-being. It's a life where each day is a new chapter in a story that's not just compelling but also profoundly inspiring.

So, as you step forward into the unfolding path of your life, remember that you're not just walking it; you're mastering it. You're not just surviving; you're thriving. And most importantly, you're not just living; you're embodying a legacy of alkaline mastery that will echo through the annals of time, inspiring generations yet unborn to embark on their own journeys toward holistic transcendence.

In this grand tapestry of life, your thread is not just a color; it's a vibrant hue that adds depth, texture, and brilliance to the entire masterpiece. So go ahead, embrace your role as a master, and let's weave a future that's not just healthy but also profoundly harmonious and deeply fulfilling.

Acknowledgments

The Invisible Hands That Shaped This Journey

A Symphony of Gratitude

As we reach the final pages of this transformative odyssey, it's essential to pause and acknowledge the invisible hands that have shaped this journey. Acknowledgments are often relegated to the back of the book, but their significance reverberates through every word, every concept, and every transformative idea presented.

The Pillars: Family and Friends

First and foremost, my deepest gratitude goes to my family and friends. You are the bedrock upon which this work stands. Your unwavering support, your challenging questions, and your endless love have been the pillars that held me up when the weight of this endeavor seemed too much to bear.

The Guiding Lights: Mentors and Teachers

To my mentors and teachers, both formal and informal, your wisdom has been my guiding light. You've taught me not just the science of alkalinity, but the art of living a life that's balanced, purposeful, and deeply fulfilling. Your teachings have transcended the classroom, spilling over into the very essence of this work.

The Heartbeat: The Alkaline Community

To the vibrant and ever-growing alkaline community, you are the heartbeat of this movement. Your stories of transformation, your questions, your challenges, and your triumphs have enriched this narrative in ways that words can hardly capture. You've proven that this isn't just a book; it's a living, breathing dialogue.

The Unsung Heroes: Researchers and Scientists

A special acknowledgment goes to the researchers and scientists whose tireless work has provided the backbone of credibility to the alkaline lifestyle. Your dedication to unraveling the complexities of human health has made it possible for us to approach this subject with both curiosity and rigor.

The Catalysts: Critics and Skeptics

Even the critics and skeptics deserve a nod. Your challenging questions have been the catalysts for deeper inquiry. You've pushed me to look beyond the surface, to question the status quo, and to present a narrative that's as robust as it is transformative.

The Final Brushstroke: The Reader

Last but certainly not least, to you, the reader. You are the reason these pages have life. Your quest for holistic health, your commitment to personal growth, and your courage to step into the unknown have made you an integral part of this journey. This book is not just a monologue; it's a conversation, one that I hope will continue long after you turn the final page.

The Cosmic Web: An Interconnected Journey

In the grand tapestry of life, we are all interconnected, each adding our unique thread to the cosmic web. This book is a manifestation of that interconnectedness, a symphony where each acknowledgment is a note, contributing to a melody that's as ancient as time and as fresh as the morning dew.

So, as we close this book, let's carry forward the spirit of gratitude and interconnectedness into our lives, knowing that the journey to alkaline mastery is not a solo endeavor but a collective pilgrimage towards a healthier, happier, and more harmonious world.

Thank you for being a part of this incredible journey!

Printed in Poland
by Amazon Fulfillment
Poland Sp. z o.o., Wrocław